Navigating the Maze of
NURSING RESEARCH
AN INTERACTIVE LEARNING ADVENTURE

Navigating the Maze of
NURSING RESEARCH
AN INTERACTIVE LEARNING ADVENTURE

Rae W. Langford, EdD, RN
Private Practice
Research and Statistics Consultant
Rehabilitation Nurse Consultant
Legal Nurse Consultant
Houston, Texas

Illustrated

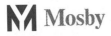 Mosby

A Harcourt Health Sciences Company

St. Louis   London   Philadelphia   Sydney   Toronto

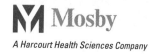

A Harcourt Health Sciences Company

Editor-in-Chief   Sally Schrefer
Executive Editor   June D. Thompson
Senior Developmental Editor   Linda Caldwell
Project Manager   Catherine Jackson
Production Editor   Jeff Patterson
Book Design Manager   Amy Buxton

Mosby, Inc.
A Harcourt Health Sciences Company
11830 Westline Industrial Drive
St. Louis, Missouri 63146

Printed in the United States of America

ISBN 0-323-00947-6

01   02   03   04   05   TG/FF   9   8   7   6   5   4   3   2   1

Rae W. Langford

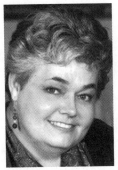

Let me introduce myself. I have been a faculty member for more than 25 years. I have taught research and statistics at the baccalaureate, masters, and doctoral levels for nursing, allied health, and education students. I have also worked with numerous practicing nurses to make research less mystifying and more readily applicable to clinical practice. During that time I have experimented with a number of ways to more clearly distinguish and optimize learning experiences for various levels of students and to make research come alive for students and practitioners alike. This learning package is, in part, a result of that experimentation.

Many of the games, puzzles, and challenges have been tested with baccalaureate students. Students found them fun and challenging. Many have commented that this approach makes research seem more real and relevant and they feel more confident in reading and making sense out of research articles. I have had faculty members in clinical courses ask me what I am doing because their students are suddenly discussing and applying research findings in their clinical situations.

The goal of this learning package is to equip students with skills that enable them to quickly find, critically read, and readily identify possible uses for relevant clinical research. It uses an interactive, multimodal approach that gets students actively involved in the learning process and provides multiple opportunities to practice and integrate newly acquired skills. I hope you find this approach as useful as my students and I have.

REVIEWERS

Margaret M. Anderson, EdD, RN, C, CNAA
Associate Professor, BSN/MSN Programs
Chair, Department of Nursing
Northern Kentucky University
Highland Heights, Kentucky

Betsy Barnes-McDowell, PhD, RN, CCRN
Associate Professor
School of Nursing
Lander University
Greenwood, South Carolina

An Important Message from Your Author!

Did you know that crossing your legs elevates blood pressure readings? (Read *Nurs Res* 48(2):105, 1999)

Do you think ear thermometers are accurate measurements of temperature? (Read the latest in *Appl Nurs Res* 11(4):158, 1998)

Does exercise adversely affect persons with rheumatoid arthritis? (Find out in *Res Nurs Health* 20(3):195, 1997)

Do you know how to assess pain in an infant? (Check out *Appl Nurs Res* 11(2):62, 1998)

Do you know which psychiatric in-patients are most likely to fall? (See *Appl Nurs Res* 11(3):115, 1998)

Do you know which type of gastrostomy tube works best in children who keep them in place long term? (Find out in *West J Nurs Res* 20(2):145, 1998)

Do you know an easy and inexpensive way to lower pain during the process of drawing blood? (Read *Appl Nurs Res* 10(4):168, 1997)

Answers to these questions are just a sample of the wealth of information that waits at your fingertips to help you improve the nursing care that you give everyday. If you want **to be the best nurse you can be . . .** then find out what a little judicious use of nursing research can do for you.

What does **RESEARCH** have to do with this, you ask? Well, your professional association, the **American Nurses Association,** considers research so vital to the profession of nursing that it expects **all** registered nurses, regardless of educational preparation, to be research consumers. What is a **research consumer?** A research consumer has the ability to read research articles, evaluate their relevance, and apply the findings to the practice of nursing.

This is where this learning package (textbook, CD-ROM, and website) fits in. This package is designed to enhance your skills so that you can effectively read, understand, evaluate, and apply research findings in your everyday clinical practice. It encourages you to examine what you do in the clinical area and to pose such questions as "Is this the best intervention?" or "Is this the best way to carry out this intervention?" It seeks to involve you as an active participant in this learning process. There are student activities and critical thinking opportunities featured throughout the text and interactive exercises, puzzles, and games on the CD-ROM. The more you participate in the various activities, exercises, and discussions about the identified research content, the more confident and competent you will become in using research as a tool to improve your practice.

This learning package is also designed to enhance skills so that you can find information fast and read and use it effectively. Section 1 is devoted to honing library and Internet skills, reading skills, and abstracting skills. Section 2 gives you the vocabulary necessary to read and understand research studies by introducing you to the two main types of research: quantitative and qualitative. Section 3 gives you step-by-step guidance in applying research findings to a variety of clinical situations. It also explores ways to use research results to change the way you practice and to influence the systems that you practice in.

Special Features in the Book

- Student Quote   You can probably identify with other students' feelings about nursing research.

- Abstract   Just as a research article has an abstract, an introductory paragraph that summarizes the article, so too does each chapter.

- Learning Objectives   describe what you should be able to do after reading each chapter and working the exercises.

- Chapter Outline   A list of each heading in the chapter gives you an idea of the topics covered throughout it.

- Key Terms   A list of the terms that it's important to know for each chapter.

- Student Challenge   **Try these exercises to apply what you are reading and learning.**

- Hints and other boxed information   **Be sure to remember these useful tips and notes!**

- Resource Kit   **Materials to refer to for further information.**

- Glossary   **A list of all the key terms in the book is provided in the back of the book for your convenience.**

How to Use Your Learning Package

You have three integrated tools to help you make your way through this maze:

- Textbook   **As you read the textbook, you will be referred to activities on the CD-ROM and to websites accessible through links on the book's MERLIN website. In the page margins you will see icons referring you to the activities on the CD-ROM** and the website activities found on the MERLIN site.

- CD-ROM   **The CD-ROM provides over 40 interactive exercises that cover all 12 chapters in the book. It includes activities such as word scramble, multiple choice, cryptograms, and many other fun and challenging exercises. A special icon appears in the margin of the book when there is a corresponding CD-ROM exercise, signaling you to go to the CD-ROM.**

- MERLIN website   **The website, located at www.mosby.com/MERLIN/Langford/maze provides links to Internet sites that correspond to activities on the CD and other websites relevant to the nursing research. Each activity in the book that sends you to the Internet is indicated by this symbol. Also included on the website are Frequently Asked Questions about nursing research, Teaching Tips for faculty members, and other pertinent information.**

You may find that you not only learn how to effectively use research in your nursing practice, but that you also gain greater abilities to read and think critically, to analyze situations, and to better use and manage available resources. I invite you now to begin the first step in your journey to navigate the maze that is nursing research.

Rae Langford

CONTENTS

One

FINDING IT FAST AND READING IT WELL

Taking Advantage of the Information Explosion and the Miracles of Modern Technology

...Be Prepared

We live in a time where information is available on just about any subject you can dream up, and more is produced everyday. Unfortunately, many of us fail to take advantage of this wealth of information and have little idea about how to find and use it when we do need it. Maybe we are overwhelmed by the abundance and cope by ignoring it all. Unfortunately, ignoring the problem breeds ignorance. To be information literate is essential to our personal and professional well-being, but how do we achieve this? We must recognize when we need information and hone the skills necessary to find, evaluate, and use that information. Both the library and the Internet offer excellent readily available resources. This section discusses how to use the library and the Internet and describes how to effectively read and summarize essential information. It will help you develop skills to take advantage of and harness the information explosion.

Learning Objectives

1 Describe the organization and functions of libraries.

2 Describe relevant library components and services.

3 Locate components and services in a specified library setting.

4 Discuss the purpose of library filing systems.

5 Distinguish between manual and computerized information retrieval systems.

6 Discuss the differences between cataloging and indexing systems.

7 Compare and contrast sample indexes available to access nursing- and health care–related information.

8 Describe how to conduct an information search using library resources.

9 Conduct a search at a specified library setting, using available library search tools.

10 Evaluate the results of a search effort for an identified topic.

Chapter Outline

Do You Need This Chapter?
What Is a Library?
  Types of libraries
  Classification schemes
What's in the Library?
How Do You Use the Library?
  Catalogs
    Manual catalogs
    Electronic catalogs
  Indexes and abstracts
    Manual indexes and abstracts
    Electronic indexes and abstracts

Comparing manual and electronic indexes
How Do You Successfully Search for Information?
  Clearly define your mission
  Choose the appropriate resources
  Choose the appropriate indexes
  Define your search parameters
  Place limits on your search
  View your search results

Getting the Most Out of the Library

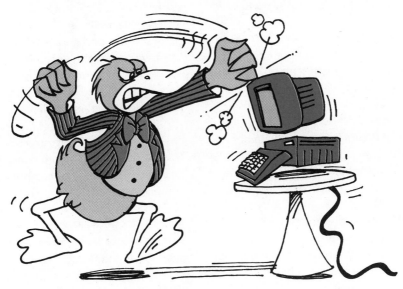

Whatta ya mean there's no articles about tear ducks?

Student Quote   *"The library used to be so overwhelming. I'd avoid going because I could never find what I needed anyway. Who knew it could be so useful?"*

Abstract   Libraries collect, store, and organize information and make it readily accessible for use. Materials are organized using a classification system and are arranged on shelves by call numbers. Materials are located by using catalogs and indexes. These filing systems are available in print and electronic form. Successful searches for information about a particular subject demand certain skills. These include the ability to define the topic of interest, select appropriate search resources, refine search skills, and selectively review materials produced by a search.

KEY TERMS

Library Lingo

Abstract A short summary of an article.

Abstracts Special type of indexes that include citations and summaries of articles.

Archive A collection of older materials that have some historical value.

Book (monograph) A volume about a single subject or related subjects published once (later editions may update material).

Call number (classification number) A number or letter-and-number combination that is assigned to each book and/or journal to indicate where it is shelved in a library.

Catalog A list of all books owned by the library with a citation and call number for each book.

CD-ROM A compact disc containing one or more electronic databases, programs, or images.

Circulating Materials that may be checked out of the library.

Citation Bibliographical information about books or journals (e.g., author, title, source, date of publication).

Collection All materials owned by a library.

Database A collection of related information such as a catalog, index, or abstract.

Dissertation (thesis) A research paper written by a graduate student as part of the degree requirement.

Electronic database A database that is accessed for a search by computer.

Holdings The specific volumes or issues of periodicals owned by the library.

Index A list of periodical citations arranged by subject or author. Indexes are usually organized around a specific subject area or field of study.

Interlibrary loan A library service that allows books and copies of articles to be borrowed from other libraries for use.

Microform Materials that have been reduced and placed on photographic film (e.g., microfiche, microfilm).

Noncirculating Materials that cannot be checked out of the library.

On-line Materials that are computerized and accessed by other computers (e.g., a computer network).

Periodical A journal or magazine.

Reference collection Noncirculating materials that are meant to be used as reference rather than read through (e.g., indexes, encyclopedias, dictionaries).

Search Use of indexes, abstracts, and catalogs to find information about a specified subject.

Stacks Library bookshelves.

Volume A single book or a bound sequence of issues of a periodical.

I've heard many nurses admit that they have not darkened the door of a library since they finished school. I've taught senior students who have no library skills. I'm afraid some of them don't even know where the library is located. Why? The first excuse given usually has to do with lack of time or with the library's shortcomings (e.g., "They never have what I want," or "I can never get any help.") Further exploration with students and practicing nurses alike, however, usually reveals feelings of being over-whelmed, of not knowing where to start or who to ask. In short, a trip to the library results in a frustrating and unpleasant experience. If you find libraries a little intimi-dating or if you need a refresher course in how libraries work, this chapter is for you.

Do You Need This Chapter?

Take the following little quiz to find out if you need to read this chapter:
1. Do you know what libraries are available in your area?
2. Do you know what kinds of materials they have and what kinds of services they offer?
3. Do you know where they are located, when they are open, and who can use them?
4. Do you have library privileges? Are they current?
5. Have you used a library in the last month?
6. Do you find it easy to find what you're looking for when you do use a library?
7. Can you operate the manual and/or computerized search systems? (Hint: If you don't know what a search system is, you need this chapter.)
8. Do you know how much it costs to make a photocopy of a needed reference?
9. Could you identify a reference librarian if he or she weren't behind the refer-ence desk?
10. Do they know you by name at the circulation desk?

If you can answer yes to most of these questions you may want to skim this chapter. However, if you've ever said to an instructor, "There wasn't any informa-tion about (*fill in the blank*) available," then you definitely need to read this chap-ter and complete the student challenges.

What Is a Library?

A library is a place where large amounts of information are available on various subjects. More specifically, a library is a **collection** of materials that has been organized for ease of use. The key terms here are "collection" and "organized." We usually think of a library collection as consisting of **books (monographs)** and journals, but it might also be a collection of art or maps or audiovisual materials. What is collected often determines the library type.

> A library is a collection of materials that have been organized for use.

Types of Libraries

There are three basic types of libraries that may prove helpful to you: public libraries, academic libraries, and special libraries. Public libraries are provided through public funds for public use. They collect information of interest to the community being served. These may be local or national libraries, and they may have several hundred to several hundred thousand available items. If you live in a large urban area, the public library is probably divided into numerous neighborhood branches with a main library located in the downtown area. The main library houses the most extensive part of the available collection of materials.

Academic libraries are connected with academic institutions above the secondary level and collect information of interest to faculty and students. The types of materials collected are strongly associated with the major degree areas offered at that academic institution. The size of the student body and the sources of funding influence the size and quality of the collection. Many large universities have more than one library on campus. One of these is usually designated as the main library, and the others tend to be specialty libraries.

Special libraries are formed by organizations with specialized information needs. They collect information on specific topics dictated by the needs of the organization that funds them. These may include business and corporate libraries or professional libraries, such as law or medical center libraries. The information collected is based on the needs of the special population being served. If you are located in a health science center, you may have access to a health science center library, which is usually a cross between an academic and a specialty library.

Classification Schemes

Shelves of haphazardly collected books do not constitute a library. Fortunately, libraries don't keep their books organized like we do at home. Can you imagine going into a library and the librarian saying, "You want a copy of *Mosby's Handbook of Diseases*? Let's see, I seem to remember that it is pocket-sized and has a blue cover with a pink drawing. I know it's around here somewhere." Libraries actually use very precise systems to organize all the information they collect. These organizing systems are called classification schemes. Libraries use two major classification schemes: the Dewey Decimal Classification (DDC) and the Library of Congress classification.

The DDC was devised in 1876 by an American librarian named Melvil Dewey. He used a system of categories and decimal numbers to indicate subjects of books. This meant that one place in the library would contain all the books on a particular subject category. Dewey devised 10 main categories that are numbered in segments of 100. These main categories each contain 10 subcategories with number segments of 10. These subcategories are infinitely expandable to additional subcategories using a combination of numbers, decimal sets, and letters. This classification scheme was 12 pages long in 1876. It is now more than 3,500 pages long and continues to expand (ALA, 1986).

The Library of Congress system also classifies information by subject matter using main categories and subcategories. However, its 21 main categories are designated by letters of the alphabet. Subcategories are formed by adding a second letter and/or a series of numbers. This system is more flexible and more readily revised than Dewey's system (Feather and Sturges, 1997).

Both systems use number-letter combinations to label their collections. These labels are called **call numbers.** Some libraries put call numbers on all their materials, while others label only books. Each book has a unique call number, and ranges of call numbers are clearly marked on library shelves to make finding a particular book or a range of books about a specific subject easy to locate. As a rule of thumb, most public libraries use the DDC, and most academic libraries use some form of the Library of Congress classification. Special libraries may use a scheme adapted to handle large volumes of materials in relatively few subject areas. Medical libraries often use the National Library of Medicine classification system, adapted from the Library of Congress system. The key point is that all of the material in the library is carefully organized to make it easy to find and use.

> The key point is that all of the material in the library is carefully organized to make it easy to find and use.

What's in the Library?

Every library is arranged differently, but they usually have common features. The main section of the library typically contains a circulation desk, an information desk, a reference desk, and an area for catalogs, indexes, and abstracts. Other key areas include a **reference collection,** a current periodicals section, a bound periodicals section, and the stacks. Most libraries also have a media or audiovisual center, microforms section, reserve section, and special collections.

The circulation desk is where you check out books and other **circulating** materials to use outside the library setting. The information desk is the place to go when you don't know where to look for needed materials or when you have questions about various library services and resources.

> **Hint:** Many libraries have pamphlets on library use and locations of materials. Read them. However, if you can't find what you need within 10 minutes, don't hesitate to ask a librarian.

The reference desk is staffed by a reference librarian who can help you find specialized or hard-to-find resources. Some libraries combine the functions of the information and reference desks. Some floor area is set aside for the catalog and indexing systems that serve as search tools. These systems list all of the library's materials and let you know where to find them.

The reference collection contains materials such as encyclopedias, dictionaries, statistical reports, directories, handbooks, and other materials that are handy for quick reference. Some libraries also put periodical indexes and abstracts here. These materials are referred to as **noncirculating** because they are intended for use on the premises and may not be checked out or removed from the general reference area.

The current **periodical** section has the newer issues of journals and magazines, displayed and organized alphabetically by title or call number. These issues frequently start with the first issue of the current year and contain all the issues for the year to date. The bound periodicals section contains journals and magazines for previous years. They have been bound together in a book form called a **volume.** The number of years contained in a volume depends on the size of the journal and number of issues published annually. Typically, 1 year of a journal constitutes a volume, and the specific volumes or issues of periodicals the library owns is referred to as its **holdings.** This section is also arranged alphabetically by periodical title.

The **stacks** are the library's main bookshelves. They usually contain books and occupy the most space in a library.

Hint: Some libraries store bound periodicals in the stacks rather than in a periodical section. If this is the case, the periodicals are given a call number and are stored by subject.

The media or audiovisual center contains films, videotapes, audiotapes, and computer software. Some libraries also house CD-ROMs here. The **microform** section contains microfilm and microfiche and the machines that allow you to read them. Microfilm and microfiche are inexpensive methods to store large amounts of printed material in a small space. You may find back issues of newspapers, magazines, theses, maps, and other materials stored on microforms.

The reserve section contains materials placed aside by the library staff or faculty for special use. These materials typically can only be checked out for 1 or 2 days or may not be checked out at all. These materials are often heavily used, and a reserve system allows access to a greater number of people.

Special collections, or **archives,** contain rare materials that may not be replaced easily. These might include collections of such things as government and professional documents; old, rare, or one-of-a-kind books; or materials of historical importance. Access to these materials may be restricted, and they may not be checked out.

Chances are that you have at least visited your university or health science center library. However, if you have only a sketchy idea about where things are located and how things are operated, please take time to do the following Student Challenge. It can save you a lot of time and energy when you need to use the library and want to locate the materials or services you need quickly.

ADVENTURE
CD
1-2

STUDENT CHALLENGE Exploring Library Layouts

Make a trip to your university or health science center library. Allow an hour for this experience.
    Wander around, explore, and browse.
    Pick up any handouts that are available to users as helpful hints or guides.
    Sit for awhile and people watch.

Continued

STUDENT CHALLENGE Exploring Library Layouts—cont'd

Skim the brochures you've collected.

Become comfortable with the space and with the idea of being there, then do the following tasks:

1. Make a map of the physical layout. (Hint: The library may have a ready-made map for users.) Locate and physically visit each of the following areas:
   a. circulation desk, information desk, reserve desk, reference desk
   b. search tool section (e.g., indexes, abstracts, and catalogs); find available computerized and manual versions.
   c. list of periodical holdings
   d. current periodicals
   e. bound periodicals
   f. book stacks
   g. reference collection
   h. special collections and archives
   i. government documents
   j. theses and dissertations
   k. media center
   l. audiovisual aids (microfilm, microfiche, videotapes, and audiotapes)
   m. copy machines, change machines, vending machines
   n. study areas, lounges, rest rooms, and telephones
   o. computers for word processing
   p. any other services

2. Find out about library operations.
   a. What hours are the library open?
   b. When are library staff available to help?
   c. Are library tours and/or classes in library use available?
   d. What are the policies for checkout and return of materials?
   e. How do you get checkout and interlibrary loan privileges?
   f. Is this library connected with other libraries that you can use?
   g. Can you access computer search tools from computers in other locations on campus or from your home computer?

3. How is the library collection classified?

4. Where are the nursing materials located? Nursing books? Nursing journals? Professional documents from the American Nurses Association (ANA), National League for Nursing (NLN)? Statistics about nurses and nursing?

5. What nursing journals do they own? What nursing research journals do they own?

How Do You Use the Library?

To find specific materials and retrieve the information you seek, you must understand the library's filing system. This means knowing how to use catalogs, abstracts, and indexes to help you locate the materials you're interested in. These resources may be in manual (printed) or computerized form. Most libraries offer combinations of both options. If you want to get a feel for how a catalog or index is organized, you may want to sit down with a manual system and skim it. If you are doing a search, however, the computer is generally much quicker and more versatile.

ADVENTURE CD
1-3

Catalogs

The **catalog** lists books and sometimes other materials that are available in a specific library. Books are listed with bibliographical information, call numbers, and checkout status. Title, author, or subject matter can be used to locate a needed book. The titles of periodicals and other library materials, such as government or professional documents, may also be listed, but information about the specific content contained in those periodicals or documents is usually not in the catalog.

MANUAL CATALOGS

If the library has a manual cataloging system, every book is listed on a 3 × 5 index card and stored alphabetically in wooden file drawers. There are at least three cards for each book: one is listed and filed by book title, one by the author's last name, and one or more by the subject matter of the book. Some libraries have separate filing cabinets for each type of card—a title catalog, an author catalog, and a subject catalog. Others integrate all the cards in one large cataloging system. Each card lists all bibliographical information plus the call number and related classification subject headings. An example is shown in Figure 1-1.

Some libraries still have all their books on a manual card system. Most, however, use a computerized system of some kind. Some libraries have both systems in place with older books on the manual system and newer books on the computer system.

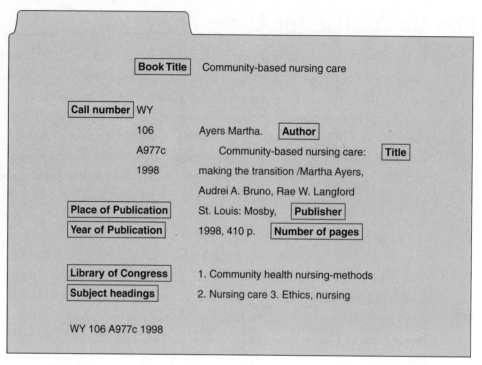

Fig. 1-1   Sample card catalog on 3 × 5 index card listed by book title.

ELECTRONIC CATALOGS

A computerized cataloging system may be on **CD-ROM** (compact disk-read only memory) or directly **on-line.** A CD-ROM catalog disk looks just like a music compact disc except it contains information on books or other materials located in the library. You access that information by putting the CD-ROM disk into the CD-ROM drive of a personal computer located in the reference or main section of the library. Directions will pop up on the screen that tell you how to search for a book by title, author, or subject matter.

On-line catalogs require you to use a computer terminal or personal computer that has a connection to the computerized **database,** which lists books and other library materials. The entries and directions look similar to those on the CD-ROM. The advantage of computerized systems (CD-ROM, on-line) over manual systems is that you may do a subject or title search using any of several key words, which affords you more flexibility. On-line systems offer the added advantage of providing the latest information on all new materials coming in to the library. CD-ROMs must be replaced with new versions and may be as much as a year behind in listing new materials. On-line systems usually also carry additional information such as whether a book is on the shelves or has been checked out and, if so, when it is due back. They may also give you information about resources in other nearby libraries.

If your library has a computerized catalog, do the following challenge:

STUDENT CHALLENGE Scanning Computer Catalogs*

1. Sit down at one of the computer terminals in the library.
2. Examine and try the different options available on the computer screen.
3. Use the on-line catalog to locate one of your nursing textbooks by using a keyword in the title.
4. Now try locating it by author.
5. Then try locating it by subject matter.
6. Which way was easiest for you? Did any of these give you problems? How did you solve them?
7. Now go locate the book in the library. What information did you use to find the book?

---

*Note: Catalogs list book citations; indexes list periodical citations.

Indexes and Abstracts

Indexes list citations to periodicals and other publications such as newspapers and government or professional documents. **Abstracts** are simply indexes that also include a short summary of each citation. These **citations** are arranged by subject matter and/or author. Several different indexes exist for a wide variety of specialty areas. The library will not own all of the materials cited in a particular index, but it may have access to them through **interlibrary loan.** Look for a list of the indexes and abstracts available in a particular library to aid in your search abilities. A list of some common and useful indexes and abstracts is found in Box 1-1.

Two indexes—*Cumulative Index to Nursing and Allied Health Literature* (CINAHL) and *Index Medicus*—serve as major search tools for materials in nursing and medicine. CINAHL contains indexed citations for over 1,200 journals in nursing, medicine, and 15 other allied health disciplines. Over 500 of the journals have **abstracts**—short summaries of articles—included with the article citation.

Box 1-1   List of Sample Indexes/Abstracts

Journals:
Cumulative Index to Nursing and Allied Health Literature (CINAHL)
Cumulative Index of Nursing Research—no longer in print
Index Medicus (MEDLINE)
Hospital and Health Administration Index
International Pharmaceutical Abstracts
Current Index to Journals in Education (ERIC)
Psychological Abstracts (PsycLIT)
Social Sciences Citation Index (SSCI)
Sociological Abstracts
Social Work Abstracts

Magazines:
Magazine Index
Newsbank
Reader's Guide to Periodical Literature

Newspapers:
Los Angeles Times Index
Newspaper abstracts
New York Times Index
Wall Street Journal Index

Government/Professional Documents:
Index to Current Urban Documents
Index to U.S. Government Periodicals
Monthly Catalog of U.S. Government Publications
Public Affairs Information Service (PAIS)
Statistical Abstract of the United States
American Statistics Index
National League for Nursing Publications
American Nursing Association Publications

Dissertations:
Dissertation Abstracts

Computers:
Directory of On-line Databases
Guide to Use of Libraries and Information Services

Electronic version noted in parentheses.

These abstracts are generated by professional abstract writers. CINAHL also indexes material from consumer health and alternative therapy sources. Abstracts of nursing **dissertations,** educational software, and audiovisuals are included. *Index Medicus* contains indexed citations from over 3,900 journals in medicine, nursing, dentistry, veterinary medicine, and preclinical sciences. Author-generated abstracts are available for articles in most of these journals (PubMed, 1999). CINAHL covers nursing, allied health, and psychosocial issues better than *Index Medicus*, but coverage of medicine is more comprehensive in *Index Medicus*. Most major nursing journals can be found in either index.

MANUAL INDEXES AND ABSTRACTS

Indexes are available in both printed and computerized formats. The printed indexes and abstracts are bound in large volumes arranged by different areas of specialty. They are usually stored on tables so that you may use them in the same location that you find them. Many libraries have printed indexes for older periodicals (i.e., before the mid-1980s) and computerized indexes for newer periodicals. To become familiar with printed indexes, try the following Student Challenge.

STUDENT CHALLENGE Perusing Printed Indexes

1. Select a printed volume of any one of the indexes available in your library.
2. Skim through it. What do you see?
3. Locate the listing of subject heads. (Hint: The listing of subject heads is located at the front of the index.)
4. Examine it. Try finding a topic or two in this listing.
5. Was the topic there? If you couldn't find it, did you try a synonym for the word you were looking for?
6. Look through the listings. Note that some major headings have pages and pages of listings, while subheadings have fewer listings.

ELECTRONIC INDEXES AND ABSTRACTS

Electronic databases are either available on CD-ROM or on-line. They often offer access to a wider range of information than their print counterparts. For example, CINAHL on-line offers proceedings from nursing conferences, standards of practice, and many statistics about nurses and nursing in addition to the indexed journals, professional publications, and nursing dissertations. Electronic indexes may have different names, such as MEDLINE, which is the electronic version of *Index Medicus*. Many electronic indexes combine two or more print index titles. For example, ERIC is an education electronic database that incorporates the *Current Index to Journals in Education* (CIJE) and *Resources in Education* (RIE) print indexes. Various electronic databases are available, and each operates in a slightly different fashion. The introductory computer screen and help feature will guide you in your search, but if these aren't sufficient, be sure to consult a reference librarian for additional help.

> **Hint:** When you click on the "help" button, it gives you information that corresponds to functions you are currently trying to perform.

CD-ROMs usually contain one or two indexes per disk for a certain year span. These disks are replaced each time an update occurs. Updates may range from once a month to once a year. Thus, you might use a MEDLINE Professional CD-ROM disk to view the *Index Medicus* for 1994 to the present. MEDLINE Professional is updated every 2 months. The library may have their CD-ROM collection already stored on the computer. If so, simply click on the CD-ROM listings and then click on MEDLINE to get access to that particular index.

On-line systems allow you instant access to a wide range of electronic indexes and abstracts. These indexes are kept on a master computer in a central site and are accessed by the computers in your library. You will find a listing of available on-line indexes by viewing a listing on the screen of one of your library computers. The advantages of an on-line system over a CD-ROM are that updates occur more frequently, and user-timely messages may be posted on the site.

Try the following Student Challenge to get a feel for using electronic indexes and how they differ from using computerized catalogs.

Comparing Manual and Electronic Indexes

You have probably noticed some differences in printed and electronic indexes. This section explores some of those differences. A printed index can be touched,

Sit down at one of the computer terminals in the library.

1. Does the same terminal allow you to do catalog and index searches? If so, how do you go from one type of search to the other?
2. Look at all the indexes available either on CD-ROM or on-line. Which ones look like they would be relevant to nursing or health care?
3. Explore at least two indexes that you consider relevant to nursing. Can you locate a description of the index? Can you find a list of the journals that are indexed?

picked up, and perused. It takes up physical space and you can see the whole thing at once. Print indexes have fixed entries listed under a set of preestablished headings and subheadings. When conducting a search in a printed index, you must first know the precise terms (known in library lingo as "controlled vocabulary") used in the index. If multiple terms describe your topic, you then have to look up each term separately and read all the entries listed in an attempt to eliminate nonapplicable articles. This elimination process is based largely on the title. For large topics, index entries may be endless, and the process of elimination is time consuming and confusing.

In an electronic database, you see only those things that you have specifically requested by the search parameters you set up. However, you don't have to know the specialized vocabulary on which the index is based. The computer will guide you in the terms to use. You can search for keywords or parts of words or combinations of words in any part of the article. You can do a cross search by entering several terms at once and instructing the computer how to use these terms. You can place limits on the search by instructing the computer to look only for certain groups of articles, certain types of journals, or certain publication dates. After you enter these parameters, the search results appear with the touch of a button. You can change the limits or terms instantly and rerun your search as many times as you wish. This makes the search process more flexible, less time consuming, and generally more productive.

If you have access to both the printed and electronic versions of CINAHL or *Index Medicus* (MEDLINE), try the following Student Challenge.

STUDENT CHALLENGE Comparing Printed and Electronic Indexes

Do a search of the nursing literature in the year 1997 for articles that give you information about nursing care of females with colostomies following treatment for colon cancer.

1. Use the print index first.
2. Time each search.
3. What difficulties did you encounter with each search method.
4. What did you like about each method?
5. Compare your results. Are they similar? Which method produced the best materials?

How Do You Successfully Search for Information?

A **search** is conducted using indexes, abstracts, and catalogs to find information about specific subjects. As you have probably discovered, searching for a known book or article by title or by author is fairly easy. Searching for unknown materials on a subject you're interested in is a little more complicated. If you have ever done a search and received a message that says, "there are 2,346 matches," or "there are no matches meeting your search parameters," you know what I mean. This section is designed to help you make your searches smoother and more productive.

Clearly Define Your Mission

What is it that you expect to find from your trip to the library? What is your subject area? What are key concepts and subconcepts for that subject? Which concepts are most important? What information do you already have? Reading your own textbooks or reference books for baseline information before you go to the library can help focus and direct your search. Look at the references listed in these books. You might find sources on your topic that you can look up in the library.

> **Hint:** It helps to read your own textbooks or reference books for baseline information before you go to the library.

Choose the Appropriate Resources

Books tend to give you standard accepted information and practices. They provide good baseline data on a subject, particularly if the subject area is new to you. If you have a working baseline and are looking for current information, then skip the books and go straight to the journals. Journals provide more current information than that found in books. They report changing trends and practices. Research journals provide the results of the latest research studies. Do you need definitions, statistics, trends, or professional or government standards about a topic? These are usually found in reference materials or the special documents sections of the library. Dictionaries and encyclopedias can give you quick definitions and overviews of your subject matter.

Choose the Appropriate Indexes

Ongoing research in the field of library science found that most users know very little about various indexes and made less than optimum selections about 75% of the time (Varlejs, 1991). When skimming the list of available periodical indexes, some choices are obvious. You don't look in the literature or philosophy indexes for a nursing topic. But there are several indexes for nursing journals, including CINAHL and *Index Medicus* (MEDLINE). There are also indexes from other disciplines that might have information about a related topic in nursing. For example, you might locate articles for case management in the *Social Work Abstracts*. Each index has a primary area of focus and advantages and limits. A description of the purpose of a particular index and a list of included journals is usually readily available in the library. These descriptions may be available in print and/or from the computer. Reading these descriptions can help you decide which database to use.

Define Your Search Parameters

If you're using print indexes, remember that each index uses a special preset vocabulary to list entries. So, before you begin your search, look at the directory of indexing terms for that database. (Hint: This is usually in the front of the first volume of a given index.) This allows you to make sure you're using the right terms in your search.

Electronic databases also operate with a special vocabulary. However, the computer helps you define the preferred terms to use in a search. If you enter a term, it will supply alternative terms for use. It will also let you view the entire directory if you want to see how it is organized. Different databases use different listings of terms. MEDLINE uses a medical subject-heading (meSH) directory. CINAHL uses it own specialized thesaurus. Many other databases use Library of Congress headings or their own specialized subject directories.

Place Limits on Your Search

You want to make your search as precise as possible. If you have several key terms, use them. Set other limits such as gender, age, and/or time factors if you know them. You can always lift some of the limits if you don't find what you want. Let's say, for example, that we want to find out the latest information on the effects of menopause on individuals with diabetes mellitus. If we enter the word "diabetes" to search MEDLINE, for example, we would come up with 147,316 different citations. If we use the words "diabetes mellitus" we come up with 133,554 citations. The words "diabetes mellitus AND menopause" narrow it down to 379 citations. If we narrow the search to include only adult females, we get 309 citations. If we further limit the search to articles written in English and published from 1997 to 1999, we get 57 citations. That's a number we can handle.

All computerized search databases have rules for use. The more you know about these rules and how to use them, the more successful your search will be. Most databases use something called Boolean operators. These operators are just words (e.g., AND, OR, NEAR) that help you link key terms together to get certain results. Look at the diabetes-menopause example in Table 1-1. As you can see OR is

Table 1-1 Example of Boolean Search

CONNECTOR	EXAMPLE	WHAT HAPPENS
or	Diabetes mellitus <u>or</u> menopause	Retrieves all citations containing the words diabetes mellitus or the word menopause in an article.
and	Diabetes mellitus <u>and</u> menopause	Retrieves all citations containing both the words diabetes mellitus and the word menopause in an article.
near	Diabetes mellitus <u>near</u> menopause	Retrieves all citations containing both the words diabetes mellitus and the word menopause in the same sentence of the article.

the least restrictive link and NEAR is the most restrictive link. Other operators may be used to place limits on such things as age, gender, type of journal, years of publication, and so on.

A few databases use a technique called *probabilistic searching,* which gives you a list of articles ranked from most to least likely to be relevant, based on a set of supplied search terms (e.g., diabetes mellitus, menopause, female, adult). Articles containing all the terms would be high on the list, and those containing one term would be at the bottom of the list. You can even weight the terms to indicate which are more important in the search (e.g., the terms *diabetes mellitus* and *menopause* could be more heavily weighted than female or adult).

The best way to become proficient at using search operators is through informed practice. Studies have shown that most users do not make full use of the electronic system capabilities (Varlejs, 1991). Read the materials available on conducting a search. Ask for assistance if you aren't finding anything or if you're finding too much. Explore various search options and see what happens. Most importantly, practice, practice, practice. (Hint: Make sure you correctly spell all the terms that you enter for a computerized search.)

View Your Search Results

Once you have defined and run your search, you'll want to view the results. The first viewing screen usually contains each citation with the option to view an abstract or full text if available. Simply looking at article titles or journal names helps you eliminate more articles from your search. If a citation looks promising, you may want to look at the abstract.

In the example about menopause and its effects on diabetes, a preview of the 57 citations led to 21 articles that looked like useful possibilities. I asked the computer for the abstracts on these 21 articles and found that five of the articles looked promising. I then went to the shelves and skimmed the full texts of those five articles. Three were useful, so I made copies of them. Looking at the citations may also give you clues about making a search narrower. For example, when I did the search using just the word "diabetes," the very first citation was about diabetes insipidus, leading me to add "mellitus" to the term "diabetes."

Now that you have had a little practice, try the following Student Challenge and do another search, using the computer and whichever electronic resources you deem most appropriate. Use the information from the successful search sections and the knowledge gained from the previous Student Challenges to assist you.

STUDENT CHALLENGE Putting It All Together

Search for updated information on a basic nursing skill (such as handwashing, blood pressure readings, or temperature taking).

1. Define what you're looking for.
2. What resources will you use? Why did you choose them?
3. Describe how you conducted your search. What parameters did you use? How did you limit the search?
4. How many different searches did you do? What guided your decision-making processes during the search process? What worked and what didn't work about your search approach?
5. Print the end results of your search. Locate the articles you think most pertinent to your selected topic. Did they contain the information you needed?

Resource Kit

Library help guides—Many libraries offer printed help guides designed to make library use easier. Collect them, read them, use them.

HELP! Button—Electronic databases all come with a Help button. It is designed to help you make the best use of that database. Click on it whenever you are stuck in an electronic search process and need guidance.

Librarians—Don't forget to use these helpful resources. Don't be shy. They field all kinds of seemingly dumb questions.

 Visit the book's MERLIN website at **www.mosby.com/MERLIN/Langford/maze** for further information.

 Check out the puzzles, mazes, and games on your **CD-ROM.**

References

American Library Association (ALA): *ALA world encyclopedia of library and information services*, ed 2, Chicago, 1986, American Library Association.

CINAHL information systems: *About CINAHL*, on-line at www.cinahl.com/data, May 5, 1999.

Feather J and Sturges P: *International encyclopedia of information and library science*, New York, 1997, Rutledge.

National Library of Medicine PubMed: The NLM PubMed project overview, on-line at www.ncbi.nlm.nih.gov/pubmed/overview, May 5, 1999.

Varlejs J: *Information literacy: learning how to learn*, Jefferson, NC, 1991, McFarland.

Learning Objectives

1   Describe the Internet and relevant Internet components and services.

2   Use three different approaches to web navigation.

3   Send and receive electronic mail with attachments.

4   Explore listservers, newsgroups, and/or chat rooms.

5   Discuss possible applications of FTP and Telnet.

6   Access library filing systems (indexes, catalogs) over the Internet.

7   Use professional databases available on the Net.

8   Locate print and electronic journals available on the Net.

9   Discuss professional communication and education opportunities available via the Internet.

Chapter Outline

What's This Chapter All About?
What Is the Internet?
What Does the Internet Offer?
  World Wide Web
  Communication tools
  Traditional services
How Do You Use the Internet?
  Navigating the web
    Uniform resource locators
    Hypertext links
    Search engines

Communicating on the net
  E-mail and listservs
  Newsgroups and chat rooms
  Audio and video possibilities
Trying traditional tools
How Do You Use the Net for Professional Purposes?
  Information access
  Communication possibilities
  Ongoing educational opportunities

Surfing the Internet

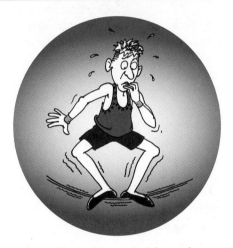

It feels like walking a tightrope to me.

Student Quote   *"I feel like an explorer setting out in uncharted territory . . . It's exciting and scary all at the same time."*

Abstract   Technology and the Internet are changing the way we find, use, and share information. The Internet is a worldwide, interconnected network of computers. You can tap into stored information and databases and send and receive communications from individuals or groups. To use the Internet you need a computer, a connection source, and a service provider. All Internet locations are identified by an address (i.e., the uniform resource locator [URL]). Navigating the Net is enhanced by the use of web browsers and search engines. Library catalogs, indexes, and other resources are available on the Internet, including various health-related databases, such as MEDLINE and CINAHL. Full-text print journals and electronic journals are increasingly available. The Internet provides instant communication to professional colleagues from across the globe. You can take a course, search for a job, or hold a meeting over the Internet. It holds new hope in the quest for information literacy.

KEY TERMS

Net Nomenclature

Bookmark A way to mark and easily access a favorite or frequently used website in Netscape Navigator (referred to as "favorites" in Internet Explorer).

Browser A program that opens and displays pages on the World Wide Web.

Download Transferring a file from the Internet to your computer.

E-mail Electronic mail; postage-free messages sent via the Internet from one computer to another.

File attachment A file that is added to an E-mail message.

File transfer protocol (FTP) A program that allows you to transfer files from the Internet to your computer.

Home page The first or base page for a website. It often serves as a map, directing you to places of interest on the site.

Hypertext An electronic document format that permits links to other web pages or other related websites. The link is underlined and can be accessed by a mouse click on the link.

HyperText Markup Language (HTML) The codes and instructions used to control the appearance and function of a website. It inserts links, graphics, and other multimedia objects on the web page.

HyperText Transfer Protocol (HTTP) The language used to transfer web pages over an Internet connection. The first letters in a URL for a site on the World Wide Web.

Internet service provider (ISP) A company that provides a connection to the Internet (e.g., AT&T Worldnet, Microsoft Internet, Sprint Earthlink).

Listserver (listserv) An electronic mailing list.

Log off Disconnecting from the Internet.

Log on Connecting to the Internet.

Navigate Moving from site to site on the Internet.

Newsgroup Discussion via posting messages on an electronic bulletin board.

On-line Active connection to the Internet.

On-line service A commercial network that provides a wide range of on-line services including access to the Internet, news, games, travel information, and so on (e.g., CompuServe, AOL, Prodigy).

Search engine Tools to find and retrieve specific information on the Web (e.g., Yahoo!, Lycos, Go.com, Altavista, Excite).

Server (host) A computer that offers an information service over the Internet.

Telnet Software that lets users log onto another computer from a remote site. It shows text only, no graphics or pictures.

Uniform resource locator (URL) The address system used by the Internet to assist in locating a web page or file.

Upload Transfer of a file from your computer to another computer using the Internet.

User A client that communicates via computer and uses Internet services offered by servers or hosts.

User name The name you use to identify your computer to another computer or computer system.

Web page One screen on a website.

Website A sequence of web pages created by an individual or organization for conveying information.

World Wide Web (www) A collection of computers on the Internet that are interconnected by hypertext and store websites.

ADVENTURE CD 2-1

Easy access to ever more affordable, powerful, and user-friendly microcomputers has forever changed the way we interact with the world around us. The computer revolution is in full bloom, and it has spawned the Internet. This information highway can instantly link us to people and resources around the world. It is changing the way we work and play. We can buy a car or shop for groceries without leaving the house. We can meet and chat with newfound friends in Australia or Japan or Brazil. We can send or receive reams of material at the push of a button. We can tap into the latest information available about almost any subject imaginable. The Internet is erasing boundaries of time and distance. It allows us to explore new worlds and ideas, to sail into uncharted waters, and to become players in an exciting adventure.

What Is This Chapter All About?

You have explored the library as a resource that can help you become and remain informacion literate. This chapter introduces you to another way to keep up with the rapid information growth of our times. We take a tour of the Internet and explore its potential, investigating what it is, what it can offer, and how to use it. We focus on the Internet as a tool for locating and accessing information resources. The ability to use the Internet can extend and enhance your library skills and make finding needed professional information easier, less time consuming, and more convenient. Picture this: It's 11 PM, and you're all ready for bed. In a panic, you realize that you have a paper due in 2 days, and you haven't even started on it. The library is closed so you can't even do a literature search. Now imagine conducting a search from your bed, in your pajamas, on your laptop, at midnight. Fantasy? No, it's courtesy of the Internet. If this sounds like a tool you would like to exploit, read on.

> Hint: If you are already an accomplished Internet user, you might want to skim the first part of this chapter and concentrate on the section that addresses use of the Internet for professional purposes.

What Is the Internet?

The Internet is, in the broadest sense, a microcosm of our world. It reflects a vast variety of cultural and societal views and allows people across this planet to share ideas on a personal level never before possible. In a more literal sense, the Internet is a huge network of interconnected computers located all over the world. These computers are linked together by a series of networks. Some of the computers in the network are known as hosts, or **servers,** because they "serve" information in various ways to computer owners known as clients, or **users.**

> The Internet is a huge network of interconnected server and user computers located all over the world.

Anyone with a computer, a modem, and an account can access the Internet and communicate with all the other participating computers. This means that you, as an Internet user, can interact with people from around the world. You also have access to a vast array of information and resources stored on those computers. The Internet currently connects millions of computers and is more than doubling in size every year.

> Anyone with a computer, a modem, and an account can access the Internet.

The Internet, or "Net" for short, began as a highly specialized network of computers designed by the United States military in the 1960s. Other governmental agencies, universities, and research institutions began to use it to exchange scientific and technical information in the 1970s. In the 1980s, libraries and other professional associations began using the Internet to exchange scholarly information. Then, an explosion occurred in the personal computer industry. The easy availability of personal computers allowed individuals access to the Net.

The 1990s marked a rapid evolution of the Internet. It has become a personal communication exchange and commercial marketplace, as well as an information resource. Local, state, and national governing bodies; professional and community associations; educational and research institutions; and businesses and individuals use the Net. It is used for learning, research, business, and pleasure and remains relatively lacking in structure and control. There are few rules and no central organizing concept. Even the "experts" struggle to keep up with the changes.

The potential of the Internet seems limitless, but that very potential also presents challenges (Box 2-1). The biggest challenge when using the Internet is learn-

Box 2-1   Some Issues Encountered When Using the Internet

Confusion and Chaos: The Internet operates in a freewheeling culture with few rules, limits, or boundaries. No entity exercises control over Net offerings, and there is little regulatory control over Net transactions.

Needle in a Haystack: The number of Internet websites is growing at an incredibly fast pace. No single search device has been devised that allows efficient access to everything on the Net. Sometimes you have to wade through a haystack of useless and irrelevant junk to find the needle that you need.

Time Drain: Although touted for its instant access and speed, it is easy to spend hours moving and scrolling through various web pages on the Internet with little to show for the effort.

Questionable Reliability of Information: Anyone is free to post information. This leads to a dilemma about the accuracy and reliability of such information. The exact source and that source's credibility are often hard to track on the Internet.

ing to **navigate** the Net efficiently and effectively. Think of it as an adventure because it can be a powerful tool for communication, information retrieval, and learning.

What Does the Internet Offer?

There are many services on the Internet. The World Wide Web (www) and electronic mail (E-mail) are probably the best known, but other applications include listservs, newsgroups, chat rooms, audio and interactive video, file transfer protocols (FTP), and Telnet. Each of these is described in the following section.

World Wide Web

The **World Wide Web (www)** or "the Web" is the most rapidly growing portion of the Internet. The terms "Internet" and "World Wide Web" are often used interchangeably. However, the Web is a subset of the Internet. The Web is a huge, loosely organized collection of documents on thousands of topics stored on various computers worldwide. The collection is located on various **websites,** each containing numerous **web pages** of material. These web pages use a variety of multimedia resources with a mixture of text; sound; graphics; color; and, sometimes, videos.

The pages are linked together by **hypertext,** which allow you to move from one page to another or from one website to another by clicking on a highlighted word with your computer mouse. This is often termed "surfing." For example, you might be on a website about the care of diabetes mellitus and discover links to a diabetic diet, insulin, or foot care. More about navigating the Web later.

Communication Tools

There are a number of ways to communicate with others over the Internet. These range from electronic mail to chat rooms, newsgroups, and videoconferencing. A discussion of communication tools follows.

Electronic mail (**E-mail,** for short) allows you to send and receive messages over the Internet. You can even attach and send computer files, called **file attachments,** with your message. The message travels postage-free and arrives at its destination in a matter of seconds. As a student, you can send and receive messages from faculty members, or you can send a term paper or care plan by attaching them to a message. You can converse with nursing students in other universities around the world. E-mail also allows you to send a message to multiple people simultaneously. A **listserv** is an E-mail list that is organized around a particular area of interest. To use a listserv, simply send an E-mail message to the owner of the list, who then distributes the message to all the members of a particular interest group that have subscribed to the list.

Newsgroups are electronic message boards that allow you to post and receive messages from participants in that newsgroup. Chat rooms are similar to newsgroups, except that you can carry on typed conversations with people who are currently logged on their computers and are tuned into a particular chat room. So, feedback in a chat room is immediate, whereas feedback in a newsgroup is delayed.

If you have the right hardware and software, you can use the Internet as a telephone and actually speak to people through an Internet connection. If you add special video equipment, you can hold video conversations and actually see the person as you talk. You can even hold videoconferences. As technology continues to improve, this use of the Internet will become more common.

Traditional Services

Two older or more traditional systems on the Internet that you may still see in action are **Telnet** and **file transfer protocols (FTP).** Telnet connects a text-only computer to one or more remote locations via the Internet. It requires special software to establish a connection. Some universities and libraries still use Telnet systems.

FTP is a particular process used to transfer files across the Internet. Typical files include public domain software, lesson plans, electronic books, research reports, and graphics.

How Do You Use the Internet?

To use the Internet you need access. This requires a computer, an Internet connection, and an on-line service or Internet service provider. The most common connection is through a modem. Satellite dishes, cable television, and digital subscriber lines (DSL) also offer Internet access in some locations. The modem is used to dial up a commercial **on-line service** such as America On-line, CompuServe 2000, or Prodigy or to connect to an **Internet service provider (ISP)** such as AT&T Worldnet or Sprint Earthlink. These services typically charge a subscription rate. Some ISPs provide free connections, but you are likely to be subject to a barrage of advertisements. (The Resource Kit at the end of the chapter lists several on-line services and ISPs).

Once you have a connection, you are ready to **log on** to the Net. However, you need a program that will let you take advantage of the resources on the Internet. Two popular programs, Internet Explorer and Netscape Navigator, provide you with the ability to browse the Web, send and receive E-mail, access newsgroups and chatlines, use an electronic telephone, and edit web pages. Even though they allow you to access multiple Internet resources, they are often called web **browsers.** One of these programs may have come with the purchase of your computer, or your ISP or on-line service may have provided it to you. Both systems look similar and operate very similarly (Fig. 2-1), and both are available for Macintosh and Windows computer operating systems.

ADVENTURE
CD
2-2

Navigating the Web

The browser that is built into the Internet Explorer or Netscape Navigator program serves as your guide to the World Wide Web. As you will discover, it is easy to lose track of where you are on the Web. A browser allows you to track the websites you visit, to track and revisit previous sites, and to save favorite sites so that you can find and visit them easily.

When you first connect to the Internet, you will automatically connect to the front page of your on-line or Internet service provider and to your Web browser

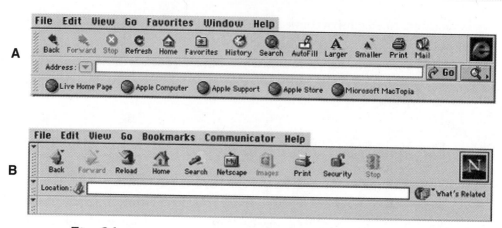

Fig. 2-1 **A,** Internet Explorer toolbar. **B,** Netscape Navigator toolbar.

program. Your screen will display a **home page** from your service provider with the browser toolbar and menu at the top.

UNIFORM RESOURCE LOCATOR

There are three major ways to move around the Web from that initial page. The first is by entering the address of a particular site that you wish to visit. Each place on the Internet has a **uniform resource locator (URL),** which is an address for a specific location on the Internet. For example, http://www.wnba.com is the URL for the Women's National Basketball League website.

If you know the address, you can enter it on the location line of your web browser, and it will take you directly to that site. Various print, CD-ROM, and on-line directories list website addresses. They often resemble telephone directories. There is even a website yellow pages. You will also notice that an increasing number of businesses, newspapers, and television programs are posting their URLs.

> **Hint:** You must type the URL exactly as it appears. If you add a space, omit a dot, or misspell a word, the site can't be located. However, you can omit the "http://" at the beginning of a web address. The web browser will automatically insert it for you.

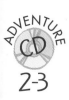

ADVENTURE
CD
2-3

Examining a URL can tell you something about the site. Figure 2-2 presents the elements of a URL. To see how URLs work, try the following Student Challenge.

STUDENT CHALLENGE Using URLs

If you have Internet access, try the following:

1. Collect three or four URLs you've seen mentioned in a newspaper, magazine, on television, or in another source.
2. Connect to your ISP and web browser.
3. Enter one of the URLs in the address or location text box on the browser. (Hint: On most browsers, the text box to type in the URL is located right below the toolbar and above the page viewing area.) You may have to erase an existing URL before entering the new URL.
4. Highlight the URL you have entered and click on it, or hit the "Go" button to the right of the text box, or hit "Enter" on your keyboard.
5. You should now be looking at the first page of the site that you entered the address for.
6. Now enter another URL and repeat the procedure described above. You have now moved to another specified site.

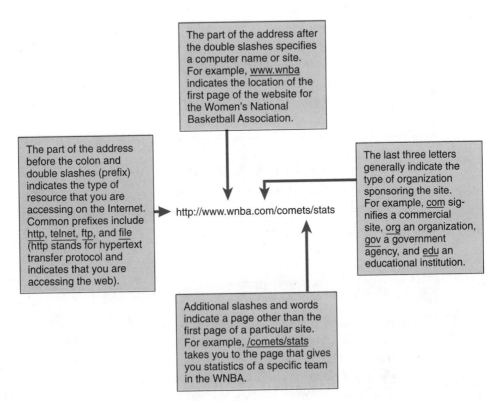

The part of the address after the double slashes specifies a computer name or site. For example, www.wnba indicates the location of the first page of the website for the Women's National Basketball Association.

The part of the address before the colon and double slashes (prefix) indicates the type of resource that you are accessing on the Internet. Common prefixes include http, telnet, ftp, and file (http stands for hypertext transfer protocol and indicates that you are accessing the web).

The last three letters generally indicate the type of organization sponsoring the site. For example, com signifies a commercial site, org an organization, gov a government agency, and edu an educational institution.

http://www.wnba.com/comets/stats

Additional slashes and words indicate a page other than the first page of a particular site. For example, /comets/stats takes you to the page that gives you statistics of a specific team in the WNBA.

Fig. 2-2   Elements of a uniform resource locator (URL).

HYPERTEXT LINKS

A second way to move around the Web is by clicking on the highlighted web links or icons (little pictures) found on each web page. These are known as hypertext links. When your mouse pointer moves over a link, the pointer will change form (e.g., my pointer changes from an arrow to a hand). This alerts you to the presence of a link. These send you instantly to other pages within that site or to other related sites. For example, I might click "games" on my ISP home page. It will send me to a listing of games.

STUDENT CHALLENGE Leafing Through Links

Using one of the sites that you found by using a URL, try the following:
1. Look at the web page. Note that some of the text is highlighted and underlined. These are hypertext links. Click on one of these links. You have just moved to another web page.
2. Check the address window on your web browser. Note how the URL has changed. If the address has been added to, you have moved to another page. If the information right after "www" has changed, you have accessed a new site.
3. Explore the pages for this website by clicking on various links and viewing several web pages.
4. Try clicking on icons and boxed text. These may also be links.
5. Play around, enjoy the feeling of moving from link to link and page to page. When you are done, don't **log off** (disconnect). Do the next challenge first.

By now you have probably discovered that you can become lost in the forest, so to speak, rather quickly. This is why a web browser is a useful tool. The web browser can help you leave a trail of bread crumbs to mark where you have been. Try the following Student Challenge.

STUDENT CHALLENGE Trailblazing or Trial Browsing

You should be using the results of your click-and-link exercise.
1. Locate the web browser toolbar at the top of your screen. Click on the "Back" button on your web browser tool bar. This will move you back one web page. Click on the "Back" button again. Do it again. Great! Now click on the "Forward" button. This will move you forward one web page

---

STUDENT CHALLENGE Trailblazing or Trial Browsing—
cont'd

with each click. You have just discovered a basic way to retrace your path when you want to revisit a previous page or advance to the next page.

2. Next, if you have Internet Explorer, click on the "down" arrow located to the right of the "Back" button on your browser toolbar. A list of the pages you just visited will appear. Click on one of these pages. You go right to it. This can save you multiple clicks on the "Back" button.

3. Now, click on the "down" arrow to the right of the address or location window. Note it lists the URLs for the sites you have visited most recently. Note it lists only the site. It doesn't list the various pages in a site. Click on one of these sites.

4. Do you want a comprehensive record of where you have been on the web? If you have the Internet Explorer browser, click the "History" button. Click on the week and the day that you're interested in. Click on the site you're interested in. It provides a trail of all the pages you visited in that site. If you have Netscape Navigator, open the "Communicator" menu and choose "History" to produce the history list.

5. Do you want to save a site or a page you really like and want to visit again? To **bookmark** a website, bring the site or page up on your screen. If you have Internet Explorer, open the "Favorites" menu and click on "Add to Favorites." Your page is permanently saved for you. Anytime you want to access it, just click the "Favorites" button on the toolbar and then click on the saved web page of your choice.

    If you have Netscape Navigator, open the "Bookmarks" menu located to the left of the location box and click on "Add Bookmark." To get a bookmarked page just click the "Bookmarks" menu and select the web page of your choice.

6. Explore the other buttons on your web browser toolbar. Can you figure out what they do? Open up the various drop down menus for your browser. Check out the help menu. Don't be afraid to try out buttons and menu options. Have fun, explore, and play.

SEARCH ENGINES

A third way to navigate the Web is by using a search engine. **Search engines** are tools that allow you to search for information by using keywords. You will find that they resemble the search tools you used in Chapter 1 when doing index searches. Various search engines are available to help you do a search of websites. Some of the most commonly available engines are described in Box 2-2.

Navigate the Web by:
1. Entering the URL of the website
2. Clicking on hypertext links
3. Using search engines

Box 2-2   Sample Search Engines

The website for each of the following search engines is accessible through this text's MERLIN website at www.mosby.com/MERLIN/Langford/maze.

Alta Vista is a very comprehensive search engine with a large and reliable index. It has basic and advanced search capabilities. You need to have search parameters fairly narrowed down or you will get an overwhelming response to your search query.

Excite may be helpful when you're not quite sure what term or terms to use in a search. It uses a method known as *concept searching*. This means it will not only look for the key words entered, but it will also look for materials based on the idea the terms convey. It will also suggest related terms to use. If you find a source you like, Excite also has a feature that lets you search for similar sources by clicking on the "more like this" option.

Hotbot is a comprehensive search engine that is very user friendly. It will guide you through the process and allows you to search by date or by domain type (e.g., you can limit your search to educational sites or delete commercial sites).

Go.com allows you to search other Internet sites in addition to websites such as news stories from the newswire services. It also has a special feature called "imageseek" that lets you look for pictures or graphics.

Lycos uses probabilistic searching and lists search results in rank order of relevancy to your search. It also has a browseable index.

Magellan not only does a search, but also it rates and reviews many of the sites located. You can search the entire Magellan database or limit your search to the reviewed and/or top quality sites.

Northern Light is one of the latest "in" search engines because it will directly link you to full text resources and a way to order them on-line.

Yahoo! allows you to use a subject index or keyword search approach. You can even conduct a key word search within a selected index category. Yahoo! also has hypertext links to other search engines. For these reasons, many people consider Yahoo! to be the best overall search engine available.

MERLIN
Activity
1

Many other search engines also exist. Some are very specialized and search only certain segments of the web. These may be helpful to narrow a technical or specialized search. For example, some search engines search only news or health sources or reference resources. Others, known as "metasearch" tools, allow you to use a number of different search engines at once for a more global search. Although metasearch tools permit a wide search, they seldom offer you the ability to refine a search. Box 2-3 presents examples of specialty and metasearch tools. We explore professional health care search indexes later in this chapter.

You have access to all of these engines through your ISP or by using the URL address of the particular engine. Each of these search engines uses slightly different search methods and different indexing systems. This means you need to rely on the

Box 2-3   Specialized Search Engines

The website for each of these is accessible through the book's MERLIN website at www.mosby.com/MERLIN/Langford/maze.

Specialty Search Engines

My Virtual Reference Desk is an electronic source for locating many of the same materials you would find in the reference section of a library, including dictionaries, encyclopedias, and quick facts.

Internet Public Library permits you to search for many resources that you might find in a public library. It leads you to many full-text references and sources.

News Index lets you search for current news stories worldwide.

Achoo helps web browsers look for medically related topics for consumers.

Health A to Z is a search tool for heath-related topics for consumers.

Metasearch Tools

Cyber 411 searches 16 search engines simultaneously with one set of terms and removes duplicate entries. It allows use of Boolean operators.

Dogpile allows you to use up to 25 different search engines in any sequence you designate for one set of key search terms. It also has a link to Metafind.

Metafind allows you to search several engines sequentially and sort your results while the search engine remains running in the background.

Inference Find lets you do parallel searching. It filters out duplications in your search efforts and clusters your results for you.

MERLIN
Activity
2

help feature when first using a particular search system. This allows you to get a feel for how that system operates. A perfect search system would help you find all the relevant information about your topic that is available on the web. Such a search engine does not exist. If you use several different search engines for the same topic, you will get differing results. Some engines use Boolean search logic, and others use probabilistic methods. Each has a unique indexing system. Some allow you to search only by key words. Others allow you to search by key words or to use a subject index.

If you want further information on search engines and how they work, log on to the book's MERLIN website at www.mosby.com/MERLIN/Langford/maze and link to the Spider's Apprentice website. This site explains how search engines work, gives you tips on conducting and refining a search, provides ratings for several popular search engines, and even lets you try out several search engines.

Ultimately, the best way to view the way that search engines work and to see the difference in results is to use and explore a few of them. Try the following Student Challenge.

STUDENT CHALLENGE Sampling Search Engines

Decide on a specific subject area you're interested in. Get adventurous and have fun. Explore the art of breadmaking, caring for your cat, or old movies. Use your imagination. Once you have an area of interest, log on to your ISP and web browser. Then do the same search using three or four different general search engines.

1. Note the rules for searching for each search engine that you try.
2. Note the different special features that are available.
3. Compare the results from the various searches.
4. Which search engine was the easiest to use? Which gave you the best results?
5. Try a specialty topic and use a specialty search engine.
6. Try out one of the metasearch tools.

Communicating on the Net

A number of communication opportunities await you on the Internet. You can send and receive electronic mail with individuals and groups. You can post messages, chat on-line, use the telephone, or hold videoconferences. With a little basic information, you will be a confident communicator in no time.

E-MAIL AND LISTSERVS

To send E-mail over the Internet, you need an Internet mailing address and electronic mail software. Several Internet sources provide free E-mail accounts and E-mail software. Chances are, however, that you already have E-mail access, since it is one of the services included when you subscribe to an on-line service or an ISP. An E-mail feature is also included with the Netscape Navigator and Internet Explorer web browser packages. All of these services provide help to use the E-mail program feature. You will get guidance in setting up an E-mail account and obtaining an E-mail address.

An E-mail address consists of two basic parts: the **user name** and the host name. These two parts are connected by an "@" symbol. You determine the first part of the address. The second part of the address is dictated by the service that supplies your Internet account. Examining an E-mail address reveals information about the location of the account (Fig. 2-3).

Once you have a functioning E-mail account, you are ready to send and get mail. Sending or receiving a message is easy. First, you connect to the Internet. Then you call up your E-mail software program. If you subscribe to an ISP or on-line service, you can connect by using the icon or link that appears on the opening page immediately after you connect to the Internet. It will be labeled something like "message center" or "mail center." If you are using your web browser's E-mail capabilities, the Netscape E-mail program is called "Netscape Messenger" and the Internet Explorer E-mail program is called "Outlook Express."

All E-mail programs look slightly different and have a slightly different menu system. However, all of them have common features. They allow you to compose and send messages to anyone with an E-mail account (provided you know their E-mail address) and to read and save or print messages sent to you by others. They also let you keep an E-mail address book. All of these features are easily accessible through various menu options or toolbar buttons. Many programs offer several features that enhance sending and receiving mail: (1) you can attach and **upload** one or more files when sending a message; (2) you can **download** files sent to you by others; (3) you can add graphics and special formatting to your messages: and (4) if you get a special digital certificate and key, you can even send and receive messages that are in code and unreadable by anyone except authorized users.

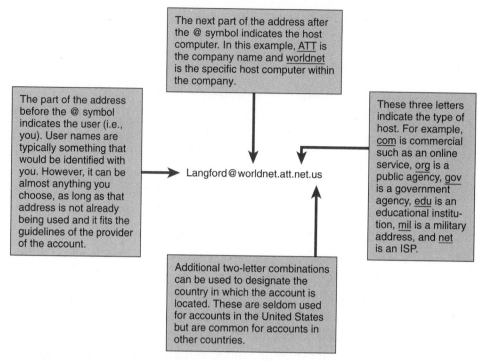

The next part of the address after the @ symbol indicates the host computer. In this example, ATT is the company name and worldnet is the specific host computer within the company.

The part of the address before the @ symbol indicates the user (i.e., you). User names are typically something that would be identified with you. However, it can be almost anything you choose, as long as that address is not already being used and it fits the guidelines of the provider of the account.

These three letters indicate the type of host. For example, com is commercial such as an online service, org is a public agency, gov is a government agency, edu is an educational institution, mil is a military address, and net is an ISP.

Langford@worldnet.att.net.us

Additional two-letter combinations can be used to designate the country in which the account is located. These are seldom used for accounts in the United States but are common for accounts in other countries.

Fig. 2-3   Elements of a sample E-mail address.

STUDENT CHALLENGE E-mail Explorations

If you have access to an E-mail account and are not yet familiar with or comfortable with using it, try the following.

1. Have the E-mail address of one or more friends or fellow students handy.
2. Get on the Internet and access your mail center. Explore the various menu options and toolbar buttons. If you are unsure about what they're for, use the help feature.
3. Try to compose and send a message to your friends. In the message, instruct them to reply by E-mail to your message.
4. Check your E-mail address book. It should automatically have the E-mail addresses on those people you just sent messages to.
5. When you have finished exploring and sending, log off. Come back later and check for messages. When you have messages, practice opening them and reading them. Try printing them out. Try saving a message to a file. Try deleting a message.

STUDENT CHALLENGE E-mail Explorations—cont'd

6. If you are having difficulty with either sending or receiving, and the "help" function is no help, try asking a friend who is an E-mail user to demonstrate for you. Or purchase a basic book on Internet use. Suggestions are available in the Resource Kit at the end of the chapter.

7. If you are feeling comfortable with your E-mail prowess, try attaching and sending files. Have someone attach and send a file to you. Try downloading the file to your computer and opening it.

As an Internet user, you have access to listservs that allow you to send E-mail to an entire group of people who share a common interest. To do this you simply subscribe to that particular listserv (subscriptions are free) and send an E-mail message to the listserv address. This message is then sent to the other subscribers of that listserv. You also receive E-mail messages from other subscribers. If you want to receive lots of E-mail, just join a listserv. Thousands of listservs are available. If you're interested, you can access a listserv directory on the Web such as Liszt Select. (This site is accessible through the MERLIN site.) Over 250 health-related listservs are listed in this particular directory. This site also contains links to other listserv directories.

MERLIN
Activity
4

NEWSGROUPS AND CHAT ROOMS

Newsgroups and chat rooms also allow you to communicate over the Net. Over 20,000 newsgroups or bulletin board sites are available on the Internet. On this type of site you can post messages for any subscriber to read and respond to. Messages and replies are clustered together to establish a conversational flow. Like listservs, newsgroups revolve around particular interest areas. Some of these newsgroups have a moderator or manager who sorts through messages and makes decisions about what is posted. Others are totally uncontrolled, and all messages are posted. If you're interested in newsgroups, most search engines allow you to search for them. You can also tap into a website specifically devoted to newsgroups. They have search mechanisms and category links. One such site is Deja, which you can access through the MERLIN site. If you find a newsgroup of interest, you subscribe to it at no charge. You may even post messages and ask people to reply privately via your E-mail address rather than responding on the bulletin board.

MERLIN
Activity
5

You can also communicate with one or more people by typing back and forth to each other in a chat room. The main difference between chat rooms and list-servs or newsgroups is that you are holding a running conversation with others who are on-line at the same time you are. If you're interested, you might want to visit Yahoo! (remember this search engine?), because it also offers a number of chat rooms. It will also allow you to search for other chat rooms. Chat rooms are also available from your on-line service or ISP.

AUDIO AND VIDEO POSSIBILITIES

With the right equipment and an Internet phone program you can talk to anyone else who also has the right equipment and software program. You can also place conference calls. Technology that even allows for videophone calls and videocon-ferencing is available. These relatively recent technological innovations are not in common use. However, the price is decreasing, and use is expected to expand rapidly.

Trying Traditional Tools

FTP is still a very useful process for transferring files from one computer to another over the Net. It has now been incorporated into use of the Web, and you can per-form this procedure with the help of your web browser. However, it is not a web ap-plication. FTP is often used to obtain updated versions of software programs and Internet tools that you are already using. You can also use FTP to transfer *shareware* (free or nominally priced software programs).

To perform a file transfer procedure you need a web browser and the URL of the file you want to receive. You simply connect to your web browser, type the URL in the address or location box and click on the URL. A file directory will appear. You scroll through the directory and click on the file you want and it will appear on your screen. You can then save the file to whatever location on your computer that you choose.

If the file that you are transferring is a compressed or *zipped* file (a large file that has been condensed for easier storage and transfer), you will need a special piece of software to decompress or unzip the file to read or use it. Your web browser or ISP usually provides you information that allows you to directly download such a pro-gram for use. Winzip is a common unzipping program that can be purchased for a nominal fee.

Telnet allows you to log onto a specific computer on the Internet from a computer at another site. You may wonder why this is important in light of all you have just learned about the Web. Some computer information and services are not currently available on a website. Access is only possible through a Telnet connection. To log on to another computer site, you must have some type of Telnet software and the Telnet URL for the computer you wish to access. Telnet URLs start with telnet://. Some libraries have Telnet connections that allow you log on to their library computer and use their catalog and indexes. You may want to check and see whether your library uses Telnet. If so, you may want to investigate how you can use it.

How Do You Use the Net for Professional Purposes?

Many professional uses have already been alluded to in this chapter. I'm sure such ideas came to you as you completed the student challenges. You may already be using some of the ideas we are about to cover. If so, good for you. This section examines some of the ways that you can make the Internet work for you to enhance your professional life. Our focus is on the information and communication capabilities of the Internet.

Information Access

Many professional information sources are available on the Internet. You have access to a wide variety of databases, patient and nursing education resources, as well as some full-text and virtual nursing journals. One of the most helpful things I have discovered is the ability to conduct a library search from my own personal computer in the comfort of my study at anytime I choose. I have two primary avenues for this type of activity: a user account via the Internet to my local health Science Center Library and direct web connections to search indexes and databases offered by other libraries or commercial services.

My health science center library has an Internet website that library cardholders can access from any personal computer with the use of a special password. This means that I can use all of their electronic indexes and the electronic catalog. I also have direct access to all their on-line materials, including reference materials such as dictionaries and encyclopedias, a large number of medical textbooks, and a variety of health care journals with full-text articles. Unfortunately, most of these full-text sources are currently medical, but the librarian has assured me that more nursing materials will soon be available electronically. There are also hypertext links to other libraries and to other health care information sites.

I also have access to a number of library services, including photocopying and delivery of library materials for a fee. Thus, it is possible for me to conduct a library search and request that my research results be copied and delivered to my doorstep. This can be very helpful when I need only two or three articles. For a large amount of source material, I can still conduct a complete search before making a trip to the library. When I arrive at the library, I can then immediately pull, evaluate, and copy or check out what I need.

You may also have such remote access. Explore this possibility with the following Student Challenge.

STUDENT CHALLENGE Making the Most of Library Resources

Check with your library to see what kind of remote access you have to their electronic resources. Explore the requirements for use of remote library access.

1. Is such access possible?
2. Is it available to you?
3. What are the procedures for requesting access?
4. What equipment and software are needed?
5. Is a special password required?

If you don't have remote capabilities through your local academic or health sciences library, don't despair. You can also conduct index searches by accessing MEDLINE or CINAHL through other websites. MEDLINE is produced by the National Library of Medicine (NLM) and is available free of charge through a number of websites. Two of the more well-known access sites are PubMed and Internet Grateful Med. (Links to these sites are accessible through the MERLIN site.) The National Library of Medicine sponsors both of these sites. MEDLINE is also avail-

MERLIN
Activity
6

able through commercial vendors for a fee. Many of these vendors have enhanced this service and made the search mechanisms more user friendly.

PubMed is the NLM search mechanism that allows you to search MEDLINE and PREMEDLINE databases. PREMEDLINE is a fairly new service that allows you to search basic citation information and abstracts before the full citation record is generated and added to MEDLINE. This means you can find the most current material available. New records are added to PREMEDLINE everyday. Internet Grateful Med provides assisted searching for MEDLINE and 14 other health-related databases, including AIDSLINE, Health STAR, POPLINE, and TOXLINE.

CINAHL is also accessible from a website. (This site is available through MERLIN.) However, because CINAHL is a commercially maintained index, an access fee is charged to use the search mechanism. They do offer student discounts. Your membership gives you on-line full-text access to approximately 17 print nursing journals, as well as the CINAHL database. Most of the current full-text offerings for these journals begin with 1997 or 1998 issues and are available for published articles at least 6 months to 1 year old. A listing of these journals and their tables of contents are accessible on the website free of charge. You may wish to locate the website and explore it to determine whether a subscription would be helpful to you.

MERLIN
Activity
7

Electronic journals and on-line versions of print journals are beginning to appear in nursing. CINAHL offers access to an electronic journal entitled *On-line Journal of Clinical Innovations*. This journal focuses on research reports and clinical innovations. There is an annual subscription fee, and the journal is produced quarterly. Articles from this journal can be downloaded and printed out for no additional fee.

Another electronic nursing journal, *On-line Journal of Knowledge Synthesis for Nursing*, is sponsored by Sigma Theta Tau. (This site is accessible through MERLIN.) This journal provides full-text critical reviews of current research as it pertains to clinical nursing practice. Check to see whether your library carries subscriptions to one or both of these electronic journals. If so, you may have remote on-line access through connection with your library Internet site.

MERLIN
Activity
8

Other electronic nursing journals include the *On-line Journal of Issues in Nursing*, sponsored by Kent State University. This is a peer-reviewed journal with an interactive format. You may view and download all articles at no charge. Penn State University also offers an on-line nursing journal called *On-line Journal of Nursing Informatics*. Journal subscription is free.

Full-text articles from six print journals in nursing are available on-line at the Nursing Center website. Table of contents and abstracts of articles are free. However, a hefty charge to view and/or download a single article may make a trip to the library worthwhile. Mosby also offers the table of contents and abstracts for eight print nursing journals, as well as a number of medical, dental, and allied health journals. On-line subscriptions are available for the medical journals. However, on-line subscriptions for the nursing journals are not yet available. Slack offers on-line subscriptions to nine print nursing journals.

A wide range of health care–related databases and professional sites are available to you via your computer and an Internet account. A brief sampling of such databases can be found in Box 2-4.

MERLIN or Mosby's Electronic Resource Links and Information Network will link you to a special website set up just for this learning package. It contains hypertext links to related areas of interest, content updates, author information, and more. If you have not already done so, take a minute to use MERLIN and log on to explore the website. Try the following Student Challenge.

STUDENT CHALLENGE MERLIN Magic

1. Log on to the MERLIN website at www.mosby.com/MERLIN/Langford/maze.
2. Add the website to your Favorites or Bookmarks list.
3. Explore the site and see what is offered.
4. Find out a little about me (your textbook author).
5. Read up on some frequently asked questions.
6. Check out available links, then log off and insert your CD-ROM for this text.
7. Note the MERLIN button, located at the bottom of the main menu and submenus. It allows you to go directly to the MERLIN site from the CD. Try it out.

Communication Possibilities

Communication capabilities on the Net open a wide range of professional possibilities, including interaction with fellow students and faculty at your university via E-mail. You can also turn in assignments to faculty using E-mail attachments. You

Box 2-4 Selected Professional Websites and Databases

The website for each of these is accessible through the book's MERLIN website at www.mosby.com/MERLIN/Langford/maze.

Hardin Meta Directory of Internet Health Sources—A metalisting with links to indexes that index health care sites. A huge listing of nursing indexes is found here.

Nursing Net—Just one of the indexes from the Hardin site. This is a good electronic guide for nursing journals and other publications and references as well as continuing education sites and employment postings. It even links you to an on-line discount bookstore.

Nursing World—The website for the American Nurses Association (ANA). You can link to state nursing association sites, check nursing and health-care policy, read up on credentialing issues, and do much more.

Nursing Society—The website for Sigma Theta Tau. It contains information about the society, grants and research activities, on-line publications, and eligibility requirements, among other topics.

On-line Books—An index with links to over 9,000 full-text books that are available for on-line reading, free of charge. It has a large medical and health care section.

Journals—An index for journals, magazines, and newspapers.

Library of Congress—The on-line catalog for this government organization. Links to other library catalogs, search mechanisms, and resource help are available at this site.

Centers for Disease Control—Provides access to thousands of health-related statistics, including morbidity and mortality statistics from the National Center for Health Statistics, and government information on hundreds of health-related topics.

National Institutes of Health—The home base for several government agencies of interest, including the National Institute for Nursing Research (NINR) and the National Library of Medicine (NLM).

U.S. Department of Health and Human Services—Provides access to links for numerous health care journals, medical dictionaries, databases, listservs, and metasites. To find it, look under the Health Finder.

MERLIN
Activity
9

can send and receive messages from other professional colleagues worldwide. You can hold discussions with colleagues about patient care issues, brainstorm about solutions to clinical problems, and more by using listservs, newsgroups, or chat rooms. A number of professionally-related discussion groups already are available on the Net. You could even start your own.

ADVENTURE
CD
2-4

STUDENT CHALLENGE Communication Contingencies

1. Explore professional listservs and newsgroups on the Net. (Hint: Remember Liszt Select, Deja, and your search engines.)
2. See if your school or university is the Web. If so, check to see what discussion groups they have available.

Ongoing Educational Opportunities

The ease of access to the Internet and the Web has also opened new avenues in education and learning opportunities. It is now possible to take courses over the Net. Many of these offerings feature interactive classrooms where you can talk with the instructor and fellow classmates on-line through audio or videoconferencing capabilities. The concept is known as *distance learning*. Many universities are starting remote site campuses to offer classes in areas with little access to university settings. Continuing education opportunities abound on the Internet. Although these opportunities are relatively new, they are growing rapidly. It may someday be possible to earn a college degree by completing most or all of your degree requirements on-line. We are entering a new millennium that is filled with possibilities and promise for taming the information revolution.

Resource Kit

Checking Out On-line Services

Several of the largest on-line companies are
America On-line
Compuserve 2000
Microsoft Network
Prodigy

Finding Internet Service Providers

If you have a computer with Microsoft Windows, you can find out about major ISPs by using the Internet Connection wizard located in your Internet Explorer program. The wizard can also help you download the software required to set up your chosen ISP and then make the connections to run the ISP.

Resource Kit—cont'd

You can also find local ISPs in the telephone Yellow Pages under the heading Internet Services.

Easy-to-Use Guides to Help You Log on to and Use the Internet

B Eager: *Internet Quick Reference,* Indianapolis, Que, 1999.

Quick reference, visually-oriented, economical.

Levine JR, Baroudi C, and Young ML: *Internet for dummies,* IDG books, 2000.

More comprehensive reference, easy to follow, economical.

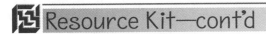 Visit the book's MERLIN website at **www.mosby.com/MERLIN/Langford/maze** for further information.

 Check out the puzzles, mazes, and games on your **CD-ROM.**

References

Berkman R: *Find it fast,* New York, Harper Perennial, 1997.

CINAHL website at www.cinahl.com, May 6, 1999.

Finding medical help online, *Consumer reports* 62(2):27-29, 1997.

Heide A and Stilbourne L: *The teacher's guide to the Internet,* ed 2, New York, Teachers College Press, 1999.

Internet Grateful Med User's Guide at http://igm-01.nlm.nih.gov/splash/IGM. survival.guide.html, April 30, 1999.

Lybecker C: A nurse explores the Internet, *AJN* 97(6):42-50, 1997.

NLM PubMed: The NLM PubMed project overview, on-line at www.ncbi.nlm.nih.gov/ pubmed/overview, May 5, 1999.

Sigma Theta Tau website, www.nursingsociety. org, May 26, 1999.

Trimble E: Strategies for searching, *Consumer Reports* 62(2):30-31, 1997.

Understanding E-mail Addresses, www. powerup.com.au/htmlxp/emailadd.htm, May 21, 1999.

Learning Objectives

1 Describe the components of effective reading.

2 Discuss factors that influence reading rate and comprehension.

3 Examine personal reading skills.

4 Explore strategies to increase reading effectiveness.

5 Define summarization/abstraction.

6 Describe steps necessary for competent summarization.

7 Apply abstraction skills to selected materials.

8 Describe the factors that influence the quality of information.

9 Discuss ways to evaluate the quality of information.

Chapter Outline

What Is This Chapter About?
What Is Effective Reading?
   Reading rate and comprehension
   Reading more effectively

What Is Summarization/Abstraction?
How Do You Evaluate Information?
   Factors affecting information quality
   Evaluation skills

CHAPTER 3

Reading Faster, Reading Smarter: Managing Information Wisely

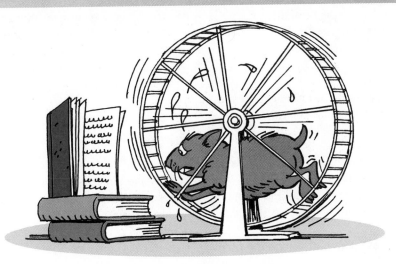

This speed reading is hard work.

Student Quote   *"Breaking the highlighter habit has made me focus more when I read."*

Abstract   Efficient use of information requires the ability to effectively read, competently summarize, and critically evaluate the various sources we locate. Speed and comprehension—the cornerstones of effective reading—are affected by factors such as difficulty level, reading level, subject familiarity, mechanical skill, and various internal and external environmental factors. A consistently used and organized reading strategy can increase reading effectiveness. The ability to summarize and restate what has been read ensures a greater understanding and grasp of the subject matter. As the quantity of available information increases, we must be able to quickly evaluate the quality of such information. Several factors help determine quality of information including accuracy, adequacy, balance, currency, presentation, and reliability.

KEY TERMS

Reading Rhetoric

Abstract A summary of the essential characteristics of something more extensive.

Advance organizers Preselected mental landmarks that serve to organize materials as you read. They are often provided by bold headings, outlines, and so on.

Comprehension Ability to perceive and understand concepts or ideas.

Effective reading rate The number of words that can be read in a minute while maintaining a high level of comprehension.

Reading level The readability of a specific piece of written material.

Reading rate The number of words that can be read in a minute.

Reading strategy (method) A system that breaks a reading assignment down into manageable parts that are more readily processed.

Speed reading Reading at an increased rate through techniques that encourage fewer eye fixations on the page.

Summary A concise recapitulation of previously stated information that captures the main ideas.

Evaluation Expressions

Accuracy Conformity to existing facts and the truth as we know it.

Adequacy Sufficient scope and depth of information presented for a specific audience.

Balance Presentation of competing points of view.

Currency Addresses the immediacy of presented information.

Presentation Manner in which information is displayed.

Reliability Dependability and trustworthiness of information.

What Is This Chapter About?

Now that you have learned how to effectively gather information, the next step is to efficiently dissect and use that information. This includes the ability to effectively read, competently summarize, and critically evaluate the information at hand. Some of you are probably good readers and may view reading as enjoyable. Others of you may see reading as a necessary chore. Still others may find reading a frustrating experience. Whatever your feelings, there are ways to improve your abilities and make the time you spend reading more productive. This chapter discusses effective reading, competent summarization, and critical evaluation issues and examines ways to improve your skills in each area. You can practice these skills through use of the Student Challenges and the CD-ROM games and puzzles.

What Is Effective Reading?

Reading can be broken down into two basic types: fun reading and learning-related reading. Each type requires differing levels of focus. Fun reading is reading for pleasure and may include browsing the latest *People* magazine, scanning the morning newspaper, or curling up with a good mystery novel. Reading for fun does not require the same level of preparation, attention, or thought as reading to learn. This chapter focuses on reading to learn.

Effective reading is the ability to quickly read and comprehend the materials at hand. Your reading rate and comprehension are key factors in reading effectively. These two components are closely related. Your ability to grasp relevant ideas as you read increases your reading speed. Speed without comprehension is of little value. However, a slow, plodding, laborious approach to reading can lead to frustration and loss of your train of thought.

Reading Rate and Comprehension

Reading rate is defined as the number of words that can be read in a minute. An **effective reading rate** is defined as the number of words that can be read per minute while maintaining a high level of comprehension. **Comprehension** is defined as the ability to grasp ideas and to understand the concepts being presented.

3-1

Reading rates and comprehension are affected by a number of factors that emanate from the material, the reader, or the environment. These include the difficulty level of the material, the reading level at which the material is presented, the reader's familiarity with the subject area and mechanical reading skills, and internal and external environmental distractions.

FACTORS AFFECTING SPEED AND COMPREHENSION
Source Factors
   Difficulty level
   Reading level
Reader Factors
   Familiarity with subject
   Mechanical skills
Environmental Factors
   Internal distractions (fatigue, hunger, illness)
   External distractions (noise, temperature, light)

Information comes in varying degrees of difficulty or complexity. Complex and abstract concepts require more thought and a more careful reading. This slows the rate at which they are read. Some subjects that are more complex are harder to grasp and apply than others. Materials that contain highly specialized and/or technical information have a higher level of difficulty. This is true even if the reader is familiar with the subject being presented. For example, a nursing research article that is filled with statistical notations and tables is harder to read than an anecdotal journal article on a patient experience.

Reading level refers to the readability of a given piece of written material. It is affected by the number of syllables in words and the number of words in sentences. The higher the average number of syllables per word and words per sentence, the greater the reading level. As reading level rises, comprehension requires more effort and reading rate slows. When material is loaded with 3-syllable words and 22-word sentences, the brain tends to struggle. However, very low reading levels result in a dull and monotonous presentation. A succession of 6-word sentences full of monosyllables can be mind numbing. Do not confuse readability with difficulty. Difficulty refers to the idea being presented, whereas readability refers to the presentation of the idea. Even simple ideas can be made hard to read, and difficult ideas can be presented in reader-friendly form.

> Do not confuse readability with difficulty. Difficulty refers to the idea being presented, whereas readability refers to the presentation of the idea.

Reading level is usually calculated and expressed as some form of index. These indexes typically report a value that corresponds to the educational level required to read a particular document with ease (e.g., fifth grade versus twelfth grade). Generally, the higher the number of the index, the harder the material is to read. If you use the Microsoft Word (versions 95, 97, or 2000) word processing package on your computer, you can calculate a readability score on any document you write. It is located under the "Tools" menu under grammar options. One of the most popular readability indexes is the Gunning Fog Index, and it is fairly easy to calculate by hand. The steps are presented in Box 3-1.

If you're having trouble reading a particular piece of information, you might want to check to see the reading level at which it is written. Try the following Student Challenge.

STUDENT CHALLENGE Reading Readability

1. Using selected samples (a paragraph or two) from each of the following sources, calculate a reading level.
   a. this textbook
   b. one of your other textbooks
   c. an article from a popular magazine
   d. a source you considered very difficult to read and understand
   e. a student paper or assignment that you have written
2. Compare the results from the various samples. How do they compare? What did you learn?

Box 3-1 Calculation of the Gunning Fog Index

Step 1: Select a sample.
   Choose a 100-word (to the nearest sentence) sample from the material to be analyzed.
Step 2: Determine the average number of words per sentence.
   Divide the total number of words in the sample by the total number of sentences in the sample.
Step 3: Determine the percentage of words with three or more syllables.
   Divide the number of three-plus syllable words by the total number of words. (Do not count the following as three-syllable words: Capitalized words, hyphenated words, or words for which the addition of an "es" or "ed" make the third syllable)
Step 4: Calculate the grade level index. Add the result of step 2 to step 3 and multiply by 0.4.
   Example:
   Step 1: 110-word passage
   Step 2: 110 words in 11 sentences 110/11 = 10
   Step 3: 21 three+ syllable words out of 110 words 21/110 = 19%
   Step 4: Add average words (10) to percent of polysyllable words (19) and multiply by 0.4 (10 + 19 = 29 × 0.4 = 11.6).
   Result: Reading level is the eleventh to twelfth grade in high school.

From Gunning Fog Index,1999; Smye, 1999.

Familiarity with the subject and the vocabulary used greatly affects reading rate and comprehension. If you have insufficient background in a particular subject, you are handicapped when you try to read about it. The unfamiliar concepts and ideas require additional thought. Words may be foreign or used in specialized ways for various topics. Vocabulary is particularly important to reading because the words on the page are actually tools for building thoughts. It is difficult to formulate or extract ideas from your reading if you are unfamiliar with several of the words being used to present those ideas.

A lack of familiarity with the words on the page also greatly slows your reading rate. A nurse researcher can read most nursing research articles with relative speed and high-level understanding. As a nursing student, you might arrive at a lower level of understanding after a much greater time investment. As a nurse, you need to be equipped with a good general vocabulary and specialized vocabularies from several fields, including chemistry, biology, physiology, pharmacology, medicine, and nursing, to read effectively.

Reading requires certain mechanical skills. If the reader is lacking some of these skills, both reading rate and comprehension can be affected. These skills include the way the eyes focus when reading, the way words are viewed on the page, the way the eyes fix on and sweep a page, and the smoothness or flow of the process. Focus in reading means that you read for ideas rather than words. You are tuned into the meaning behind the words. You have a purpose for reading such as understanding a key point or looking for an answer to a question or a solution to a problem. Words are viewed as thought clusters rather than as single entities. Eyes sweep the page with few fixations (pauses as the eyes move across the page). You take in groups of words at a time. The lips are still, and reading is silent. If reading mechanics are lacking, then the reading rate slows. A sufficiently slow rate affects comprehension. It is difficult to pick out key ideas if you are concentrating on seeing and reading each word.

There are courses that actually teach you to increase your rate and comprehension by improving your reading mechanics. They are often known as **speed-reading** courses. They teach you techniques that allow you to take in large groups of words on a page while controlling your eye movements. These techniques force you to see and consider several words as a single unit. Although you will never read technical material at a high rate of speed, it is a valuable skill to be able to view words in groups rather than as single entities.

Internal and external environmental factors can also affect your reading speed and comprehension. If you are tired, anxious, sick, hungry, or otherwise distracted, your ability to focus and read effectively is affected. Likewise, if the room is too noisy, too hot, too cold, too dark, or the site of other activities, your ability to concentrate and read is affected. You may have discovered that there are times when you are more alert and better able to concentrate. If so, take advantage of these times. For example, I can focus and engage my brain much better from 10 AM to 3 PM than at any other time. So I schedule tasks that require focus and creative thought at those times.

Reading More Effectively

An organized approach to reading can help you read more actively and understand what you are reading. A good **reading strategy** breaks the reading assignment down into manageable parts and helps you process one part before moving on to the next part. A number of reading strategies have been advocated to increase reading effectiveness. Several of these are listed and described in Box 3-2. If you do not already have a proven reading strategy, you may wish to read further about some of the described strategies and try out one or more of them. See the Resource Kit at the end of the chapter for references. Having a reading strategy is more important than the particular strategy you choose. The reason a systematic approach is effective is because it allows you to organize and focus your reading.

As you look at Box 3-2, you'll note that all of the strategies have common tactics. They all advocate that you first survey or preview the material to get an overview of what you are about to read. This means paying attention to advance organizers. **Advance organizers** are things such as the table of contents, preface,

---

Box 3-2 Effective Reading Strategies

SQ3R- **S**urvey, **Q**uestion, **R**ead, **R**ecite, **R**eview- Devised in the 1940s by Francis Robinson for students at Ohio State University, this system has been used for years, and a number of variations have come from this original work.

SQ4R- A variation of the above method, SQ4R adds a record step to the process in which the user records key ideas on paper or note cards.

OK5R- **O**verview, **K**ey ideas, **R**ead, **R**ecord, **R**ecite, **R**eview, **R**eflect- This strategy offers yet another twist on the basic strategic formula.

SSS- **S**kim, **S**crutinize, **S**weep up- By now you should be seeing a pattern.

PRR- **P**review, **R**ead actively, **R**ecall. This reading strategy is endorsed by several university study skills programs.

chapter outlines, learning objectives, titles, subject headings, abstracts, introductions, and summaries. These are placed in material specifically to help you organize your thoughts. They prepare you to read by giving you a road map to the presented material. They tell you in advance what points are important and help you establish ties between major information segments.

These reading strategies also ask the reader to examine or scrutinize what is being read. This means identifying main ideas and key points and asking how they relate to other key points. It means getting a firm understanding of what you are reading and addressing points that are confusing or unclear. It means looking for signs that indicate how the information is organized or what is important. These signs include information that is set off by highlighting or boxes. Words such as "first or second," "for example," "in summary," or "finally" also serve as signals.

Finally, these strategies ask the reader to review what has been read. When you finish reading the material, you need to gather all the key ideas and summarize what you have gleaned from the material. Check your summary of key points against the authors' by rereading the summary, key points, or abstract of the material. Now is the time to note and clear up points of confusion. It's also a good time to physically make notes of the key ideas and points that you have pulled from the material.

Do not use a highlighter or underline phrases in the material. This encourages lazy thinking. Highlighting does not require you to pull out and examine relationships between key ideas. Many people also use highlighting as an escape tactic to delay the hard work of thinking about what they are reading. They highlight anything that looks important, with the promise that they will read and make sense of it later. I have seen student texts with entire pages highlighted. Something about having to write down your thoughts encourages you to more clearly refine your understanding. The physical act of writing also serves to lodge the idea more firmly in your memory bank.

Hint: Do not use a highlighter when reading. It encourages lazy thinking.

Try the following Student Challenge and see if you have some system in place for effective reading.

STUDENT CHALLENGE Strategic Strategies

Respond to the following questions and directions using this textbook as your example.

1. Did you examine and survey the general text layout before beginning your first reading assignment (e.g., preface, table of contents, glossary, appendices, special supplements)?

2. Do you know what general layout and features are included in each chapter?

3. Did you preview the outline and learning objectives for this chapter before you began reading it?

4. If not, take some time to do that survey now. What did you learn from your examination of the text ?

5. When you read, do you ask yourself what the central point is in each paragraph? Do you make use of the abstract that is provided with each chapter?

6. Do you pay attention to the boxed materials? Figures? Tables? Charts? Diagrams?

7. Did you make note of the defined terms?

8. Did you try out the Internet sites listed on MERLIN for the professional databases in Box 2-4 in Chapter 2?

9. Are you doing the Student Challenges? CD-ROM exercises?

10. When you finished the first two chapters, were you clear about the key points? Did you have any questions? If so, did you actively seek and find answers?

11. If your reading skills need refining, then find a reading strategy and incorporate it in your reading sessions. (Hint: Your library probably has a number of resources filed under effective reading or effective study.)

Box 3-3 Tips on Effective Reading

1. **Prepare your environment.** Banish as many distractions as possible. Find a quiet, comfortable, well-lit place to read. Have all the necessary supplies such as pens, note paper, and other resources before you begin.
2. **Prepare yourself.** Select times of the day when you are alert and at a mental peak. Schedule reading times in advance and keep the appointment. Read in manageable chunks. Remember, concentration requires energy. If you find your mind wandering or you're having trouble seizing on the key ideas, take a 5-minute break.
3. **Read actively.** Think about what you are reading. Read with a purpose. Actively search for key points and ideas. Look for examples or illustrations of those ideas. See if you can think of other examples. Make connections between the ideas being presented. Get a picture of the whole idea in each paragraph, each section, and each chapter.
4. **Use tools to increase understanding.** If you are unfamiliar with the subject, you may want material that provides background before tackling material that addresses specific issues on a subject. If you are unfamiliar with the vocabulary, use a dictionary as you read and apply what you find back to the materials you're reading.
5. **Increase your mechanical skills.** (1) Read phrases rather than individual words. Very few ideas are expressed in single words. They come in units of words. Reading in phrases allows you to better follow the meaning of the material. (2) Eliminate reading out loud, word pronunciation, and lip movements. These are indications that you are reading words rather than phrases, which means you are focusing on the words themselves rather than the ideas they represent. (3) Reduce rereading to a minimum. Often the next phrase or sentence will offer an explanation making rereading unnecessary. Reread only if the point is still unclear after you complete a section.

There are other tactics that you can employ to read more effectively. These are listed in Box 3-3.

What Is Summarization/Abstraction?

The ability to understand and condense what you have read into a few well-chosen words is an important skill. Summarization is the ability to capture the key ideas or main points in a clear concise form. A **summary** briefly states the essence of what has been previously presented. I am reminded of a comedy sketch by Father Guido Sarducci on *Saturday Night Live*. He summarized entire fields of knowledge for his 4-minute university. For example, economics was reduced to "supply and demand" and theology was summed up as "God is love." A bit extreme perhaps, but you get the point.

An **abstract** is a synonym for summary. It is often placed at the beginning of a chapter or article, while a summary is most frequently placed at the end. We are using the word abstract in this text because it is the term you will see most frequently when reading research articles. You also find an abstract at the beginning of each chapter in this text.

The ability to competently summarize any material requires that you have a fundamental understanding of the concepts being presented in that material. You can use the following questions to test your understanding of the material you're reading.

1. Can you grasp the ideas being expressed and distinguish key ideas from secondary points?
2. Can you express key ideas in words different than those used by the author?
3. Can you identify supporting evidence for a particular point?
4. Can you give examples to illustrate that point?

If you're having difficulty separating out the main or key points as you read, remember to use the cues presented by the material. Check for advance organizers. Look for bold topical or section headings. Search for signal words. If you find that you cannot express the author's ideas in your own words, then you are having trouble comprehending what is being said. You may need to reexamine the paragraph. Is the concept foreign? If so, seek additional resources. Are some of the words unfamiliar? If so, consult a dictionary. Are you tired, distracted, or not thinking clearly? If so, take a break and reread it when you have a clearer focus.

To provide supporting evidence, you must see the relationships between and among the points being presented. The same mechanisms you use to pull key ideas also help in visualizing secondary and supporting ideas. When you think the concept is clear, test yourself by coming up with a specific example of the concept. If you have difficulty with this, scan the material and see if a sample example was provided.

Let's use a paragraph from this chapter as an example in the art of summarizing.

Effective reading is the ability to quickly read and comprehend the materials at hand. Your reading rate and comprehension are key factors in reading effectively. These two components are closely related. Your ability to grasp relevant ideas as you read increases your reading speed. Speed without comprehension is of little value. However, a slow, plodding, laborious approach to reading can lead to frustration and loss of your train of thought.

The paragraph's main idea is that good reading has two interconnected elements—speed and understanding. Its first sentence tells you what the two elements are. Note that the second sentence repeats this same idea using different words. The author then tells you that the elements are related and uses supporting examples to expand on the relationship of the two elements. This paragraph also sets up the following paragraphs, which discuss reading rate and comprehension in more depth.

Let's look at another example.

Now that you have learned how to effectively gather information, the next step is to efficiently dissect and use that information. This includes the ability to effectively read, competently summarize, and critically evaluate the information at hand. Some of you are probably good readers and may view reading as enjoyable. Others of you may see reading as a necessary chore. Still others may find reading a frustrating experience. Whatever your feelings, there are ways to improve your abilities and make the time you spend reading more productive. This chapter discusses effective reading, competent summarization, and critical evaluation issues and examines ways to improve your skills in each area. You can practice these skills through use of the Student Challenge exercises and the CD-ROM games and puzzles.

This is the first paragraph in this chapter. The main idea is to inform the reader that this chapter addresses ways to use information by examining abilities to read, summarize, and evaluate. This paragraph not only serves to link the previous two chapters to this one, but also it serves as an advance organizer. It tells you what general topics to expect in this chapter. It also reminds you that student learning activities are available to help master the content.

Now put your summary skills to the test with the following Student Challenge.

ADVENTURE CD
3-3

STUDENT CHALLENGE Summary Skills

Select several (at least five) paragraphs from this chapter. Summarize each selected paragraph in one sentence.

1. How did you decide what the main idea was? Did you make use of advance organizers? Signal words?
2. Do your summary sentences use your own words? If not, try restating the summary again.
3. Can you think of a way to illustrate the main idea? Cite an example for two or three of your summaries.
4. Did you have any trouble understanding what was being said? If so, what did you do to help you understand?

How Do You Evaluate Information?

As greater amounts of information become more easily accessible, it becomes increasingly difficult to separate the good stuff from the bad. Your brief excursions on the Internet should have already tipped you off to this problem. So one of the critical issues facing us in this "age of the information explosion" is how to assess the quality of the information we are exposed to. Chapters 1 and 2 addressed the issue of finding information. Now we are going to talk about how to decide whether the information we locate is adequate.

Factors Affecting Information Quality

Several factors—accuracy, adequacy, balance, currency, presentation, and reliability—affect the quality of information. **Accuracy** is associated with the content of the material. Accurate information is the result of an active effort to confirm or verify and shows conformity to existing facts and the truth. **Adequacy** refers to the scope and depth of information presented. Adequate information provides the reader with materials that are sufficient in scope and depth for the specific purposes of that reader. **Balance** deals with acknowledgment and presentation of competing points of view. Lack of balance leads to bias. **Currency** addresses immediacy of the material and whether it accurately reflects ongoing changes in a particular field of study. **Presentation** has to do with whether the content is presented in a well-organized manner. **Reliability** is often connected with the source of the material. Reliable information is consistently dependable and comes from a generally proven and trustworthy source.

FACTORS AFFECTING THE QUALITY OF INFORMATION
Accuracy
Adequacy
Balance
Currency
Presentation
Reliability

Evaluation Skills

Several considerations can help you make judgments about the quality of the information you are using. The first consideration is the source of the material. If you have tapped into materials from published textbooks, reference books, or recognized journals, there is a reasonable expectation that the material has been reviewed and edited by authorities in the area. You may wish to check this out. Many text and reference books list contributing authors and/or reviewers and their credentials in the front matter of the book. Journals may be refereed or peer reviewed (i.e., the article is sent for critique by one or more experts in the field before being accepted for publication). This is an additional sign of quality. So most traditional sources (textbooks and journals) have been adequately reviewed and evaluated by a reputable publisher and are generally trustworthy.

However, if you have pulled the information from the Internet, evaluating the source requires more effort. Look first at the three letters in the URL that tell you what type of organization is sponsoring the site. (Note: Some sites don't use this identifier). If it is a commercial organization (.com), ask yourself what they are selling and whether this might bias their presentation of data. In other words, treat the information like you treat advertisements. If the address is for a nonprofit organization (.org), ask yourself what their purpose and agenda is and what audience materials are geared for. Government (.gov) and educational (.edu) sites are generally good sources for reliable information.

Whenever possible, check the author's credentials and affiliations. This is often difficult on the Internet. However, I have found that the more reliable sources usually provide this information on the site. Because there are no editors or quality checkpoints for much of the material on the Internet, you need to exercise greater caution and skepticism about the information you find. (Note: Some sites, particularly professional sites, have editorial or peer review. When this is the case, it is clearly stated on the site.)

The second thing you can do is evaluate the types of materials you're using. Is the information from a primary or a secondary source? A *primary source* is the original source of the data. A *secondary source* secures the data from the primary source. The secondary source should cite the primary source when securing such data. This allows you, the reader, to access the primary source, if you wish, for more information about a specific point. (Note: Footnotes or cited references tell us when data is from another source.) Is the material intended for a professional or lay audience or the general public? This often changes the presentation manner, breadth, and depth of coverage. You need to decide whether the material contains enough information for your purposes.

Third, evaluate the timely nature of the information. Check the publication date and see how current the information is. If you are seeking information in a rapidly changing field or subject, this step is crucial. Remember that information in a book is already 3 to 5 years old when it is first published. Information in journals tends to be from 6 months to 2 years old. The Internet with posted conference proceedings, electronic journals, and professional forums may provide the most current resources available. If it is an Internet site, check to see when the information was last updated. This is usually posted on the site home page. (Hint: Page info on Netscape Navigator also provides this information.)

Finally look at the content of the material itself. Is it presented in a well-organized and straightforward manner? Are major points adequately illustrated and explained? Are arguments backed up with supporting material? Is the presentation balanced, and does it include alternative points of view. Does the material make sense? Is the material logical? Is the material adequate, or does it leave the reader with partially answered or unanswered questions? Compare the content with other sources. Look for similarities and differences. How do various sources agree or disagree? What common ground can you find?

Try the following Student Challenge and see what you discover.

ADVENTURE CD
3-4

🔲 STUDENT CHALLENGE Checking Sources

1. Check the front of this text and see if you can spot the listing of the author and reviewers and their credentials.

2. Look at two or three nursing journals and locate their policies for manuscript acceptance. Did you find any that were peer reviewed? If not, check *Image* or *Nursing Research*.

3. Check out some of the health-related websites on the Internet. What information was available about the source of the information? Could you distinguish professional and academic sites from general sites? Could you tell how current the data were?

4. Check out one of the Internet sites that posts professional conference proceedings. Find a newsgroup or other forum on the Web that is for health care professionals. Explore it and see what it has to offer. Did you find any breaking information?

Much of the evaluation process requires that you think critically about your resources. That means not taking material at face value. Just because it is in written or electronic form does not make it so. You need to ask questions, cross-check resources against one another, and bring a healthy amount of skepticism to your reading. For example, it's quite possible that segments of material in your current nursing textbooks are no longer valid because they are outdated.

This is particularly true of information that is time sensitive. When a text cites statistics, make a habit of looking at the date of the reference material. When the text describes certain procedures or tests, ask yourself whether that material is the most current or if other technology has replaced that which is described. Ultimately you must make a judgment about whether a particular resource can be trusted to provide the quality information that you need. I can almost guarantee that some of the material in Chapter 2 about the Internet is now outdated because the technology discussed is rapidly changing. Thus, information that was up-to-date as of June 2000, has probably changed since then.

Activity
10

 Resource Kit

Reading Strategy References

Robinson, F: *Effective study*, ed 4, New York, Harper and Row, 1970.
This book is out of print but can still be found in many academic libraries and can be located at used bookstores through the Amazon.com website. A link to Amazon.com can be found on the book's MERLIN site.

Wahlstrom C, Williams B and Dansby C: *The practical student*, Boston, Wadsworth, 1999. This resource has several good study skills in addition to a chapter on effective reading that examines the SQ3R system.

Johnson D and Johnson C: *Learning power*, New York, Simon and Schuster, 1998. Another general study reference with a chapter on the SSS reading strategy.

 Visit the book's MERLIN website at
www.mosby.com/MERLIN/Langford/maze
for further information.

 Check out the puzzles, mazes, and games on your **CD-ROM.**

References

Grammar checkers, reading ease and other faery tales, website at www.writepage.com/ writing/gramchek.htm, 1999.

Gunning Fog Index at http://isu.indstate.edu/ bminnick/asbe336/Powerpoint/fog-index. htm,1999.

Microsoft Word: Readability scores, Microsoft Word 97 Help menu, 1997.

Peake T: *The Flesch factor*, web site at http:// peake.home.mindspring.com/tfy5/flesch.htm, 1997.

Robinson F: *Effective study*, ed 4, New York: Harper and Row, 1970.

Smye R: *Readability indexes*, web site at www. sheridanc.on.ca/~randy/rap.dir/Cutfog.html, 1999.

University of Houston, Clear Lake Campus: *How to read more efficiently*, CTS Study Skills Program materials, University of Houston, 1999.

University of Houston, Clear Lake Campus: *Time saving tips for text reading*, CTS Study Skills Program materials, University of Houston, 1999.

TWO

TALKING THE TALK

Learning the Language, Defining Research, and Exploring Quantitative and Qualitative Perspectives

... Jump In

Health care and health care technology are becoming increasingly complex and expanding at a rapid rate. The practice of nursing changes on a daily basis. How do we cope? How can we keep our knowledge base and our practice current? Research is the key. It provides a solid foundation on which to base our practice. This means that we as nurses need to incorporate nursing research findings into our practice settings. To do this we must be able to read, understand, and apply the research literature that is available. This section defines research, explores quantitative and qualitative research methodologies, and provides you with the vocabulary and tools to read and understand research articles.

Learning Objectives

1 Explore preconceived self-notions about research.

2 Define the terms "research" and "nursing research."

3 Describe ways to acquire knowledge.

4 Discuss why nursing research is important.

5 Describe the historical development of nursing research.

6 Discuss nursing research priorities.

7 Delineate future directions for nursing research.

8 Describe the research expectations of nurses from various educational levels.

9 Discuss perceived barriers to the use of research findings in the clinical area.

10 Identify efforts to facilitate research.

Chapter Outline

How Do You Feel About Research?
What Is Research?
   What is knowledge?
     Tradition and custom
     Authority
     Trial and error
     Personal experience
     Intuition
     Reasoning
     Research
   What is nursing research?

Why Is Research Important?
   Why is nursing research important?
Where Has Nursing Research Been and
   Where Is It Going?
   A historical look at nursing research
   The future of nursing research
Who Is Involved in Nursing Research?
   Consumers and producers
   Research barriers and facilitators

Research: What, Why, Where, and Who?

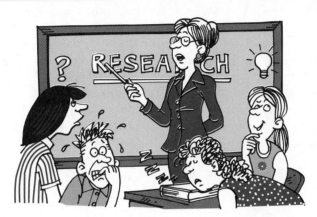

Now class, "research is the systematic, controlled, empirical and critical investigation of hypothetical propositions about presumed relations among natural phenomena" (Kerlinger, 1973).

Student Quote   *"At first, I thought this course [Research] was going to be a total waste of time; now I'm pumped because I'll be giving the very latest in [nursing] care to my patients."*

Abstract   Research is one way that we acquire knowledge. Others include tradition, authority, trial and error, personal experience, intuition, and reasoning. All of these methods provide viable options to make sense of the world. Research offers us a systematic way to confirm existing knowledge and to build new knowledge. Nursing research explores issues important to nursing to refine and expand the body of nursing knowledge. Although research in nursing was slow to develop, it has become an institutionalized force and plays an increasingly vital part in the practice of nursing in this complex and rapidly changing society. Nursing continues to grapple with ways to better facilitate the use of nursing research findings in the clinical practice setting.

KEY TERMS

Knowledge Nomenclature

Authority Knowledge gleaned from the expertise of others.

Bias Any influence that may alter the outcomes of a research study.

Clinical nursing research Nursing research that has direct impact on nursing interventions with clients.

Deductive reasoning A logical system of thinking that starts with the whole and breaks it down into its component parts.

Inductive reasoning A logical system of thinking that begins with the component parts and builds them into a whole.

Intuition Insight into the whole of a situation without possessing readily supportable or confirming data.

Knowledge Essential information about the world around us that allows us to function more effectively.

Nursing research Use of the research process to gain knowledge important to nurses and the practice of nursing.

Personal experience Knowledge derived from the cumulative experiences of living.

Reasoning Use of logical thought patterns to solve problems. May be inductive or deductive in nature.

Research A systematic process using both inductive and deductive reasoning to confirm and refine existing knowledge and to build new knowledge.

Tradition The handing down of knowledge from one generation to the next.

Trial and error Trying a succession of alternative solutions until one solves the problem at hand.

How Do You Feel About Research?

The first thing I do when facing a new class of research students is to pose a series of questions. Questions such as: What image comes to mind when I say the word research? What are your feelings about studying research? Is research important to nursing? Who should do or use research?

STUDENT CHALLENGE Preconceived Notions

Consider each of these questions one at a time and record your answers.

1. What image comes to mind for the word "research"? Paint a word picture or draw an image. For example, I think of a little eggheaded bald man with glasses, bent over a microscope in a tiny, cluttered back room.

STUDENT CHALLENGE Preconceived Notions—cont'd

2. What characteristics does a researcher possess? List traits you think it takes to be a researcher.
3. How do you feel about research? About your study of research? Use feeling words like happy, sad, scared, or anxious. Then try to examine why you might be feeling that way.
4. Do you think research is important to nursing? Why or why not?
5. Who do you think should do nursing research? Use nursing research? Do you picture yourself involved with research? Compare your answers with two or three classmates. Discuss similarities and differences. What do your answers tell you? Did you learn anything that might be useful to you as you begin your study?

Just about now, many of you are probably wondering why you are studying research. You may have a vague notion of what research is, but you're unsure about what it has to do with the day-to-day practice of nursing. You may think only intellectual types are attracted to research, and you may worry about whether you'll be able to understand and make sense of it all. Although you probably agree that research has a place in nursing, you may think someone else should be doing or using it and that your time could be better spent in other pursuits. Or you may be excited and curious about this course but somewhat anxious about getting started.

Let's begin with the premise that research is an important tool in the rapidly changing practice of nursing. It is a tool that can be used by all nurses at all educational levels and at all stages in their careers to do their jobs more effectively. This means that you can use research right now to improve the care that you give to patients in the clinical area. With that premise in mind, this chapter seeks to introduce the concept of research in a general context and within the specific context of nursing. It explores the ways we come to know about the world. It also looks at the importance of research in nursing and the history and future of nursing research. Finally it defines research roles and discusses obstacles to the use of research findings.

Research is an important tool in the rapidly changing practice of nursing.

What Is Research?

Research literally means to search again or to examine carefully. It employs a systematic process to ask and answer questions that generate knowledge. The research process is often compared to the problem-solving process because they are similar—both employ a systematic approach in an attempt to answer a question. However, there are several important differences. The research method is much more formal and has identified standards and conditions that guide the process. Problem solving is concerned with an immediate solution for a particular situation. Research seeks answers that can be applied to other situations. Finally, problem solving seeks to find a solution within the boundaries of what we already know, whereas research seeks to confirm or refine what we think we know or to discover new knowledge. In fact, research often occurs because existing knowledge is inadequate to solve a particular problem that has been raised.

What Is Knowledge?

Knowledge is the comprehension and understanding of facts, truths, or principles. It is the information we use to conduct our personal and professional lives. We acquire knowledge in several ways.

STUDENT CHALLENGE Thinking About Thinking

1. Either alone or with a small group of friends, brainstorm how you come to know what you know.
2. When you are finished, compare your list to the list in Box 4-1.
3. Any surprises? Did you come up with ways that are not listed?
4. Can you think of examples of how you use each of these sources of knowledge in your daily life?

We not only acquire knowledge in several ways, we may use more than one method at a time in working on a solution to a problem or the answer to a question that is troubling us. All the methods are viable options and valid at various times. Each offers us a way to deal with the world. All possess strengths and weaknesses. The ultimate task is to recognize and use them all to our best advantage. The following sections discuss each in a little more depth.

Box 4-1 Sources of Knowledge

Tradition and custom
Authority and role models
Trial and error
Personal experience
Intuition
Reasoning
Research

TRADITION AND CUSTOM

Knowledge derived from **tradition** is "truth" that is passed to us from previous generations. It is often a reflection of our culture or heritage. It involves those things that we know or do because "that is the way it has always been." We usually accept these truths as given with little questioning. This can be advantageous because it offers a common cultural ground from which to communicate and make decisions. Many practices that evolve from this kind of knowledge are ritualistic in nature. The reason or rationale for such practice may have been lost or may have disappeared over the years.

I am reminded of a story of two friends preparing dinner together. One of them took the pot roast, cut off each end, and then placed it in the Dutch oven to brown. The other asked, "Why did you cut off the ends first?" "I don't know," said the first, "It's the way my mother taught me." However, being curious, she called her mother and asked for an explanation. Her mother didn't know either, having learned to cook pot roast by watching her mother. So the woman called her grandmother in search of an answer. "Well," the grandmother said, "I used to cut the ends off the roast because the pot I cooked it in was too small to hold the whole thing."

Large segments of information and several practices in nursing are based largely on tradition. For example, we routinely take patient vital signs each shift and require daily baths and linen changes. Can you think of other examples? Many of these practices were originally instituted for good reasons. However, much like "cutting off the end of the pot roast," the reason for the practice may no longer be viable. So, it might be to our advantage to more critically examine those things in nursing that we "know" by tradition or things that we "do" because that's the way its customarily done. However, some of these practices persist even when we have evidence that the practice is no longer effective or even safe. Consider the example of nurses who put an air bubble in the syringe when drawing up medications for injection. The reason given, if one is stated, is to clear all the medication from the needle and thus ensure that the full dose is given. This was the correct technique in the days when nurses used reusable syringes. The disposable syringes used today are calibrated so that the proper dose is administered with no air bubble. Use of a bubble with a disposable syringe results in a medication overdose (Beyea and Nicoll, 1995).

AUTHORITY

We rely heavily on individuals who are "experts" in certain areas to provide us with information about various topics so that we can make better informed decisions and better learn how to perform certain functions. The first **authority** figures we encounter are our parents. When we go to school, we begin to rely on teachers and textbooks for expanding our knowledge base. We also rely on the opinions of authorities that have expertise in areas we don't. This is a natural evolution and to be expected because it would be impossible for us to be knowledgeable about everything. As we choose a profession, we look to authorities in the field to teach us what they know. When we imitate the example set by authority figures, they serve as role models. Student and novice nurses can gain confidence and competence by selecting and using faculty or expert clinicians as role models.

The caution when using knowledge gleaned from authorities or in imitating their behaviors is to pick your authorities and role models carefully. Ask yourself questions such as what makes this person an expert? What is their educational background and experience? How did they come to know? Do you accept the word of faculty or nurses without question? How well read and current are your faculty? Are they involved in scholarly activity and research? Are their clinical skills current? What about the nurses you see in the clinical area? Do they keep up with the latest discoveries in their specialty area? Do they show evidence of critical thinking in their clinical decision making or do they justify actions with "that's the way we do it here"?

Textbooks and other information sources often assume an authority role in the life of a nursing student. We tend to assign a lot of credibility to the written word. Do you take every piece of information that you read at face value? Do you know if you are learning the best information available? Do you regularly use nursing journals as information sources? Did you know that the information in most textbooks is at least 3 to 5 years old by the time it is published? I coauthored a quick reference handbook on diseases. Within 1 month of sending my work to the publisher, 6 major developments occurred that affected the content of that book. The book itself was not available until a year after I finished writing. I don't even want to count the number of changes that occurred in that 1-year period. So, view the information critically. Is it in line with other authorities in the same area. Is it backed with sound rationale? Is it clearly and logically presented? Is it current? This is particularly timely advice in the age of an information explosion in which material is readily available on every topic imaginable.

TRIAL AND ERROR

The process of **trial and error** uses a successive number of alternative solutions to a problem until one works to solve the problem at hand. It is often used when we have little frame of reference to draw from, when seemingly equal options are easily accessible and/or when we have exhausted standard approaches. This approach tends to be haphazard and results often cannot be reproduced a second time. Did you ever try to reproduce a dish that you just sort of threw together with a little of this and a little of that and have it actually turn out to be tasty?

We may also wind up using one option when another would work better. This occurs because the selected option adequately solves our problem, leaving the better option unexplored. I am never more aware of this consequence, than when I have played around in a trial-and-error fashion to produce a certain result with my computer. I proudly show the results of my handiwork to a more computer-literate friend. She then shows me how to get the same result in one or two key strokes or mouse maneuvers, rendering my solution laughable and needlessly convoluted.

Using a system of trial and error may also entail a certain amount of risk. Using trial and error to learn to play "Commando" on the computer is acceptable. If your character gets blown up, you just start over. Using trial and error to find the correct dose of medication for a patient could spell disaster. However, trial and error can bring about surprising results. When you approach an obstacle from a "let's try this and see what happens" perspective, you are not bound by the restraints of logic. This type of exploration may provide solutions that might not even have been attempted with a more "logical" approach.

PERSONAL EXPERIENCE

Knowledge derived from the cumulative experiences of living is familiar and powerful. It comes from seeing, hearing, touching, tasting, feeling, and doing it ourselves. It is first-hand knowledge. We know it because we were there. We know it because we have been there before. We are intimately acquainted with this form of knowing. We trust it and highly value it in our decision-making process. It is personal. We witnessed it while it was happening. It affects how we adapt and integrate knowledge that we have not experienced on a first-hand basis. The more experience we gain in a situation, the greater our comfort and skill in that situation. As the number and variety of our experiences increase, we transfer, adapt, and extend knowledge learned from previous situations to fit new situations. As the depth and breadth of our experience grows, our operating knowledge base becomes increasingly complex. **Personal experience** is individual and is often hard to translate or explain to others, particularly those who have no similar experience.

Personal or first-hand experience is also a useful tool in the professional arena. Patricia Benner (1984) describes five levels—novice, advanced beginner, competent, proficient, and expert—a nurse goes through in developing clinical expertise. Movement from one level to the next occurs with experience. Experience is only gained when previous knowledge is refined or challenged by actual clinical evidence. The novice nurse begins with knowledge gained in large part from authoritative sources and from the ability to reason and problem solve based on that body of knowledge. Experience is then added to the equation. Expertise develops over time when the nurse tests out and refines her body of knowledge in actual real-world situations. Thus according to Benner, experience is a necessary prerequisite for developing expertise.

INTUITION

Intuition is a "gut hunch" or feeling about a situation that is not readily explained or easily backed up logic or facts. It is an insight or understanding of the whole seen apart from its component parts. Intuition is closely tied to personal experience. Extensive personal experience allows an ingraining of knowledge so that it becomes second nature. Acting on this deeply imbedded knowledge often occurs automatically and quickly as a flash of insight, an immediate recognition of the whole. It is often difficult to even recall or recount what produces this insight. Intuition has long been discounted because it is not easily examined or readily categorized. It also appears to occur apart from consideration of available facts and use of a reasoning process. So, in a society that holds logic at a premium, intuition is labeled as magic or as a lucky guess.

Benner (1984) describes intuition as perceptual awareness. Intuition in her estimation is not a lack of knowledge or a lucky guess. Rather it is deep knowledge derived from long hours of clinical observation and experience. It is being attuned to very subtle shifts that may be important only in the case of a specific patient. Benner (1984) documents several instances where expert nurses recognized impending warning signs of a life-threatening situation long before the so called "objective signs" revealed that something was going wrong. This type of clinical knowledge needs greater study so that it can be more clearly understood and taught.

REASONING

Reasoning is the use of logical thought patterns to solve problems. It can be broken into two broad subcategories: inductive and deductive reasoning. **Inductive reasoning** begins with several specifics or facts and builds a larger picture or whole that incorporates the smaller pieces. The accuracy of such reasoning rests with which pieces of information are chosen to build the larger whole. **Deductive reasoning** starts with the big picture or the whole and tries to break it down into its smaller parts. Reasoning allows us to try out alternatives in our mind and to preselect the one that seems to best fit the situation. It can, however, stifle creativity and overlook viable alternatives that may appear logically inadequate. No evaluation mechanism is built into the reasoning process. Much of the utility of our reasoning process is tested through experience in real-world situations.

RESEARCH

Research is a combination of deductive and inductive reasoning processes. It is a systematic process used to confirm and refine existing knowledge and to build new knowledge. Inductive reasoning allows us to generate new concepts and theories; deductive reasoning allows us to test out those concepts and theories. Quantitative research is used to describe, explore, explain, or predict observable or measurable conditions. Qualitative research allows us to identify, examine, and explain subjective experiences of an individual or group. We talk in depth about these two types of research in later chapters.

Research has built in checks and balances as well as evaluation mechanisms. It seeks to acknowledge and reduce **bias.** However, all sources of knowing are influenced by personal bias. All that we learn is filtered by our own set of views, and we have a tendency to use incoming knowledge to confirm those preheld views. Thus, when filtering information, we tend to note and remember those things that support our views and ignore or deny those that are contrary to our views.

> Research is a systematic reasoning process used to confirm existing knowledge and build new knowledge.

Is research then a magic bullet, an answer to all questions, a solution to all human problems? Of course not. It is a very specific set of processes designed to examine only those problems that can be directly or indirectly seen, touched, heard, tasted, or smelled. Research cannot be used to produce answers about fundamental moral or ethical issues such as whether abortion is good or evil or whether cloning is right or wrong. It cannot take the place of philosophical debate about the meaning of life or the existence of God. The research we conduct is only as good as the limits of the study and the way the study is designed, and all studies have limits or flaws. Some explorations using the research process are even out of reach because we haven't yet invented the instruments that would allow us to measure what we want to study. Results obtained from the research process provide us with reasonable or plausible answers. The knowledge gained is never final or absolute. It is, in fact, always subject to ongoing investigation and scrutiny. Research is a tool, albeit a very powerful tool, to explore the world around us.

> Research is a tool to explore the world around us.

What Is Nursing Research?

Nursing research is simply research that addresses issues that are important to nurses and the nursing profession. Nursing research uses the research process as a tool to search for, develop, refine, and expand a body of knowledge that shapes and enhances the practice of nursing. Research can be classified as nursing research anytime the research endeavor produces knowledge relevant to nursing. This includes the areas of clinical practice, education, and administration, as well as various professional issues. The focus in this text is on nursing research that has direct impact on nursing interventions with clients. This is often referred to as **clinical nursing research.**

> Nursing research uses the research process as a tool to search for, develop, refine, and expand a body of knowledge that shapes and enhances the practice of nursing.

Why Is Research Important?

The ultimate importance of research is found in its definition. It generates knowledge. This in turn allows us to make better-informed decisions and choices. It may validate existing practices built through experience, intuition, and personal experience. It may examine tried and true practices and make them more efficient, less expensive, or less complicated. It may explore ways to tackle newly evolving problems in an increasingly complex world.

Why Is Nursing Research Important?

Nursing research serves several purposes for nursing as a profession and for nurses as individuals. It provides a standard and reliable knowledge base upon which to build the practice of nursing. This in turn ensures that the care given to clients is the best possible at that given moment in time. So nursing research plays an important role in guiding and improving the delivery of nursing care to clients.

Professions are commonly judged by the body of knowledge they generate. A clearly defined knowledge base built on a strong research foundation lends credibility to nursing as a distinct profession. The more defined this knowledge base, the clearer the role of the nurse in the delivery of health care. If nurses can more clearly define their role, then they can more clearly articulate distinctions and similarities between their own roles and those of other health care professionals. This in turn allows consumers of health care and potential clients to better see and value the contributions of nurses and nursing as a profession.

The practice of nursing in today's litigious society demands increasing accountability for one's actions. Consumers demand reasons for nursing interventions. Thus nurses need sound rationale for their decisions and actions. A knowledge base grounded in the findings of sound research provides such rationale. Individual nurses must keep their knowledge base current in order to keep their practice current and to be responsible and accountable to the consumer.

Nurses are increasingly called on to document cost effectiveness of the nursing care that is given. Many health care facilities have tried to reduce the bottom line by substituting untrained personnel for nurses. In part, this is because nursing services consume such a large part of an institution's budget. Research can demonstrate that effective nursing care leads to fewer patient complications, shorter hospital stays or fewer readmissions, and that nursing cutbacks actually increase overall institutional costs.

Where Has Nursing Research Been and Where Is It Going?

This section takes a look at the past lives of nursing research and then peers into the future of nursing research.

A Historical Look at Nursing Research

Research is a relatively new addition to nursing's tool bag of knowledge sources. While the first research efforts can probably be traced back to Florence Nightingale, little formal research was carried out by nurses on the behalf of nursing until the late 1940s. The progress of nursing research is closely tied to the development of nursing and nursing education.

Research was slow to develop in nursing. Schools evolved from military and religious roots and stressed order and obedience. Inquiring minds had little place in this system of education. Instead, dedication to hard work and submission to authority were valued. Training was viewed as an apprenticeship with long hours and rote repetition the order of the day. Nurses had little free time and little say in their own training or work. The traditional subservient role of women in society reinforced the values promoted by hospitals and hospital schools of nursing.

Only when nursing began to move toward advanced education and affiliation with university settings did research begin to emerge. Ironically, it was research by investigators in other disciplines that exposed the deficiencies in the preparation of nurses and urged better educational opportunities and a move to university settings. Sociologists found the study of nurses and nursing as a work culture particularly fascinating. As a female-dominated occupation, nursing held special appeal for sociological investigation. Nursing work, habits, roles, and attitudes were dissected and reported for decades in sociological literature.

World War II increased the demand for nurses and sparked interest in nursing as a profession. Nurses and nursing were in the spotlight. Funds for development were suddenly available from government and private sources. There was a push for basic and advanced education in university settings. Nursing research got a major boost. A nursing research center and a nursing foundation were established to promote nursing research. A journal was created to publish the results of that research. More nurses were receiving advanced degrees and had expertise in research. Unfortunately, most of these degrees were in fields other than nursing. Thus, early research efforts by nurses tended to ask questions about the education, psychology, or sociology of nurses.

The number of nurses with advanced degrees and research skills continued to increase in the 1960s and 1970s, and a push for doctoral preparation in nursing was begun. Formal support mechanisms for research and research funding in nursing increased and stabilized. Nursing practice was becoming more standardized, complex, and specialized. Nursing education at the master's level became more common and emphasized specialization in rapidly emerging specialty areas. Research was carried out to establish standards for specialty practice. Nurses began to turn to nursing care and clinical practice to provide questions for research. The focus shifted from the study of nurses to the practice of nursing. Nursing theories evolved that attempted to describe and explain the practice of nursing. These theories began to be tested by nurse researchers. Practice-related research flourished and by the end of the 1970s, two new research journals were launched to handle the nursing research explosion.

By the 1980s there was a critical mass of nurses with doctoral degrees and research skills. The computer revolution was getting into full swing. Focus in the research arena turned to improving the quality of research. Questions about research methodology and statistical treatment were raised. The manner in which data were collected and the analysis of that data became important. A National Center for Nursing Research was federally mandated and funded under the National Institutes of Health (NIH). It was later named an Institute in its own right. Centers for nursing research proliferated in numerous hospital and university settings. The quality and quantity of nursing research continued to grow, and two more research journals were launched to help disseminate nursing research findings. Clinical practice specialty groups increasingly funded, promoted, and published research in their respective specialty areas.

The 1990s have been dedicated to refining and expanding nursing research efforts. There are now more than 50 doctoral programs in nursing in the United States, and the use of qualitative research methodologies has gained wide acceptance. The issue of better use of findings by those in clinical practice is a burning one. The Internet is being explored as a tool for increased dissemination of results. It is an exciting and optimistic time for nursing research. Box 4-2 presents some highlights in the development of nursing research in the United States.

Activity

11

STUDENT CHALLENGE Netting the NINR

1. Log on to the Internet and check out the National Institute for Nursing Research. Or you can access the NINR site through the book's MERLIN site at www.mosby.com/MERLIN/Langford/maze.
2. Explore the history of NINR and discover its central mission.
3. Do you think it is important for nursing to have its own governmental institute? Why or why not?
4. Who is the current director of NINR? Do you think she or he is qualified for the job? What did you base your evaluation on?

The Future of Nursing Research

A national nursing research agenda was a priority for the newly formed National Center for Nursing Research (NCNR). A conference of 50 nurse scientists was held to develop broad research priority areas for the profession of nursing. The information generated from that conference served as the raw material used by an NCNR subcommittee to delineate a set of seven priority areas for nursing research for a 5-year period from 1989 through 1994. A second conference established five research priorities for 1995 through 1999. These priorities served to guide government research grant funding in nursing. Box 4-3 delineates the priorities from the first two conferences.

Shortly after the second conference, it became evident that the national nursing research agenda needed to be more responsive to the current state of nursing science, to present health care needs, and to rapidly shifting future health challenges. The 5-year approach was abandoned, and a more flexible approach was initiated to identify emerging areas of research opportunity. Input comes from the National Research Roundtable, regional research societies, and an annual forum. Areas of research opportunity are generated and released on an annual basis. They may be revised if the state of nursing science shifts or a pressing need arises (O'Neal, 1999). The areas of opportunity for 2000 are listed in Box 4-4.

Box 4-2 Nursing Research Highlights in the United States

1872 First hospital-based school of nursing established
1900 *American Journal of Nursing* started
1909 First university-affiliated school of nursing
1912 Founding of American Nurses Association (ANA)
1923 *Goldmark Report*—detailed deficiencies in nursing education
1924 First doctoral program in nursing
1927 First nurse to receive a doctoral degree
1936 Sigma Theta Tau began funding nursing research
1948 *Brown Report*—a 3-year national study reemphasizing deficiencies in nursing education and urging move to university setting
1948 First manual detailing how to conduct nursing research
1950 5-year master plan for nursing research published by ANA
1952 *Nursing Research* journal started
1955 American Nurses Foundation formed and dedicated exclusively to promoting nursing research
1956 United States Public Health Service (USPHS) began awarding grants for nursing research
1957 Department of Nursing Research established at Walter Reed Army Institute of Research
1959 National League for Nursing established Research and Studies Service
1959 First research grants awarded to nursing faculty
1962 ANA issued a blueprint for nursing research
1962 Graduate training grants begun to train nurse scientists
1965 ANA began sponsoring conferences in nursing research
1971 ANA started Council of Nurse Researchers
1974 ANA called for nursing practice research priorities for next decade
1976 ANA recommended research preparation be included in undergraduate, graduate, and continuing education programs
1978 *Research in Nursing and Health* journal started
1979 *Western Journal of Nursing Research* started
1980 ANA Commission on Research set research priorities for the 1980s
1986 National Center for Nursing Research established at the National Institutes for Health
1988 *Applied Nursing Research* and *Nursing Science Quarterly* journals started
1988 National Center for Nursing Research sets nursing research priorities
1990 *Qualitative Health Research* journal started
1991 *Clinical Nursing Research* journal started
1993 National Center for Nursing Research became National Institute of Nursing Research
1993 On-line computer library and the *Online Journal of Knowledge Synthesis* started by Sigma Theta Tau
1996 Nursing Information and Data Set Evaluation Center started by ANA

Box 4-3 NINR Research Priorities

Conference One (1989-1994)

Prevention and care of low-birth-weight infants
Prevention and care for HIV infection
Long-term care for older adults
Symptom management for pain
Using nursing informatics to enhance patient care
Health promotion for children and adolescents
Dependence on technology across the lifespan

Conference Two (1994-1999)

Development/evaluation of community-based nursing models
Assessment of effectiveness of nursing interventions in AIDS
Development/evaluation of remediation approaches for cognitive
    impairments
Evaluation of interventions for coping with chronic illness
Identification of biobehavioral factors/evaluation of interventions to
    promote

From National Institute of Nursing Research (NINR): *NNRA process, developing knowledge for practice*, Washington, DC, 1993, NINR.

STUDENT CHALLENGE Foraging for Future Research

1. Log on to the Internet and check out the National Institute for Nursing Research strategic plans for the twenty-first century. Refer to the previous Student Challenge to access the NINR website.
2. Compare the areas of research opportunity for the year 2001 with those cited in Box 4-4. How did they change?
3. Have areas been posted for 2002?
4. Discuss the delineated areas. What relevance do they have with what you see in the clinical area?

Box 4-4 NINR Areas of Research Opportunity for Year 2000

Chronic Illness or Conditions
Enhancing adherence in diabetes self-management
Managing asthma symptoms in children

Behavioral Changes
Biobehavioral research for effective sleep
Acute care of children with posttraumatic brain injury

Compelling Public Health Concerns
Enhancing end-of-life care
Collaborating with clinical trial networks

From NINR: *2000 NINR areas of research opportunity*, website at www.nih.gov/ninr/2000AoRO.htm, 7/12/99.

The future for nursing research promises to be bright and challenging as we prepare for the twenty-first century. Priorities are likely to remain directed at nursing practice. There will be an increased emphasis on building on the results of completed studies. This includes repeating studies using various subjects in a variety of settings (replication). There will also be an ever-greater push to find ways to ensure that nurses use the results of all this nursing research in the course of their day-to-day practice.

Who Is Involved in Nursing Research?
Consumers and Producers

All levels of nurses have roles to play as either consumers or producers of nursing research. Consumers of nursing research are responsible for reading current research and adapting useful findings in their practice. Producers design and implement research studies and disseminate the study results for consumers to use. The American Nurses Association has delineated various levels of research participation by educational level (Table 4-1). Note that as an associate degree or baccalaureate degree graduate, you are viewed primarily as a research consumer. Your priority is to read and use research results in the clinical setting.

Table 4-1 Research Participation by Educational Level

DEGREE	PARTICIPATION IN RESEARCH
Associate degree	Uses research findings in practice with supervision of nurses with advanced credentials. Assists with data collection within a defined protocol. Assists in identifying clinical problems that need to be researched.
Baccalaureate degree	Critically reads research studies and uses applicable results in practice. Promotes understanding of ethical principles of research. Identifies clinical problems, collects data, and implements findings. Assists investigators in gaining access to clinical sites.
Masters degree	Collaborates with experienced researchers to develop and conduct research. Creates a climate in the practice setting that supports the conduct of research and provides leadership in the integration of research findings.
Doctoral degree	Conducts research aimed at theory testing and theory generation. Acquires public and private funding for conduct of research. Disseminates research findings to scientific community, clinicians, policy makers, and lay public.

Adapted from American Nurses Association: *Education for participation in nursing research*, Kansas City, Mo, 1994, ANA.

Research Barriers and Facilitators

It is perhaps surprising that the application of research findings to nursing practice remains such a problem in today's health care climate. Research is being funded and carried out on a wider scale by more qualified nurses than ever before. At least eight nursing research journals and countless nursing specialty journals publish research articles. On-line sources provide abstracts of and present research results. Numerous health care institutions have nursing research committees. Opportunities for continuing education and participation and involvement are countless. Yet, application of research findings by those providing nursing care continues to

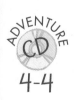

ADVENTURE
CD
4-4

be a problem. Studies have been done for more than 40 years that have identified perceived barriers to research use. Lack of time, insufficient knowledge base, discomfort with the material, inaccessibility of relevant literature, and lack of institutional support continue to be the major reasons cited for nonuse of research results (Camiletti and Huffman, 1998; Carroll et al., 1997; Rutledge et al., 1998).

There is evidence that certain factors facilitate use of research findings. Studies have shown that nurses with advanced degrees read and use research findings in practice a greater percentage of the time (Brown, 1997). Specific clinical models and programs that actively target research use in practice have been shown effective in increasing the use of research in the practice setting (Warren and Heermann, 1998; Radjenovic and Chally, 1998). If clinical institutions view research integration as important and structure clinical settings to encourage such practices, use of research findings also increases. Some clinical settings have initiated journal clubs in which practicing nurses come together on a regular basis and discuss research articles that are relevant to their areas of practice. Others provide resources for nurses to attend research conferences. Some have newsletters that present timely and pertinent research abstracts. Others have research committees that look at integration of research into policies and procedures. This issue of integration of research findings into practice becomes increasingly critical in this age of rapid change and complex health care challenges.

STUDENT CHALLENGE Checking out Barriers and Facilitators

1. Conduct a MEDLINE or CINAHL search for recent articles on perceived barriers and facilitators to the use of research findings in nursing practice. Try the key terms "nursing research utilization." Summarize the results.
2. Interview five nurses prepared at the associate degree or baccalaureate level. Ask them what they see as their role in nursing research. Ask them if they subscribe to or read any nursing research journals on a consistent basis. If they do not, ask them why they do not. Ask them about what might induce them to read and use research. If they do subscribe to a nursing research journal, ask them what they do with the information they read.

Continued

STUDENT CHALLENGE Checking out Barriers and Facilitators—cont'd

3. Compare your search results with your interview results. What are the similarities and differences in perceived barriers and facilitators. Share your results with some of your fellow classmates.
4. What suggestions do you have for ensuring better use of research findings in practice?

This learning package is designed to aid you in becoming an informed consumer of nursing research. It will provide you with tools to critically read and apply research findings in your everyday nursing practice. This role of informed consumer is a critical one. Nurse scientists can conduct numerous research studies that have potential impact for the practice of nursing. They can publish those findings in leading research journals and present findings at research conferences. However, the practicing nurse is the key for ensuring that those findings become an integrated part of nursing practice.

Resource Kit

Nursing Research Journals

Nursing Research
Research in Nursing and Health
Western Journal of Nursing Research
Applied Nursing Research
Nursing Science Quarterly
Clinical Nursing Research
Image: Journal of Nursing Scholarship
Scholarly Inquiry for Nursing Practice

 Visit the book's MERLIN website at
www.mosby.com/MERLIN/Langford/maze
for further information.

 Check out the puzzles, mazes, and games on your **CD-ROM.**

References

American Nurses Association: *Education for participation in nursing research*, Kansas City, Mo, 1994, ANA.

Benner P: *From novice to expert: excellence and power in clinical nursing practice*, Menlo Park, Calif, 1984, Addison-Wesley.

Beyea S and Nicoll L: Administration of medications via the intramuscular route: An integrative review of the literature and research based protocol for the procedure, *App Nurs Res* 8(1):23-33, Feb 1995.

Brown DS: Nursing education and nursing research utilization: Is there a connection in clinical settings?, *J Contin Educ Nurs* 28(6):258-262, 1997.

Camiletti YA, Huffman MC: Research utilization: Evaluation of initiatives in a public health nursing division, *Can J Nurs Adm* 11(2):59-77, 1998.

Carroll DL, et al: Barriers and facilitators to the utilization of nursing research, *Clin Nurs Spec* 11(5):207-212,1997.

Kerlinger FN: *Foundations of behavioral research*, ed 2, New York, 1973, Holt Rinehart and Winston.

National Institute of Nursing Research (NINR): *NNRA Process, developing knowledge for practice*, Washington, DC, 1993, NINR.

NINR: *2000 NINR Areas of research opportunity*, website at www.nih.gov/ninr/2000AoRO.htm, 7/12/99.

O'Neal D, Chief Officer of Science Public Policy and Public Liaison, NINR: Conversation with the author, 7/12/99.

Radjenovic D, Chally PS: Research utilization by undergraduate students, *Nurs Educ* 23(2):26-29, 1998.

Rutledge DN, et al: Barriers to research utilization for oncology staff nurses and nurse managers/clinical nurse specialists, *Oncol Nurs Forum* 25(3):497-506, 1998.

Warren JJ, Heermann JA: The research nurse intern program. A model for research dissemination and utilization, *J Nurs Adm* 28(11):39-45, 1998.

Learning Objectives

1 Define quantitative research.
2 Describe quantitative research classifications.
3 Discuss the phases of the research process.
4 Describe steps involved in conceptualizing a study.
5 Describe steps involved in designing a study.
6 Describe steps involved in conducting a study.
7 Describe steps involved in analyzing a study.
8 Describe steps involved in using study results.
9 Discuss the relationship among phases of the research process.
10 Cite examples of steps and phases of the process.

Chapter Outline

What Is Quantitative Research?
Quantitative Research Classifications
   Reasons quantitative research is conducted
   Time span and point of data collection
   Purpose
   Research design
What Is the Research Process?
   Phase 1: Conceive the study
     Identify the problem
     Review the literature
     Define a theoretical framework
     Formulate variables
   Phase 2: Design the study
     Select research design
     Identify sample and setting

     Select data collection methods
     Evaluate instrument quality
   Phase 3: Conduct the study
     Get approval to use human subjects
     Recruit subjects
     Collect data
   Phase 4: Analyze the study
     Describe the sample
     Answer the research questions
     Interpret the results
   Phase 5: Use the study
     Recommend further research
     State implications for practice
     Disseminate results

Quantitative Research: Summing It Up

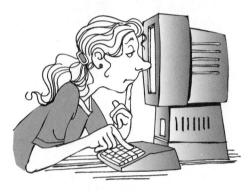

Hmmm! There has to be a statistic here somewhere that will make my results come out with the right answer.

Student Quote *"Once you understand what all those terms mean and learn that there is a very set structure and defined process for doing a (quantitative) research study, it's not so hard to follow what's happenin'."*

Abstract Quantitative research is a systematic logical process used to answer questions about measurable concepts. It can be classified in numerous ways, including via the stated goals of the research or by the choice of research design. The research process is a circular one comprised of an orderly series of five phases that move the researcher from formulation of researchable problems to discovery of probable answers. The phases begin with conceptualization and crystallization of the problem. This problem is grounded in a literature base of previous research and theory. A study plan is then developed that specifies a research design, the subjects to be studied, and the instruments to be used for measurement. The study is implemented and data are collected using a set of ethical guidelines. Data are statistically analyzed, and research questions are answered and placed in a theoretical context. The findings are examined for their relevance to nursing practice and future research. Results are communicated to research consumers.

KEY TERMS

Quantitative Connections

Concept A mental picture of an object or phenomenon. Concepts may be concrete or abstract.

Conceptual definition Statement attaching a specified meaning to a word (e.g., what the word means for a particular research study).

Conceptual framework A loosely related collection of concepts that have not yet been tested.

Constant A characteristic that does not vary for a particular research study.

Control Mechanisms used by the researcher to reduce the influence of extraneous variables.

Data Measurable bits of information collected for purposes of analysis.

Data collection Gathering the information necessary to address the research problem.

Dependent variable Variable that is affected by the action of the independent variable.

Descriptive statistics Statistics used to describe and summarize data.

Experimental research Quantitative research in which one concept (independent variable) is manipulated to determine whether another concept (dependent variable) is affected.

Extraneous variable Variable that interferes with the relationship of the independent and dependent variables in a specified study.

Findings Results of the statistical analysis of study data.

Generalization The ability to apply study results from the sample to the population.

Hypothesis Statement of predicted relationship or difference between two or more variables.

Implication Inference drawn about the results of a research study.

Independent variable Variable that causes a change in the dependent variable.

Inferential statistics Statistics that are used to study relationships or differences among variables in a sample and infer the results back to the population.

Informed consent An agreement by a research subject to voluntarily participate in a study after being fully informed about the study and the inherent risks and benefits of participation.

Institutional review board (IRB) Committee responsible for review of research proposals to ensure that human subjects are protected from harm.

Instrument Device or technique used to collect data in a research study (e.g., biophysical instruments such as glucometers, psychological instruments such as questionnaires or interviews, behavioral instruments such as observation).

Literature review A critical summary of available theoretical and research literature on the selected research topic. It places the research problem for a particular study in context of what is currently known about the topic.

Manipulation An intervention or treatment introduced by the researcher in an experimental study.

Measurement A set of rules used to assign numbers to variables.

Key Terms—cont'd

Nonexperimental research Quantitative research in which concepts are not manipulated. They are examined as they occur naturally.

Nonprobability sample A sample selected using nonrandom techniques.

Operational definition Specifies how a variable is to be measured.

Population All known subjects that possess a common characteristic of interest to a researcher.

Probability (random) sample A sample selected using techniques to ensure that each subject in the population has an equal chance of being selected.

Problem statement Interrogative or declarative statement that describes the purpose of a research study, identifies key concepts, and sets study limits.

Quantitative research Systematic process used to gather and statistically analyze information that has been measured by an instrument and converted to numerical data.

Recommendation A statement derived from a research study to guide future research about a specified topic.

Reliability A characteristic of a good instrument; the assessed degree of consistency and dependability.

Research design The overall plan for collecting data in a research study.

Research process An orderly series of phases and steps that allow the researcher to move from asking a question to finding an answer.

Research question Use of an interrogative format to identify the variables to be studied and possible relationships or differences between those variables.

Sample A subset of a population selected to participate in a research study.

Sampling The process used to select the sample.

Setting The physical location and conditions under which a research study takes place.

Theoretical framework The theoretical foundation or frame of reference for a research study.

Theory Integrated and interrelated set of concepts used to explain some phenomenon.

Validity A characteristic of a good instrument; the extent of an instrument's ability to measure what it purports to measure.

Variable A concept, characteristic, or trait that varies (e.g., takes on measurably different values) within an identified population in a research study.

ADVENTURE
CD
5-1

There are two large general classifications for research: quantitative and qualitative. They are grounded in different philosophical approaches. This chapter addresses quantitative research, and Chapter 6 addresses qualitative research. The intent of these two chapters is to provide you with working knowledge of both research approaches. This will give you the necessary background and vocabulary to recognize, read, and use the findings from the nursing research literature. This chapter defines quantitative research, explores various ways that quantitative research can be classified, and identifies and discusses the specific steps of the quantitative research process.

You may find the next two chapters difficult to read and comprehend. That is to be expected because you are learning a new vocabulary. Don't panic. Remember what you learned in Chapter 3, and use your reading strategy. Take the time to thoroughly read and summarize the material. These two chapters provide the foundation you need to enable you to read and apply research results. Take a deep breath and attack this chapter one paragraph at a time. You can do it.

> **Hint:** The Glossary contains many of the terms used in this chapter even though they are not in located in your Quantitative Connections list. So take advantage of the Glossary. It is located at the back of the book, and it is on the CD-ROM.

What Is Quantitative Research?

Quantitative research is a systematic, objective process used to gather and analyze information that has been measured by some kind of instrument. Instruments are used to convert information into numbers. Quantitative research uses statistics to manage those numbers. The statistics may describe the numbers or analyze the numbers. This allows the researcher to draw a numerical picture of the information collected, to look at how the things being measured are alike or different, and to make decisions about whether things are related or different or to determine whether one thing causes another to react in a certain way.

> Quantitative research is a systematic process used to gather and statistically analyze information that has been measured by an instrument and converted to numerical data.

Quantitative research uses a logical approach that emphasizes deductive reasoning. It has several identifiable characteristics. It begins either with an educated guess (hypothesis) about how the **concepts** to be researched might be related, or with a question (research question) about what is to be explored or described. It studies only quantifiable concepts (concepts that can be measured and turned into numbers). The process is very structured. It seeks to be objective and tries to limit or control the effects of things not being studied. This approach yields results or **findings** that are clearly defined and easily interpreted.

However, this approach does have limitations. It is not readily used to study complex issues in which a large number of factors are at play. It cannot study concepts that can't be numerically measured. Also, although objectivity is prized and strict controls are imposed to ensure this objectivity, bias is inevitable and begins with the researcher's interest in a particular area of study. It continues when the researcher makes predictions or hypotheses about the expected results. The researcher often becomes highly invested in ensuring that those predictions are supported by the study's outcomes. There have been numerous reports about researchers who resort to various conscious and unconscious means to ensure certain results. For example, a recent newspaper story told of a scientist who faked data to prove there was a relationship between electric power lines and an increased incidence of cancer (Seyfer, 1999).

Quantitative Research Classifications

Several different terms are used to describe or classify quantitative research. We explore some of the more common classifications and terms so they will be familiar to you when you encounter them in the literature. Quantitative research may be classified in the following ways: the reasons the research is conducted, the span of time in which data collection occurs, the point at which data are collected, the number of subjects sampled, the purpose or aim of the research, and the research design or statistical method used (Box 5-1). Studies may fall under several of these classification schemes. Thus, you might see a particular study described as a cross-sectional, descriptive, nonexperimental study.

Reasons Quantitative Research is Conducted

Pure or basic research is done to establish or extend fundamental concepts and theories. It is a search for "knowledge for knowledge's sake." The findings may have no immediate practical application or benefit. Applied research is conducted for practical purposes and is directed at solving an immediate problem. Applied research is often based on a foundation of basic research, and its results often suggest further areas for basic research study. Because nursing is a practice discipline, most

Box 5-1   Classification Systems for Quantitative Research

Reasons Conducted
1. Basic (pure)
2. Applied
Time Span
1. Cross-sectional
2. Longitudinal
Point of Data Collection
1. Retrospective (*ex post facto* or after the fact)
2. Prospective
Purpose or Aim
1. Descriptive
2. Exploratory
3. Explanatory
4. Predictive
Research Design
1. Experimental
2. Nonexperimental (correlational)

of the research in various nursing research journals is applied research. As a consumer of nursing research who desires to improve your clinical practice, you will be most interested in applied research.

Applied research is used to find solutions to clinical problems in nursing.

Time Span and Point of Data Collection

Research is sometimes described by the span of time used to collect the data for the study or to indicate when data were collected. Cross-sectional studies use data collected at one point in time. Longitudinal studies use data collected at several points over a longer time period. Measurements of the identified concepts may be taken many times over several months or years. Prospective studies analyze data collected on factors or events as they occur. Retrospective studies analyze data on factors or events that occurred before the onset of the research study.

Purpose

The two categories that are most helpful in describing a quantitative study are the classification by purpose and classification by design. You may recall that in Chapter 4 we said, "quantitative research was used to describe, explore, explain and predict . . . measurable conditions." Thus this particular classification scheme informs us about the general purpose of the research study.

A descriptive study does as its name implies; it *describes* the concepts under study. It may look at the prevalence, magnitude, and/or characteristics of the concept. It may classify various factors in the study. A recent example of a descriptive nursing research study can be found in an article entitled "Ventilated Patients' Self-esteem During Intubation and After Extubation" (Menzel, 1999). This study measured and described the self-esteem of patients while they were intubated and after they were extubated. Another example can be found in a study by Mimnaugh and others (1999), which described the types and intensity of sensations experienced by postoperative patients during the removal of tubes.

Exploratory studies *explore*. They are used to investigate a particular concept about which little is known. They go beyond describing concepts and begin to examine the relationships or differences between the concepts and other factors. For example, Parshall (1999) explored associated characteristics and disposition for patients who came to the Emergency Department (ED) with dyspnea. She examined diagnoses, urgency of the visit, age, and whether the person was admitted or released.

Explanatory studies *explain*. These studies try to discover why a certain concept or phenomenon occurs. They search for cause and effect or interactive relationships between concepts. They are often linked with theory and represent a way to organize or integrate the relationships among various concepts or factors. For example, an explanatory study by Carruth and associates (1997) tested a complex theoretical model with multiple factors to explain the concept of family satisfaction among caregivers of elderly parents.

Predictive studies *predict*. Once events are explainable, the next step is to try to predict what will occur with one factor if a change happens in related factors. Studies that try to predict what will occur are called predictive studies. For example, Jennings-Dozier (1999) studied whether certain factors would predict which women would get a Pap smear.

Research Design

There are two major research design categories: experimental and nonexperimental. These descriptions tell us how the research study has been designed. In **experimental research**, the researcher manipulates one concept under study to see how that manipulation will change or affect another concept under study. For example, an experimental study by Gawlinski and Dracup (1998) looked at whether positioning affected oxygen saturation in critically ill patients. The concept of positioning was manipulated to see if oxygen saturation changed (e.g., the patients' positions were changed and then their saturation levels were measured).

In **nonexperimental research,** there is no manipulation. The concepts are just studied as they occur naturally. For example, in a study about pregnant and nonpregnant adolescents and self-esteem (Connelly, 1998), the researcher did not manipulate the concept of pregnancy (i.e., she did not decide who got pregnant and who did not). She simply chose teens who were already pregnant and teens who were not. She then measured the self-esteem of both groups. Nonexperimental studies are sometimes referred to as correlational studies or nonintervention studies. Correlational is really a descriptor used to describe the type of statistic used to analyze the data.

ADVENTURE
CD
5-2

> There are two major research design categories: experimental and nonexperimental.

🔲 STUDENT CHALLENGE Scrutinizing Study Classifications

Go to the library and look up the research studies cited as examples in the previous paragraphs. Do not worry about being able to decipher them at this point.

1. Can you tell why they are classified as they are? Choose several other nursing research articles.

2. Can you pick out the studies that are quantitative? (Hint: Look for studies that have numbers and symbols and talk about various types of statistical analysis.)

STUDENT CHALLENGE Scrutinizing Study Classifications—cont'd

3. Could you determine any further classification of the quantitative studies you looked at? This can be more difficult. Some will tell you in the title or the abstract. Others give some clues but fail to identify the study classification. For example, an experimental study might talk about an intervention or use of experimental and control groups.

What Is the Research Process?

The **research process** is an orderly series of phases and steps that allow the researcher to move from asking a question to finding an answer. The answer, in turn, suggests new questions. Thus research (the act of re-searching) can be envisioned as a circular process with attendant phases and steps as illustrated in Fig. 5-1. These phases and steps guide the research process. Although they occur in the general order indicated by Fig. 5-1, the order may vary, steps may overlap, and the researcher may shift back and forth between various steps or phases. In some studies, certain steps are unnecessary and are omitted. However, we can use these phases and steps as a guide to paint a picture of the research process. This will help you understand what the researcher goes through when conducting a study.

Phase 1: Conceive the Study

The first task at hand for any researcher is to make a decision about what to study. The activities in this phase involve reading, theorizing, and thinking about the area of interest. Thus the steps of problem identification, literature review, and theoretical framework development often occur simultaneously and lead to the formulation of research hypotheses or research questions. In the following sections, we examine each step individually.

IDENTIFY THE PROBLEM

The **problem statement** describes the focus or intent of the research study. It identifies what concepts will be researched. The purpose of the study (i.e., intent, goal) is also described and limits are drawn. Some problems are stated directly and sim-

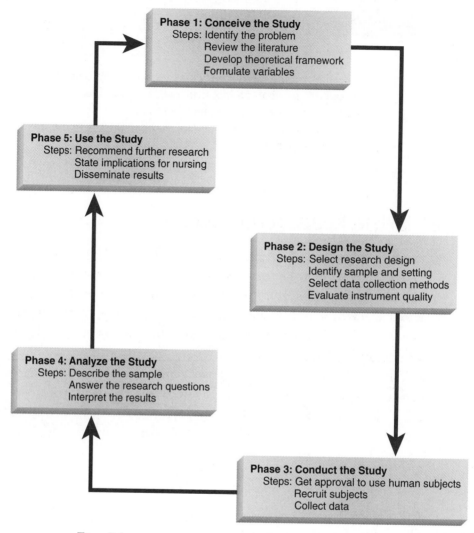

Fig. 5-1   The phases and steps of the research process.

ply in the form of a question. This is then followed by a broader description of the study's purpose or goals. Some problems are stated in a declarative form and labeled as a statement of purpose. The declarative form contains the aim (to describe, explore, explain, or predict) of the research as well as the concepts to be studied. It may also contain information about the research design (e.g., is it

Box 5-2 Sample Forms of Problem Statements*

Interrogative Form

What characteristics are common among elderly individuals who seek care in an Emergency Department?

Does parental presence affect anxiety and behavior of young children undergoing suture repair of a laceration?

Can oxygenation be improved in premature infants by use of extra-tactile stimulation?

Declarative Form

The purpose of this nonexperimental study is to describe the characteristics of elderly individuals who use the Emergency Department.

The purpose of the study is to explore the influence of parental presence on anxiety levels and behaviors of young children who get sutures for a laceration.

The purpose of this experimental study is to determine whether a stimulation protocol will improve the oxygenation of premature infants.

*Examples are taken from student thesis efforts.

experimental or nonexperimental?). Examples of both forms can be seen in Box 5-2. Many research studies include more than one problem statement or statement of purpose. This may indicate increased complexity of the study. Whether the researcher uses a problem statement or a statement of purpose or both, the intent is the same. These statements guide and focus the research.

REVIEW THE LITERATURE

The **literature review** involves a search for information that is relevant to the identified problem area. It tells us what is currently known about the area under study and places what is known in context. This allows the researcher to see how their particular study fits into a larger picture. It is much like looking at the picture on the box when trying to put a jigsaw puzzle together. The literature review also helps develop the theoretical frame of reference for the study. Finally, it may also serve to better refine and define the problem being studied. It may even provide information about the best way to design the study or the best way to measure the concepts being examined.

This sounds straightforward enough. You are already familiar with the procedures used to conduct a literature review. The card catalog and periodical indexes are used for the search and the identified concepts and related terms form the core focus of the search. Several information sources, as shown in Box 5-3 are of inter-

Box 5-3 | Information Types and Sources

Research Studies

1. Nursing research journals (*Nursing Research, Research in Nursing and Health, Western Journal of Nursing Research, Applied Nursing Research, Nursing Science Quarterly, Clinical Nursing Research, Image: Journal of Nursing Scholarship, Scholarly Inquiry for Nursing Practice*)
2. Research findings in other nursing journals (*Online Journal of Knowledge Synthesis*, various nursing specialty journals)
3. Research journals in related fields
4. Dissertations and theses
5. Research conference proceedings or paper presentations

Theoretical and Conceptual Discussions

1. Nursing books
2. Nursing journals such as *Advances in Nursing Science, Topics in Clinical Nursing*
3. Books in related fields

Facts and Statistics

1. Government documents
2. Professional documents (published by ANA, NLN, etc.)

Opinions and Anecdotes on Nursing and Health-Related Issues

1. General nursing journals (*American Journal of Nursing, Nursing, Nursing Outlook*, specialty journals)
2. Journals in related fields
3. Newspaper, Internet websites, television

est to the nurse researcher. These should look familiar to you. Research studies that have examined some of the same or similar concepts are the most helpful and form the backbone of the literature review.

The literature review should be comprehensive, balanced, and relevant. In other words, it should cover all the current theoretical and research content on the defined concepts in the problem statement. Information should be included whether or not it supports the researcher's line of thinking. The review should draw the core of information from other research efforts. It should rely heavily on primary sources of information (articles written by the person who actually conducted the research being reviewed). Secondary sources (descriptions of research studies by authors other than the researcher) should be used only to provide information about additional primary sources.

DEFINE A THEORETICAL FRAMEWORK

A **theoretical framework** uses a theory or theories to form a theoretical foundation or frame of reference for the research study. A **theory** consists of several concepts that are well integrated and interrelated and are used to explain some phenomenon. The concepts and many of the relationships have been previously tested and researched. You have probably studied many theories in the course of your nursing education. Nursing uses several theories from related disciplines (e.g., Selye's (1956) theory of stress, Maslow's (1943) theory of human motivation, Erikson's (1950) theory of development).

Nurses have also developed several theories to explain nursing practice (e.g., Orem's [1971] theory of self-care, King's [1971] theory of system transaction and goal attainment, Rogers' [1970] unitary man theory). Theories help us pull complex concepts together. They demonstrate how these concepts interact and function as a larger whole. This allows us to more effectively order our own knowledge and increase our understanding of the bigger picture.

A theoretical framework helps the researcher explain or predict study outcomes and to link those outcomes to the existing body of knowledge. Not all research studies use a theoretical framework. Sometimes, a theory is not yet available because the area of research is new. Descriptive and exploratory studies often lack a theoretical frame of reference.

In these instances, some researchers use a conceptual framework. A **conceptual framework** is a loosely related collection of concepts that have not yet been tested. However, as nursing science grows, the use of theoretical frameworks grows in nursing research. The relationship of theory and research is a circular one (Fig. 5-2). Theory supports and suggests research problems. Research findings confirm or refute theory explanations. This allows theories to be revised and provides additional avenues for research.

A researcher who is doing pure or basic research may be devising numerous research studies for the express purpose of testing and refining a particular theory. Researchers who are doing applied research can increase the usability of their research findings by relating them to theory. For example, a researcher might be in-

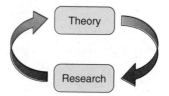

Fig. 5-2   Relation of theory and research.

terested in investigating the characteristics of individuals who consistently take
their antihypertensive medications and those who do not. If the researcher con-
ducts the study without a theoretical framework, the findings might identify
whether any characteristics distinguish medication takers from nontakers.

However, suppose the researcher decides to use Orem's self-care theory as a
theoretical framework. Now the researcher can relate the characteristics of medication takers to the concept of self-care. Those individuals with sufficient self-
care agency would be expected to engage in self-care practice (e.g., taking medication). Those with self-care deficits would be expected to need nursing
assistance. Thus research findings that identified characteristics of medication
takers versus nontakers could be seen as factors that promote self-care agency
(takers) or self-care deficit (nontakers). Nurses could then apply those characteristics to other situations in which the patient is expected to carry out prescribed
health care regimens. This might allow the nurse to anticipate when individuals
need nursing assistance to overcome a self-care deficit. This example illustrates
how use of a theoretical framework can help researchers and research consumers
expand the applicability of research findings.

FORMULATE VARIABLES

Variables are identified concepts or traits that are measured, manipulated, or controlled in a research study. A **variable** is a concept or trait that varies. These traits
may be associated with organisms or with the environment. For example, gender
is an organism variable because some organisms are male and some are female.
Weather (rain, sun, sleet, hail, and so on) is an example of an environmental variable. Almost any concept, characteristic, or trait that can be observed and/or measured can be considered a variable. When a characteristic or trait does not vary
within a given research study context, it is called a **constant**. For example if researchers wanted gender to be a constant, they might select only females as subjects

for their study. Researchers often use constants to exert control over variables they don't want to study but that might otherwise interfere with the study results.

Variables may take different forms. They may be classified by quality or quantity. Qualitative (categorical) variables change in terms of the presence or absence of a specified trait (e.g., male or not male, married or not married, blue eyed or not blue eyed). Quantitative (continuous) variables change in terms of amount or degree (e.g., income, height, weight). These variables can be described in numbers and fractions of numbers. Classifying variables as qualitative or quantitative becomes more important in a later phase of the research study because researchers choose certain statistics based on this variable classification.

Another way to classify variables is to determine whether a particular variable is acting as an independent variable, a dependent variable, or an extraneous variable in a research study. These distinctions in variables are usually used when the purpose of the study is explanatory or predictive, but they may be seen in exploratory studies in which relationships or differences are being researched.

The **independent variable** is used to explain or predict the change or variation in the **dependent variable**. For example, in a study that is researching whether a "low-fat diet" will decrease "cholesterol levels," the "type of diet" is the independent variable, and the "level of blood cholesterol" is the dependent variable. The independent variable can be considered the cause, while the dependent variable is the effect.

An **extraneous variable** can also affect the dependent variable and interfere with the relationship of the independent and dependent variables. In the previous example, the extraneous variables "exercise" and "menstrual cycle" might also affect "cholesterol levels." Can you think of other extraneous variables that might affect "cholesterol levels"? Researchers try to identify all potential extraneous variables so they can **control** them and keep them from interfering with the variables under study. The literature review helps them identify these extraneous factors. We discussed one form of control that the researcher uses by turning an extraneous variable into a constant. Sampling and statistical techniques are also used to help the researcher exert control over extraneous variables.

Once variables are identified, they must be defined. Variables are defined in two ways. The first is a **conceptual definition**. This is the type of definition that you are familiar with, the kind you look up in the dictionary. It tells what the word means in the given context of a particular study. The second definition is an

operational definition. This definition spells out how the variable will be measured. For example, the variable "anxiety" might be conceptually defined as "uneasiness or apprehension about an impending event." The operational definition might state "anxiety will be measured using the Clinical Anxiety Rating Scale." Operational definitions are often decided on in phase 2 of the study.

In a specific research study, variables come from the concepts identified in the problem statement and are specified in the form of research questions or hypotheses. The population to be studied is also specified in the research questions or hypotheses. (We discuss populations in the next phase of the research process). Box 5-4 provides examples of research questions and hypotheses as derived from the problem statement.

Box 5-4   Sample Research Questions and Hypotheses*

Problem Statement	Questions/Hypotheses
Example 1	
What common characteristics are possessed by elderly individuals who seek care in an Emergency Department?	What percent of total ED visits are by elderly persons? What are the presenting chief complaints of the elderly? Is use affected by time of day, season of year, category of ED, method of payment, gender, or age of the elderly?
Example 2	
Does parental presence affect anxiety and behavior of young children undergoing suture repair of a laceration?	Will there be a difference between the anxiety levels and disruptive behaviors of young children whose parents are present during laceration repair versus those with no parental presence?
Example 3	
The purpose of this experimental study is to determine whether a stimulation protocol will improve the oxygenation of premature infants.	Premature infants who receive extra-tactile stimulation will have higher PO_2 levels than those who do not.

*Examples are taken from student thesis efforts.

When research questions are used, the purpose of the study is descriptive or exploratory, and a theoretical framework is rarely identified. **Research questions** use an interrogative format to identify the variables to be studied and possible relationships or differences between those variables. Example 1 in Box 5-4 is from a descriptive study and shows questions used to identify and describe the variables (number of ED visits, chief complaints, time of day, season of year, ED category, payment method, gender, and age) and the population (elderly persons using the ED). In the second example from an exploratory study, a question asks about differences on two dependent variables (anxiety levels, disruptive behaviors) for two different groups of individuals (children with and without parental presence). Parental presence or absence is the independent variable and young children with lacerations are the population. Research questions serve as queries about variables and how they might interact with one another. Research questions are used when no concrete information is available to predict an answer.

A **hypothesis** is an "educated guess" about the relationships between variables and the expected outcomes of the study. It tries to predict the nature of the relationship between variables. The researcher makes these "educated guesses" based on the review of literature and the theoretical framework. The results of the research study will either support or refute the hypotheses that were established in the first phase of the study. Research studies that use hypotheses are usually either explanatory or predictive in nature.

All hypotheses contain at least one identifiable independent variable and at least one dependent variable. Some hypotheses are labeled as simple hypotheses. They contain one independent and one dependent variable. Other hypotheses are labeled complex hypotheses because they contain more than one independent and/or dependent variable. Example 3 in Box 5-4 is from an explanatory study and shows a hypothesis that predicts that one group of infants will be better oxygenated than another group. The independent variable in this hypothesis is the presence or absence of extratactile stimulation, and the dependent variable is PO_2 level. The population is premature infants.

Phase 1 can be thought of as the conceptualization phase. It lays the foundation for the research study. When done well, the foundation is firm. When this phase is not well thought out, the study rests on a slippery slope, which make the findings of the study suspect. Now that you have read about phase 1, try your hand at the next Student Challenge.

🎲 STUDENT CHALLENGE Perusing Phase 1

Select several quantitative nursing research studies from your library. Use the nursing research journals or student theses or dissertations if they are available.

Now scan these studies and see if you can identify each of the elements we have discussed in phase 1. Remember that all studies may not contain all elements.

1. Find the problem statement. Can you find examples of the interrogative form and the declarative form? Did the studies label it as a problem statement? If not, look for a statement such as "the purpose of the study was. . .," or examine the title or the abstract.

2. Was a literature review present? Did it help you better understand the context of the study?

3. Was a theoretical framework identified?

4. Can you identify the variables being studied? Can you find the research hypotheses or research questions? Can you identify independent and dependent variables? What about extraneous variables? (Hint: Look for phrases such as _____ was controlled using. . .) Did the researcher state how the variables were defined?

Were different elements easier to spot in some studies than in others? Were some elements obvious in all the studies? Were any elements missing in all the studies you looked at?

Phase 2: Design the Study

In phase 2 of a research study, the researcher makes decisions about how to conduct the study. The researcher designs the study and plans methods for conducting the study. The sample is chosen, a setting is determined, variables are operationally defined, instruments are selected and evaluated, and procedures for data collection are outlined. These decisions have implications for the credibility of the results of the study. If the research design is flawed, then findings are suspect. Let's examine each step involved in making decisions about the study design. The order of the steps may vary slightly when making decisions, but all the steps are crucial in the design process.

SELECT RESEARCH DESIGN

The **research design** is the overall plan that guides the way the study is conducted and analyzed. As we discovered when discussing classifications of research studies, there are two major categories of quantitative research design: experimental and nonexperimental. There is one important distinction between experimental and nonexperimental designs. The researcher is an active agent in an experimental study, deliberately manipulating the independent variable in an attempt to change the dependent variable. This manipulation is often labeled a treatment or an intervention. In a nonexperimental study, the researcher is an observer and recorder, and there is no manipulation or treatment.

Experimental designs are characterized by three factors: (1) manipulation, (2) use of a control group, and (3) random assignment. All of these factors allow the researcher greater overall control of the experiment and are used to ensure that changes in the dependent variable are not caused by extraneous variables. As previously discussed, **manipulation** is the treatment or intervention the researcher carries out on the independent variable to try to get the dependent variable to change.

> Experimental designs use (1) manipulation, (2) control groups, and (3) random assignment to make sure changes in the dependent variable are not caused by extraneous variables.

To make sure that the change in the dependent variable is because of the treatment (manipulation) and not some other factor (extraneous variable), the researcher puts some of the subjects into a control group and some subjects into a treatment group. The control group does not get the experimental treatment (manipulation). The treatment group does get the experimental treatment (manipulation). If the dependent variable changes for the treatment group and does not change for the control group, then the treatment is probably causing the change. Look at Example 3 in Box 5-4. This is an experimental study. The researcher had two groups of premature infants. The treatment group got the extratactile stimulation treatment (manipulation). The control group got the usual care given by the nurses in the NICU. PO_2 levels (dependent variable) were measured for both groups. The researcher was looking for an increase in PO_2 for the treatment group and no increase in PO_2 for the control group.

Random assignment is the third characteristic of experimental designs. To guard against bias, the researcher randomly assigns subjects to a treatment or control group and randomly decides which group will get the treatment and which group will not. Random assignment means every subject has an equal chance of being in either group and each group has an equal chance of being designated as the treatment group. In Example 3 in Box 5-4, the infants were randomly assigned to Group 1 and Group 2 using a table of random numbers (Box 5-5). The treatment group was then selected placing two pieces of paper with the words "Group 1" and "Group 2" in a hat. One piece of paper was drawn, and that group was designated as the treatment group.

All experimental designs use manipulation. Some, however, fail either to use a control group or to use random assignment because it isn't always possible to have a control group or to decide who should go into one group or the other. When one of these two factors is missing, it is called a quasi-experimental design. A quasi-experimental design must then use other ways to ensure that study results are valid. One way to do this is to take extra measurements of the dependent variable, or to measure the dependent variable before and after the treatment.

Nonexperimental designs do not use treatments or attempt to manipulate the independent variable. These designs use what is already occurring in a particular setting with a particular group of subjects to describe certain variables or to explore relationships between certain variables. Descriptive nonexperimental designs don't even have an identified independent variable to manipulate. Example 1 in Box 5-4 is a descriptive, nonexperimental design. The researcher is simply collecting data on several variables and describing the results. Example 2 in Box 5-4 is an exploratory, nonexperimental design with an independent variable—parental presence or absence. The researcher is looking to see if parental presence affects anxiety and behavior (dependent variables). However, the researcher did not decide when the parents would be present or absent. She simply noted whether the parents were present or absent during the suturing procedure and measured anxiety and behavior in the child.

When a study contains independent and dependent variables and the researcher chooses not to manipulate the independent variable, it is usually for one

Box 5-5 Sample of a Section of a Table of Random Numbers

77	51	30	38	20	86	83	42	99	01
19	50	23	71	74	69	97	92	02	88
21	81	85	93	13	93	27	88	17	57
51	47	46	64	99	68	10	72	36	21
99	55	96	83	31	62	53	52	41	70

of three major reasons: (1) all events have already occurred, (2) the variable cannot be manipulated, or (3) it would be morally or ethically wrong to manipulate the variable. In a retrospective nonexperimental study the researcher simply collects data on the variables after they have already occurred. Take the example of the infant stimulation study. Let us suppose that the researcher located two different hospitals—one offered extratactile stimulation as a part of routine care for all premature infants and the other offered no extratactile stimulation. Let us further suppose that the researcher collected charts of premature infants in both hospitals, looked up recorded PO_2 levels, and compared the PO_2 levels of a group of stimulated infants with a group of nonstimulated infants. This is a nonexperimental research design in which the researcher is looking at variables that have already occurred.

> When a researcher chooses not to manipulate the independent variable, it is usually for one of three major reasons: (1) all events have already occurred, (2) the variable cannot be manipulated, or (3) it would be morally or ethically wrong to manipulate the variable.

Many variables cannot be manipulated. If a researcher is interested in whether gender affects longevity, for example, the researcher cannot manipulate the gender variable. He cannot make males become females to see if that change will make them live longer. If a researcher is interested in whether aging affects calcium levels in the blood, he cannot manipulate the age variable (i.e., he cannot make someone get older). In these instances, the researcher must examine the variables as they naturally occur.

Other variables can be manipulated, but to do so would present an ethical dilemma. When researchers were studying the effects of smoking on health, they did not manipulate the variable of smoking. They did not decide who would smoke and who would not smoke because it would not be ethical to force someone to smoke. So, smoking is a variable that can be manipulated, but it is not for ethical reasons. We discuss how subjects are protected against possible unethical treatments in phase 3.

When a variable cannot be manipulated or when manipulation would cause an ethical dilemma, nonexperimental research designs must be used. This does not mean that nonexperimental designs cannot be used to explain or predict. We can use sophisticated statistical techniques to examine relationships among variables and to predict how they should function under various circumstances.

IDENTIFY SAMPLE AND SETTING

Once the research design has been established, the subjects and setting for the study must be considered. The **setting** is the physical location for and the conditions under which the study takes place. For example, the study involving children and suture repair took place in the suture room of a Level 2 ED in one children's hospital. The study involving premature infants and stimulation took place in a neonatal intensive care unit of a large teaching hospital. Premature infants from around the city are transferred to this unit, which has computerized equipment capable of continuously monitoring PO_2 levels on all infants.

The subjects of interest for a research study are known as a **population**. These subjects possess certain common characteristics or traits that identify them as a part of the population. For example "young children with lacerations that require sutures" are the subjects of interest in Example 2 in Box 5-4. Study subjects need not be human; they might be animals such as white mice, bacteria colonies in petri dishes, data such as vital signs, or objects such as charts. A **sample** is a portion or subset of a population (Fig. 5-3). Populations are usually large, so the researcher chooses a part of the population to make the study more feasible. Subjects are selected using a process known as **sampling**.

When the researcher selects the sample, he or she tries to make sure that the sample characteristics resemble the population characteristics as closely as possible so that the sample represents the population. If a sample is representative of the

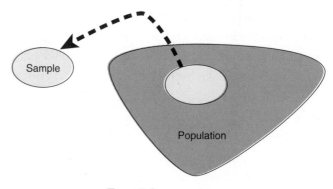

Fig. 5-3   Sampling.

population, the study results can be applied to the whole population. For example, if the children in the laceration study were less anxious during the suturing process when a parent was present, it is helpful if that finding can be applied to all children with lacerations. The ability to apply study results from the sample to the population is known as **generalization**. The type of sampling process chosen determines whether study results can be generalized from the sample to the population.

There are two major categories of samples: (1) probability and (2) nonprobability. Box 5-6 presents and defines sample categories and subcategories. Review these so that you can recognize the vocabulary used to describe sampling in a research article and can distinguish between probability and nonprobability types of samples.

ADVENTURE CD 5-4

Box 5-6   Categories of Samples

Probability Sampling—Random Selection

1. A *simple random sample* is the most basic form of probability sampling in which all subjects in a population are numbered, and a sample is selected randomly using a lottery or table of random numbers.
2. A *stratified random sample* is subdivided into groups according to some characteristic (e.g., gender—males and females; or ethnicity—African-American, Hispanic, and Caucasian) The subsets are then randomly sampled.
3. A *cluster sample* is a multistage sampling in which larger clusters (groups) are randomly selected first (e.g., hospitals) and then smaller clusters are randomly chosen (e.g., patients).
4. A *systematic sample* selects every k^{th} (e.g., every fifth or seventh or twentieth) subject from a randomized list.

Nonprobability Sampling—No Random Selection

1. A *convenience (accidental) sample* selects the most convenient subjects at hand.
2. A *quota sample* is conveniently selected according to prespecified characteristic(s) (e.g., gender or ethnicity).
3. A *purposive sample* uses subjects that are handpicked by the researcher, based on a set of defined criteria.
4. A nonrandom systematic sample selects every k^{th} (e.g., every fifth or seventh or twentieth) subject from a nonrandomized list or every k^{th} subject as they become available (e.g., every third patient admitted to the unit).

In a **probability sample**, the subjects are chosen at random. Each subject in the population has an equal chance of being in the sample. Probability samples ensure that samples are mathematically representative of the population. Therefore when researchers choose probability sampling techniques, they ensure that the results of the study can be generalized to the population. Subjects in a **nonprobability sample** are not chosen at random. There is no way to assess whether they are representative of the population. Therefore results can only be applied to the sample and cannot be generalized to the population. The sampling method used is a very important thing for you to note when you read research studies. This is because it tells you whether you can apply the study results to your situation. If a study of patients with specified characteristics used a probability sample, you can confidently apply the results of those study findings to patients with those same characteristics under your care. If a nonprobability sample was used, the results may or may not be applicable to your clinical situation.

> The sampling technique tells you whether you can apply the results in your clinical situation with confidence.

At this point, you may be asking, "If probability samples are so much better than nonprobability samples, why would a researcher ever use a nonprobability sample?" Good question! Nonprobability sampling may be preferable for several reasons—it is less expensive and requires less time and fewer resources and, sometimes, generating a probability sample is not possible. For example, it may not be possible to generate a list of every subject in the population because no comprehensive source exists. At other times, generating such a list can be prohibitive in terms of time and expense. Think about compiling and numbering a list of 1,000 or 10,000 or 100,000 subjects in a population. Access to certain subjects in a population may also be cost prohibitive (e.g., subjects in another city, state, or country). Access to certain subjects may be denied by the institutions or by the subjects themselves. Some populations are hidden and/or hard to access (e.g., stigmatized populations such as homosexuals). You will find that many nursing research studies use nonprobability sampling techniques. As computers generate ever-growing databases, as research funding and support increases for nursing research, and as the research studies and researchers grow in sophistication and complexity, this situation is beginning to change.

The size of the sample is also important in making the sample representative of the population. As a general rule of thumb, the larger the sample, the more representative it is of the population. The researcher considers several factors when selecting a sample size. These include the size of the population, the availability of the population, the characteristics of the population, and the cost and time expended per subject. The size of the sample also affects the statistical techniques that can be used. Statistics used to analyze several variables simultaneously (multivariate statistics) require larger sample sizes. When you read a research study, check the sample size. If a sample is small (under 30 subjects), particularly if it is a nonprobability sample, use the study results with caution.

> Use study results with caution when the sample is small and sampling is nonprobable.

SELECT DATA COLLECTION METHODS

To examine the proposed research questions or hypotheses, the researcher must be able to collect measurable information on the variables. These measurable bits of information are known as **data**. Data are collected using an **instrument**. Instruments that collect quantitative data can be classified by the type of data they are designed to collect. Data are generally physiological, behavioral, or psychological in nature. Physical measures generally require specialized biophysical instruments and specialized expertise on the part of the user. You are familiar with several of the biophysical measures used in health care and health care research. Examples include sphygmomanometers, thermometers, manometers, pulse oximeters, glucometers, ECG machines, EEG machines, transducers, and so on. We regularly use these instruments in clinical practice. Researchers also use them to measure physiological variables.

Behavioral data (observable actions of the subject) are generally collected through observation. In quantitative research these observations are evaluated and assigned numeric values. For example, degree of uncooperative behavior was observed and rated in the study of young children who were being sutured for a laceration. The nurse observed the child's behavior and assigned ratings at several predetermined intervals during the suturing procedure. The scale is presented in Table 5-1.

Table 5-1	Uncooperative Behavior Scale
SCORE	BEHAVIOR
0	No crying or physical protest
1	Mild verbal protest (e.g., ouch) or quiet crying
2	More prominent verbal protest/crying with movement of body parts; still complies with physician request
3	Protest and movement makes the procedure difficult
4	Protest stops the procedure and behavior is addressed before procedure can be reinitiated
5	General prolonged protest verbal and body movement with no compliance

Adapted from Venham L et al: Interval rating scales for children's dental anxiety and uncooperative behavior, *Pediatric Dentistry* 2(3):195, 1980.

Psychological measures are used to collect data about knowledge, feelings, and attitudes. Because these variables cannot be directly observed, an instrument is used that asks the subject to self-report on these variables. Such instruments include questionnaires and interviews. Questionnaires pose a series of questions for the subject to answer. In a quantitative study, the questions are usually closed ended. This means that the subject is asked to select from a given a range of choices. Box 5-7 contains several closed-ended questions that might appear on a questionnaire. You have probably responded to many questionnaires. Questionnaires are easy to administer; relatively inexpensive; can be mailed to a large, widely dispersed sample; and offer anonymity to the respondent.

Questionnaires used in research generally contain some type of scale designed to measure a certain psychological variable. Scales are instruments that assign numerical values to a set of responses on a series of questions or statements. These numbers are then added together for a score. This score is used as a measurement of the variable. The most common scale type is the Likert scale. Subjects are given a series of statements and several ranges of agreement or disagreement to choose from. Box 5-8 gives an example of a few items from a Likert scale measuring the variable commitment to nursing. The response to each item is assigned a number and the numbers from all the items are added to reflect the overall degree of agreement with the concept being measured.

Box 5-7 Sample Questions on a Questionnaire

Please circle the answer that best describes you.
1. Are you
    a. Male
    b. Female
2. Are you currently
    a. Single (never married)
    b. Married
    c. Separated
    d. Divorced
    e. Widowed
3. What is your birth order?
    a. Only child
    b. Oldest child
    c. Middle child
    d. Youngest child

Box 5-8 Sample Likert Scale

SA = Strongly Agree
A = Agree
U = Uncertain
D = Disagree
SD = Strongly Disagree
    Please circle your degree of agreement or disagreement with the following statements:

1. My most common reaction to nursing is enthusiasm.	SA	A	U	D	SD
2. I am disenchanted with nursing.	SA	A	U	D	SD
3. I consider nursing a rewarding profession.	SA	A	U	D	SD
4. I cannot imagine being in any other profession.	SA	A	U	D	SD
5. Nursing plays a major role in my life.	SA	A	U	D	SD

Adapted from Langford R: *The relationship between student sense of commitment to the profession of nursing and their perceptions of powerlessness in the academic setting,* doctoral dissertation, Houston, 1979, University of Houston.

Interviews used to collect data in a quantitative study usually consist of a series of highly structured questions that are later assigned numbers for statistical analysis. A structured interview is much like an oral questionnaire. However, it offers the advantage of allowing the interviewer to clarify responses and to ensure that all questions are answered. The chief disadvantage is the added time and expense involved in the interview process.

Appropriate instruments must be selected to measure each variable being studied. This includes desired descriptive variables (e.g., gender, education level, marital status), independent and dependent variables, and pertinent extraneous variables (e.g., variables that must be controlled using statistics). Choices are made based on criteria such as the category of data (e.g., physiological, behavioral, psychological) and the cost, availability, and skill required to administer the instrument. It is important that the instrument chosen is appropriate for the data category and the best the researcher has access to.

EVALUATE INSTRUMENT QUALITY

Instrument quality plays a big role in the selection of an appropriate instrument. The researcher is looking for "good" instruments to measure the variables in the study. What is a "good" instrument? A good instrument is one that is valid and reliable. A **valid** instrument measures what it is supposed to measure. A **reliable** instrument measures the variable consistently, dependably, and accurately. If an instrument is not reliable it cannot be considered valid. Box 5-9 lists types of validity and reliability. Familiarize yourself with these terms.

Instruments used in research studies should be evaluated for reliability and validity before use in the study. Reliability and validity issues should be addressed in the written report of the study. Biophysical measurements are generally accepted as valid measures of the variable. However reliability is an issue. Reliability can be addressed by ensuring that these instruments are calibrated and that the operators have sufficient expertise. Questionnaires, scales, interviews, and observations all need to be assessed for some form of reliability and validity to ensure the quality and credibility of the data collected. If the data are suspect, then the study results are suspect.

Now that we have covered what is involved in phase 2 of a research study, take some time to complete the following Student Challenge.

STUDENT CHALLENGE Scrutinizing Phase 2

Look again at the quantitative nursing research studies you examined for phase 1. Scan these studies and see if you can identify each of the elements we have discussed in phase 2.

1. Can you identify the research design as experimental or nonexperimental? Remember that experimental studies use terms such as experimental, quasi-experimental, treatment group, control group, treatment, intervention, or random assignment. Nonexperimental studies use terms or phrases such as retrospective, *ex post facto*, correlational, "purpose is to describe . . .," or "purpose is to explore. . . ."

2. Can you identify the sample? Can you determine what the population was? (This is harder, because it is often inferred rather than directly stated.)

3. Can you determine whether a probability or nonprobability sampling technique was used? Look for cue words such as "random" for probability samples and words such as "convenience, or accidental" for nonprobability samples. If the technique is not specified, chances are great that it is a nonprobability sample. What was the size of the sample in the studies you chose?

4. Was the setting described?

5. What instruments were used to measure the variables? Could you tell if the instruments were reliable and valid?

Box 5-9 Types of Validity and Reliability

ADVENTURE
CD
5-5

Validity

Validity is the extent to which an instrument measures what it says it measures.

   Content validity is assessed by a logical evaluation and judgment of whether the instrument adequately reflects the content of the concept. A blueprint may be used to construct the instrument, or a panel of judges may be asked to evaluate the instrument. This is a weak form of validity.

   Criterion validity is assessed using statistical measures. Instrument scores are correlated to scores on measures of selected external criteria. Also called *concurrent or predictive validity*, this is a stronger form of validity.

Continued

Box 5-9 Types of Validity and Reliability—cont'd

Construct validity is assessed using a combination of logic and statistical measures. It looks for the underlying meaning of the construct being measured. This is the strongest form of validity.

Reliability

Reliability is the degree of consistency or dependability of an instrument.

Internal consistency uses correlation statistics (e.g., Spearman's, Cronbach's alpha, or Kuder-Richardson) to measure whether the subparts of an instrument all measure the same thing. Reliability values range from 0 to 1. The closer the value gets to 1, the more reliable the instrument.

Equivalence correlates two different forms of the same instrument (also called parallel forms) or the scores of two or more raters (also called inter-rater reliability). Reliability is reported as an "r" value, with values ranging from 0 to 1. The closer the value gets to 1, the more reliable the instrument.

Stability correlates the scores obtained when an instrument is administered twice to the same group of subjects over a period of time. Reliability or "r" values range from 0 to 1. The closer the value gets to 1, the more reliable the instrument.

Phase 3: Conduct the Study

Once the study has been conceived and designed, the planning phases are over and the researcher is ready to conduct the study. This means that the researcher will now implement the study design and collect the data using the designated instruments and procedures. This is often an exciting time in the research process. The researcher begins to sense that the project is going to make it.

GET APPROVAL TO USE HUMAN SUBJECTS

When researchers use humans as subjects for study, they must protect them from harm. There have been a number of historical abuses of research subjects. The most famous might be the atrocities committed on prisoners of war by Nazi and Japanese physicians during World War II. However, unethical treatment of research subjects was not perpetrated only in foreign nations and did not cease after the war. Several famous experiments in the United States symbolize mistreatment of research subjects. One of the best known is the Tuskegee Study in which adult black males were recruited into a study begin in 1932 that examined the long-term effects of syphilis. Although penicillin became available for treating syphilis in the 1940s, subjects were not treated and continued to be followed in a research study that lasted for more than 40 years.

Unfortunately, this type of abuse was not an isolated incident. Mentally handicapped children were injected with a hepatitis virus at Willowbrook Institution in Staten Island, New York in the 1950s and 1960s. Live cancer cells were injected into elderly patients at Jewish Chronic Disease Hospital in Brooklyn, New York in 1963. Numerous accounts have surfaced of U.S. government involvement in experiments using prisoners, soldiers, and civilians to test effects of radiation, chemical, viral, and neurological agents as potential weapons.

Because of persistent reports of abuse in research, the National Commission for the Protection of Human Subjects of Biomedical and Behavioral Research was formed in the 1970s. It issued the Belmont Report (1979), which articulated three ethical standards that must be observed in the conduct of research funded by the federal government.

1. Individuals who might become subjects in a research study have the right to freedom from harm. The researcher is obligated to protect subjects from potential injury, disability, or death because of involvement in a study.

2. Individuals have the right to privacy and fair treatment. Researchers must guarantee that all identifying factors collected during the study will remain confidential. Researchers must also strive to ensure that all study participants are treated fairly, courteously, and sensitively.

3. Individuals have the right to know and choose. Researchers must fully disclose the potential risks and benefits associated with the study and allow the individual free choice in deciding whether to participate.

Institutional review boards (IRBs) are review groups that have been established by various research funding bodies and institutions involved in research to ensure that individual researchers adhere to these ethical standards. The first step then in this phase is to obtain approval for the use of human subjects from an IRB. The researcher submits a written proposal of the research study to the IRB who reviews the proposal and grants or denies authorization for the conduct of the study. When authorization is granted, the researcher can then start the process of recruiting subjects for data collection.

RECRUIT SUBJECTS

If the sample units are inanimate objects, bacteria cultures, or white mice then this step is omitted or is greatly simplified. However, since most clinical nursing studies involve human subjects, the researcher must find individuals who are willing to participate in the study. As subjects are recruited, it is the researcher's job to inform each of them about the study, the demands it will make, and the potential risks and benefits of participation. This allows individuals adequate information to make an informed choice about whether to participate in the research study. Those who opt to become subjects sign a statement that indicates they have been briefed on the study, they understand the risks and benefits, and they are willing to participate. This process is known as **informed consent.** It is very similar to the process that patients go through when agreeing to medical or surgical treatment. Box 5-10 describes the elements contained in a typical consent form. Some studies do not require written informed consent. Frequently, when written questionnaires are used, return of the questionnaire is used to imply consent. IRBs often allow researchers to conduct observational studies without consent of the subjects as long as the researcher shows strong evidence that identifying information about participants will be kept confidential.

COLLECT DATA

Once permission has been obtained from the appropriate IRBs and subjects have been recruited, **data collection** may proceed. At this point, the researcher puts the

---

Box 5-10 Elements of Informed Consent

- General statement of study purpose
- Description of study procedures
- List of potential risks and benefits
- Assurance of anonymity or confidentiality
- Statement that participation is voluntary
- Assurance that subject may withdraw without penalty
- Contact information of researcher with offer to answer any questions about the study

design into action and carries out the prescribed procedures for the study in the appropriate research setting. Treatments are conducted, instruments are administered, and data are generated and recorded. After the data are collected, the researcher organizes it into an appropriate form for analysis, and phase 3 is brought to a close.

STUDENT CHALLENGE Conduct the Study

Look again at the quantitative research studies you examined for phases 1 and 2. Look for evidence of the steps in phase 3. (Direct evidence of this phase is hard to see in published research articles. It is easier to see in theses and dissertations.)

1. Were the rights of human subjects protected in these studies? What evidence did you find to support this?
2. Is there evidence of IRB approval?
3. Was an informed consent obtained?
4. Was any information provided about what occurred during collection of the data?

Phase 4: Analyze the Study

Data cannot be reported to research consumers in raw form. Results would be too cumbersome and would not provide a very good picture of the sample or a clear answer to the research questions or hypotheses that were proposed. Thus we come to the phase that strikes fear and trepidation into the hearts of many research students—statistical analysis and interpretation of the data. Before we discuss the steps involved in this phase, a little background information is needed. To statistically analyze variables, they must be measurable. This means that the variables must be represented in number form.

Measurement is a set of rules used to assign numbers to variables. The level of measurement guides the kinds of statistical analyses that can be performed on a variable. There are four levels of measurement: nominal, ordinal, interval, and ratio. Box 5-11 presents these four levels. For statistical purposes, interval and ratio data are treated the same.

Box 5-11   Levels of Measurement

Nominal variables are broken into two or more categories and assigned arbitrary numbers. These numbers have no rank order (i.e., no sense of one category being ranked at a higher level than another).

Example:

Gender: male = 1, female = 2

Marital status: single = 1, married = 2, separated = 3, divorced = 4, widowed = 5

Ordinal measurement reflects a rank order among the categories, but we do not know how much greater than or less than.

Example:

Pain: ranked on a scale of 1 to 10 with 10 being the worst pain and 1 being no pain

Anxiety: ranked on a 5-point scale from low to high

Interval categories are made up of "real" numbers that allow us to order the numbers and to know the distance between those numbers. The intervals between the categories are equal.

Example:

Temperature: the interval between the numerical values of 76 and 77 degrees is the same as the interval between the values of 44 and 45 degrees. A degree is a precise interval. Time: hours, minutes, and seconds are precise intervals.

Ratios have the same properties as interval data, except the measurement scale for the variable possesses a meaningful zero. This means that when zero is reached on the scale, the variable is absent.

Example:

Weight, height: zero means no weight or no height.

Table 5-2 Frequencies and Percentages

VARIABLE	FREQUENCY	PERCENTAGE
Gender		
Female	82	91%
Male	8	9%
Current Marital Status		
Single	46	51%
Married	34	38%
Separated	2	2%
Divorced	8	9%
Satisfaction with School		
Very dissatisfied	2	2%
Dissatisfied	9	10%
Uncertain	18	20%
Satisfied	45	50%
Very satisfied	16	18%
Age		
19-21	16	18%
22-24	27	30%
25-27	36	40%
28-30	11	12%

$n = 90$

DESCRIBE THE SAMPLE

When analyzing the data, the researcher wants to derive a picture or description of the sample. This description is obtained through statistical analysis and the use of descriptive statistical tests. **Descriptive statistics** group the data in ways to make it easier to understand. There are four common ways to describe data using statistics: (1) frequencies, (2) measures of central tendency, (3) measures of spread (dispersion), and (4) measures of shape.

One thing we can do is count the times that scores or categories of a variable occur. Frequency counts can then be turned into percentages (number in a category divided by the number for the variable.) Table 5-2 presents sample frequencies and percentages taken from a sample of 90 nursing students.

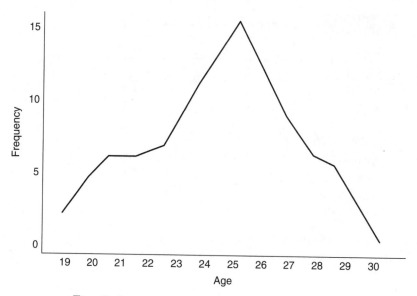

Fig. 5-4   Example of a frequency distribution.

In the examples in Table 5-2, we can see that the majority of students in this sample were single females 23 to 30 years of age who were satisfied with school. Frequencies are most useful with nominal and ordinal data. Interval or ratio data make reporting frequencies for each score a little cumbersome. So, we can group several scores together and report the frequency and percentage of the groups as we did with the variable "age" in Table 5-2. Frequencies for interval and ratio data can also be plotted on a graph to form a frequency distribution (Fig. 5-4).

We can also use statistics to describe how data are distributed along the number continuum of a frequency distribution. We can describe how data clump or cluster together, how they spread apart, and what shape the frequency distribution forms. These statistics are defined in Box 5-12. All of these statistics let us reduce large amounts of data about a variable down to a very manageable description whose meaning is commonly understood. Imagine if you tried to make sense out of the reported ages for 5,000 subjects if you had no precise way to count them, group them, or talk about how much the subjects were alike or different in age.

Box 5-12   Descriptive Statistical Measures

Measures of central tendency are statistical tests that describe how data for a variable tend to cluster together in a distribution.
1. *Mode (Mo)* is the numerical value that occurs most often for a particular variable.
2. *Median (Md)* is the middle value in a frequency distribution of numbers.
3. *Mean (M, X)* is the average of all the scores.

Measures of Dispersion are statistical tests that describe how data for a variable tend to spread out in a distribution.
1. *Range* is the distance between the highest and lowest scores for a variable.
2. *Variance (V, s^2)* is the average area of spread under a frequency distribution curve.
3. *Standard deviation (SD, s)* is the average distance of spread in a frequency distribution. It tells us how much, on the average, the scores are spread out from the mean.

Measures of shape are statistical tests that describe the shape of the distribution for a variable.
1. *Skewness* reflects the degree of symmetry or asymmetry of the distribution curve (e.g., Is the distribution symmetrical or asymmetrical?).
2. *Kurtosis* is the height of the distribution (e.g., How tall or flat is the distribution curve?).

ANSWER THE RESEARCH QUESTIONS

Once the researcher has described the sample, the next step is to analyze the data to answer the research questions or to see whether the hypothesis was true. This is the step when the researcher discovers the answer that the study was designed to uncover. If the study was a descriptive one, the researcher uses the same kinds of statistics that were used to describe the sample. Now however, the variables of interest are those from the research questions. Remember the research questions from Example 1 in Box 5-4 about elderly individuals in the ED? These questions were answered using descriptive statistics. The question "What percent of total ED visits are by elderly individuals?" was answered using frequencies and percentages. The question "What are the presenting chief complaints of the elderly?"

was answered by categorizing all the reported chief complaints and then reporting frequencies and percentages of each category.

If the study asked questions or stated hypotheses that looked at the relationships or differences between variables, then statistics that analyze those relationships or differences are used. A wide variety of statistics are available for such analysis. The easy access to personal computers with sophisticated statistical software has increased the complexity of statistical tests used. Many studies now identify and examine greater numbers of variables because analysis of multiple variables is now readily available. This means that reports of statistical analysis and study are increasingly complicated. This makes reading and understanding the results section of most studies difficult. For most studies that you will read, there is little chance that you will recognize or understand why particular statistics were selected. Moreover, you will probably have little understanding of the precise meaning of the numbers generated by those statistics.

This does not mean that you should give up without a fight. You can decipher study results with patience and armed with a few strategic pieces of information.

1. **Different statistics have different requirements for use.** Selection of the appropriate statistic is based on several factors, including the number of variables to be analyzed, the level of measurement of the variables, the nature of the question asked (e.g., testing relationships or differences), and the sampling procedure used.

2. **Research hypotheses may be translated to statistical hypotheses.** This is merely a restatement of the research hypothesis in symbol form and is used as a decision-making tool.

3. **The result of a statistical test is reported as a number.** (e.g., $t = 4.26$, $F = 3.98$, $r = .68$). The letter gives a clue about the statistical test used (e.g., t is a t test, F is an ANOVA test, r indicates a correlation). Many multivariate statistics generate a series of numbers that tell the researcher about several variables and how they vary as part of a multiple variable set.

4. **These numbers are either significant or not significant.** Significance is reported using a p value (e.g., $p = .17$, $p = .03$ $p = .01$). A p value of less than .05 is generally considered significant. Some researchers use a p value of less than .01 to decide if a value is significant. Sometimes, nonsignificance is reported by using the letters NS.

5. **A significant p value ($<.05$) means that the relationship or difference found between the variables was probably not caused by chance.** In other

words, there really is a high degree of certainty that the difference or a correlation exists between the variables tested.

6. **Statistical results are often displayed in table form.**

When you read the results section, do not panic over the numbers and the discussion of those numbers. The researcher will translate the statistical results into English at some point in the presentation of results. This is what you are looking for as you read. Search to see how the research questions or hypotheses were answered. Were the variables related or not? Was group A different from group B?

In Example 2 in Box 5-4, the research question is "Will there be a difference between the anxiety levels and disruptive behaviors of young children whose parents are present during laceration repair versus those with no parental presence?" A Hotelling T square test was used and no significant difference was found in behavior or anxiety between the group of children with parents present and the group without parents present.

Remember, we said that the effects of extraneous variables were sometimes controlled using statistics? Well in this study, age was identified as an extraneous variable that might influence whether parental presence made a difference. So, another statistical test (ANCOVA) was used to look at differences while controlling for the extraneous variable age. This analysis found that both behavior and anxiety in younger children were significantly different between those with parents present and those without. Younger children were less anxious and more cooperative with a parent present. As children became older, parental presence did not affect anxiety or behavior.

In Example 3 in Box 5-4, the research hypothesis is "Premature infants who receive extra-tactile stimulation will have higher PO_2 levels than those who do not." A t test was used to examine the differences in PO_2 between the group of infants who got stimulation and the group who did not. The resulting t value was significant. This indicated that there was a difference between the PO_2 levels of the two groups. A look at mean PO_2 levels showed that infants who received tactile stimulation had higher PO_2 levels.

INTERPRET THE RESULTS

Once the statistical analysis has been performed and the results have been examined, the researcher must interpret the results. This means making sense of the findings and how they fit into the existing research literature. Findings from descriptive studies are used to secure a tentative picture. There is very little to interpret because no relations were tested among the described variables. Findings from exploratory studies that ask questions about relationships or differences among variables provide a starting point for the researcher to explain why relationships or differences were or were not present.

Findings from studies in which relationships or differences were predicted in the form of hypotheses need the most interpretation. An explanation of the findings is straightforward if the hypothesis was supported. The researcher used theoretical evidence to make a guess about variable relations, and the guess was supported. All came out as anticipated. The study lends more proof to the underlying theoretical foundations. However, if the hypotheses were not supported, the researcher must try to explain what happened. Was there a problem with the theoretical structure for the study, or was there a problem with the research design? Answers to these questions are usually presented in a discussion section and lead to the final phase of the process.

STUDENT CHALLENGE Seeking Statistics

Examine your chosen research studies for the analyses used and the results of the analyses.

1. Can you locate a description of the sample? (Hint: Some studies include the description when discussing the sample and sampling techniques in the methods or research design section of the study.)
2. Can you find the answers to the research questions or hypotheses that were posed?
3. Can you locate how the findings were tied to the literature?

Phase 5: Use the Study

You might think that once the researcher discovers the answers to the questions posed in a study that the work would be finished. However, one important phase remains. This phase completes the research process, emphasizes its circular nature, and ensures results are shared with the research consumer.

RECOMMEND FURTHER RESEARCH

Once the findings are stated and discussed, the researcher must decide what those findings mean for future research. When the researcher examines what the next research study might be, **recommendations** for further research are made, ensure the circular nature of the process. That researcher or another researcher can accelerate the advancement of nursing knowledge by beginning another research study that builds on the one just completed.

The researcher also examines and discusses any problems encountered while doing the study. These are known as limitations. Examples include uncontrolled extraneous variables that interfered with study results, difficulties in data collection, not enough subjects, and so forth. Identifying limitations allows future researchers to correct them when repeating or doing a similar study.

STATE IMPLICATIONS FOR PRACTICE

The researcher must also decide what, if any, **implications** the study results have for nursing practice. This assists the research consumer (you and me) in making use of the study results.

ADVENTURE CD
5-6

DISSEMINATE RESULTS

The final obligation on the part of the researcher is to disseminate the results of the study. This means that the researcher must communicate what was found to the research consumer. The most common forms of communication are through articles in nursing research or specialty journals or through a presentation at a conference. An article has the most widespread effect.

STUDENT CHALLENGE Entertaining the End

1. Examine your chosen research studies for future research recommendations and implications for nursing practice.
2. Rejoice in the fact that you have now scanned entire research studies.
3. In an upcoming chapter, we walk through more studies step-by-step, so don't worry if you still feel uncomfortable with what you're reading.

Once the results have been communicated, the researcher's job is finished, and the research consumer's job begins. Nurses have an obligation to keep their practices current and grounded in a solid scientific knowledge base. This means regular reading and use of the knowledge being generated through research.

Activity
12

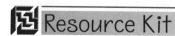 Resource Kit

Ethics and Research

Want to view a copy of *The Belmont Report?*

Want to see the official guidelines for informed consent?

Want to see what IRBs are responsible for?

Log on to the book's MERLIN website and check out the listed government website.

Research Is My Thing

If you have formed an abiding interest in the research process, you can get a more in-depth view of the process by exploring the phrase "research process" using a search mechanism on the Internet. There are even complete research courses taught on-line.

 Visit the book's MERLIN website at
www.mosby.com/MERLIN/Langford/maze
for further information.

 Check out the puzzles, mazes, and games on your **CD-ROM.**

References

Carruth AK et al: Reciprocity, emotional well being, and family functioning as determinants of family satisfaction in caregivers of elderly parents, *Nurs Res* 46(2):93, 1997.

Connelly CD: Hopefulness, self-esteem, and perceived social support among pregnant and nonpregnant adolescents, *West J Nurs Res* 20(2):195, 1998.

Erikson E: *Childhood and society,* New York, 1950, W.W. Norton.

Gawlinski A, Dracup K: Effect of positioning on SvO₂ in the critically ill patient with a low ejection fraction, *Nurs Res* 47(5):293, 1998.

Jennings-Dozier K: Predicting intentions to obtain a Pap smear among African American and Latina women: testing the theory of planned behavior, *Nurs Res* 48(4):198, 1999.

King IM: *Toward a theory for nursing: general concepts of human behavior,* New York, 1971, John Wiley & Sons.

Langford R: *The relationship between student sense of commitment to the profession of nursing and their perceptions of powerlessness in the academic setting,* doctoral dissertation, Houston, 1979, University of Houston.

Maslow A: A theory of human motivation, *Psychol Rev* 50:370, 1943.

Menzel LK: Ventilated patients' self-esteem during intubation and after extubation, *Clin Nurs Res* 8(1):51, 1999.

Mimnaugh L et al: Sensations experienced during removal of tubes in acute post-operative patients, *Appl Nurs Res* 12(2):78, 1999.

National Commission for the Protection of Human Subjects of Biomedical and Behavioral Research: *Belmont report: ethical principles and guidelines for research involving human subjects*, Washington, DC, 1979, US Government Printing Office.

Orem DE: *Nursing concepts of practice*, New York, 1971, McGraw-Hill.

Parshall MB: Adult emergency visits for chronic cardiorespiratory disease: does dyspnea matter? *Nurs Res* 48(2):62, 1999.

Rogers ME: *An introduction to the theoretical basis of nursing*, Philadelphia, 1970, FA Davis.

Selye H: *The stress of life*, New York, 1956, McGraw-Hill.

Seyfer J: Scientist faked data, feds find/No links between power lines, cancer, *Houston Chronicle* 24 July 1999, 3 Star: A20.

University of British Columbia School of Nursing: A comparative longitudinal study of gastrostomy devices in children, *West J Nurs Res* 20(2):145, 1998.

Venham L et al: Interval rating scales for children's dental anxiety and uncooperative behavior, *Pediatric Dentistry* 2(3):195, 1980.

Learning Objectives

1 Define qualitative research.

2 Describe qualitative research classifications.

3 Discuss conceptualization for various research designs.

4 Describe structural elements for various research designs.

5 Describe processes involved in conducting a study.

6 Identify methods used in analyzing various types of studies.

7 Describe the reporting of study results and conclusions.

8 Discuss the relationship among phases of the research process.

9 Cite examples of phases of the process.

10 Compare and contrast qualitative and quantitative research.

Chapter Outline

What Is Qualitative Research?
How Is Qualitative Research Classified?
  Theoretical perspective
  Research design
    Phenomenology
    Ethnography
    Grounded theory
    Historical method
    Case study
What Is the Qualitative Research Process?
  Phase 1: Conceive the study
  Phase 2: Design the study
    Setting
    Samples and sampling
    Data collection methods

Phase 3: Conduct the study
Phase 4: Analyze the study
  Methods
  Findings
Phase 5: Use the study
Using Qualitative and Quantitative Research
  Approaches Together?

Qualitative Research: The Whole Picture

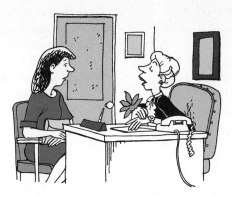

Uh, could you tell me your life story? And make it snappy. I still have a lot of people to interview this afternoon.

Student Quote   *"When I read the qualitative study we were assigned about nurses' work in the ICU, I felt like I was right there living the experience. I could really identify with what was happening."*

Abstract   Qualitative research is an objective process used to examine subjective human experiences by using nonstatistical methods of analysis. It can be classified by theoretical perspective or by research design. Research design classifications include phenomenology, ethnography, grounded theory, historical method, and case study. The qualitative research process varies across research methodologies, and the phases of the process are fluid and repetitive. The research aim provides a loosely defined boundary that guides initial data collection, which occurs predominately through observation and unstructured interview. Data collection and analysis dominate the process. Analysis dictates the direction and course of further data collection. Analysis takes place using various methodologies to manage, reduce, and synthesize data. The researcher searches for patterns of meaning in the collected narrative data. Findings are presented in a descriptive narrative format with examples from the data to illustrate key patterns and themes.

KEY TERMS

Qualitative Concerns

Basic social process A social or psychological process identified as enduring over time regardless of environmental conditions (e.g., stages of death and dying).

Bracketing A process used by the qualitative researcher to identify and set aside personal beliefs about the phenomenon under study.

Case study An in-depth research study of an individual unit (e.g., a person, family, group, or other identified social unit).

Coding Process by which data are categorized and conceptualized.

Collective case study A series of case studies that examine similar patterns about identified phenomena.

Constant comparative method Method of analysis used in grounded theory in which categories of meaning are derived by comparing collected data incidents to one another until concepts emerge.

Credibility An examination of the validity or quality of the data in a qualitative research study.

Data immersion Reading and rereading data to become familiar with its content, feeling, and tone.

Ethnography Qualitative research design that focuses on the world view of an identified cultural group.

Field A natural setting in which investigation and data collection take place in a qualitative study.

Field notes Written accounts of what a researcher sees, hears, experiences, and thinks during the course of data collection in a qualitative study.

Grounded theory Qualitative research that develops theoretical propositions about identified social-psychological processes from collected data.

Historical method Qualitative analysis of historical events to draw additional insights or inferences about how past events impact the present.

Lived experience Some dimension of daily experience for a particular set of individuals.

Phenomenology The qualitative study of lived experience to understand and attach meaning to that experience.

Qualitative research An objective way to study the subjective human experience using nonstatistical methods of analysis.

Reliability Concern with the accuracy and comprehensiveness of data collected in qualitative research.

Saturation Point at which sampling and data collection are stopped in a grounded theory study because the information being collected is redundant and repetitive.

Theoretical sampling Procedure used in grounded theory to gather additional data about emerging concepts.

Triangulation The use of both quantitative and qualitative research methodologies in a study or series of studies.

Validity Concern with the credibility of the study (e.g., does interpretation of data match the recorded description of the data) in qualitative research.

ADVENTURE CD 6-1

Qualitative research forms the second general research classification (quantitative research is the first). This chapter defines qualitative research, compares the qualitative and quantitative approaches, explores various ways that qualitative research can be classified and identified, and discusses the phases of the qualitative research process.

What Is Qualitative Research?

Qualitative research is an objective way to gain insights about the subjective and holistic nature of humans. It relies heavily on the inductive reasoning process and seeks to examine and understand the whole of a phenomenon. The focus of the research is on the process by which concepts are given meaning in a given context rather than on measurement of the concepts and their relationships. Reality is viewed as a subjective, multifaceted experience rather than as a single, fixed, objective actuality.

> Qualitative research is an objective way to study the subjective human experience using nonstatistical methods of analysis.

Qualitative research uses multiple data collection procedures that rely heavily on researcher involvement. It produces findings that are arrived at using analytical procedures that are nonstatistical in nature. (Students are frequently delighted to hear about this feature.) Qualitative researchers may seek to examine individual lives and their stories and behavior; organizations and their functioning; role relationships and intercommunications; or cultures and their conduct, interactions, and social movement.

> No singularly defined scientific approach governs qualitative research.

No singularly defined scientific approach governs qualitative research. It is driven by multiple methods across various disciplines. Therefore, many aspects of qualitative research are not as clear-cut as those for quantitative research. While traditional quantitative research has concentrated on trying to establish relationships and differences within a narrow, controlled frame of reference, qualitative research permits multiple ways to explore the depth, richness, and complexity inherent in most phenomena. Table 6-1 presents some of the differences in the two approaches.

The qualitative approach does have limitations. Because the study methodology embraces the examination of subjective phenomena, findings may be idiosyncratic to a particular situation, and it is sometimes difficult to know how to apply findings to other settings. Small sample sizes also make general application difficult. Finally, many people assume that qualitative research is easily performed and fail to receive adequate education in qualitative methodologies before embarking on qualitative studies. The truth is that conducting qualitative research studies requires every bit as much expertise as conducting quantitative research studies.

Both qualitative and quantitative approaches are needed to effectively explore questions in nursing research. The nature of the inquiry and the expertise and philosophical grounding of the researcher should guide the selection of the re-

Table 6-1 Differences Between Qualitative and Quantitative Research

QUANTITATIVE	QUALITATIVE
Focuses on small number of specific concepts and their relationships and differences.	Attempts to understand the entirety or whole of some phenomenon within a prescribed context.
Set on a predefined theoretical foundation. "Educated guesses" made about relationship of concepts and study outcomes.	No preconceived theoretical boundaries or preconceived notions about study outcomes.
Researcher controls and interprets data.	Focus on people's interpretation of events and circumstances rather than researcher's
Tends to use larger samples.	Uses smaller samples.
Uses structured procedures and formal instruments to collect information.	Collects information without formal structured instruments.
Collects information under conditions of control and manipulation.	Doesn't attempt to control the context of research, but attempts to capture it in its entirety.
Emphasizes objectivity in collection and analysis of information.	Attempts to capitalize on the subjective as a means for understanding and interpreting human experiences.

search approach. Well-defined and measurable concepts beg to be studied using a quantitative approach. Complex phenomena closely tied to the human experience are more readily understood using a qualitative approach.

> The nature of the inquiry and the expertise and philosophical grounding of the researcher should guide the selection of the research approach.

How Is Qualitative Research Classified?

Several different terms are used to describe or classify qualitative research. We explore some of the more common classifications and terms, so they will be familiar to you when you encounter them in the literature. Qualitative research may be classified by theoretical perspective or by research design (Box 6-1).

Theoretical Perspective

When theoretical perspectives are used to classify qualitative research, the label indicates the researchers' underlying belief systems. Postpositivists are closely tied to

Box 6-1 Classification Systems for Qualitative Research

Theoretical Perspective
1. Postpositivist
2. Constructivist-interpretative
3. Critical
4. Poststructural

Research Design
1. Phenomenology, ethnomethodology
2. Ethnography, participant observation
3. Grounded theory
4. Historical method
5. Case study

Adapted from Denzin NS, Lincoln YS: *Handbook of qualitative research*, Thousand Oaks, Calif, 1994, Sage Publications.

the quantitative tradition and often use language and approaches that are closely aligned with the quantitative research process. The constructivist-interpretive tradition seeks understanding of the world through lived experiences from the point of view of those who live it. Critical theorists are interested in the social construction of experience and the material resources, power dynamics, and ideologies of societies. Poststructural studies are concerned with exploring the problems of using a social context approach that does not fully represent the world of lived experience. They may be concerned with ingrained social stereotypes and prejudices. Although these designations are helpful to other researchers in a particular discipline, they offer little help to us as novice research consumers.

Research Design

Classification by research design provides us with a little more direction as to what a qualitative study might be all about. These are the classifications you are most likely to see in the nursing literature.

PHENOMENOLOGY

Phenomenology is the study of **lived experiences.** The researcher examines human experiences through interviews and descriptions that come from the people who are living in the experience. This type of research seeks to describe the total structure of an experience as it is lived and to understand the subjective meaning of the experience. It is based on the premise that the way that individuals "know" is through their perceptions. Therefore reality is perceived as subjective and unique to individuals. A prerequisite for conducting a phenomenological study is that there be no preconceived ideas, expectations, or theoretical frame of reference to guide researchers as they collect and analyze data. In fact, researchers often begin by writing down their expectations of the research and then putting those expectations aside. This process is known as **bracketing**.

Types of questions that might be asked in a phenomenological study are "What is it like to experience . . . ?" or "Tell me about your experiences of . . ." For example, "What is it like being the mother of a child in the neonatal intensive care unit?" or "Tell me about your experiences of being a nursing student at XYZ University." Interviews and observations are most frequently used to collect data. Analysis occurs by searching the data for themes and patterns. Reflections are drawn on the meaning of the whole of the experience.

A recent example of a phenomenological study can be found in an article entitled "Beyond Body Image: The Experience of Breast Cancer" (Cohen, Kahn, and Steeves, 1998). This study explores women's reactions to breast cancer and its treatment. Another example can be found in "Caring for Patients Who Experience Chemotherapy-induced Side Effects: The Meaning for Oncology Nurses" (Fall-Dickson and Rose, 1999). This study examines how nurses viewed the provision of care to chemotherapy patients.

ETHNOGRAPHY

Ethnography is the systematic study of cultures or subcultures. It has its roots in anthropology. "Culture" is a broad term whose meaning could range from study of a village in Africa to examination of a neighborhood in South Philadelphia or investigation of the culture of a hospital. Ethnography focuses on the study of the symbols, rituals, and customs of an identified cultural group. It provides a picture of that identified group through observation and documentation of interactions in their daily lives.

Research questions in ethnography focus on issues such as the following:
- What procedures does a person follow that makes them a part of a group?
- What practices do group members engage in that result in an end product?
- What kinds of work do members engage in to accomplish the goals of the group?

Ethnography focuses on group interactions and activities rather than on individual behaviors. Researchers immerse themselves in the culture or group to be studied. Data are gathered through observation and interview and analyzed for cultural patterns in an attempt to grasp the lifeways of a particular group in a particular environment.

Madeline Leininger is a prominent nurse ethnographer who has conducted a lifetime of ethnographic studies that examine the phenomenon of "caring" from various cultural perspectives. She views caring as the central and unifying theme for the practice of nursing (Leininger, 1981). Recent examples of ethnographical studies in nursing can be found in a study by Carr and Fogarty (1999) entitled "Families at the Bedside: An Ethnographic Study of Vigilance." This study examines the day-to-day experiences of families who remained at the bedside of hospitalized relatives. Another study entitled "The Experience of a Nursing Home Life" (Fiveash, 1998) uses an ethnographical approach to paint a picture of life in a nursing home.

GROUNDED THEORY

In **grounded theory** research, data are collected, analyzed, and used to develop a theoretical explanation and generate hypotheses for further research. Thus, the theory is generated from and "grounded" in the data. Grounded theory is used to examine **basic social processes** that occur in a given phenomenon. Pertinent factors, elements, and bits of data are collected. Core concepts and dominant processes that occur in interactions are identified. Then, the researcher attempts to discover explanations for these concepts and processes.

Research questions revolve around the chief concern or problem of individuals in a defined area. Examples of research questions that might be asked in a grounded theory study are "How do people prepare themselves emotionally for surgery?" or "How do cancer patients achieve hopefulness?" Data are collected using observational and interview techniques. **Coding** helps the researcher conceptualize the underlying patterns of the pieces of data collected. Categories of data are then developed. Analysis uses a process known as *constant comparison* whereby each piece of data is compared to data that are already collected. Concepts are developed as data are blended into larger and larger categories. Relationships between concepts are examined and then linked into a conceptual framework. Literature is then consulted to determine if any similar associations have already been uncovered.

Examples of grounded theory studies can be seen in "Protective Steering: a Grounded Theory Study of the Processes by Which Midwives Facilitate Informed Choices During Pregnancy" (Levy, 1999) and "Chronically Ill Children Coping with Repeated Hospitalizations: Their Perceptions and Suggested Interventions" (Boyd and Hunsberger, 1998). The titles of both studies are self-descriptive.

HISTORICAL METHOD

Historical method research examines social phenomena by studying their historical context or their past. A historical study analyzes a defined event, identifies key concepts and relationships, and draws inferences in an attempt to understand the impact of that event on the present. Historical research involves revisiting a historical event, viewing it from a fresh perspective, and searching for new meaning. Historical research is used to investigate past similar events or phenomena and derive common theoretical explanations of those events. For example, a historical study might try to explain a nursing shortage by examining past cycles of nursing shortages.

Historical researchers look at what has been, what is, and what should be. The researcher begins with an acknowledged philosophical or interpretive point of view. This is important because this point of view influences how information is gathered, read, and interpreted. Thus different researchers with varying points of view could revisit the same set of historical events and interpret them differently. Theresa Christy is nursing's foremost historical researcher. She views historical research as tool for nursing to determine its future course. She asks, "How can we . . . plan for where we are going when we don't know where we have been nor how we got there?" (Christy, 1978, p. 9).

Historical research is somewhat different from the other forms of qualitative research discussed thus far. Rather than observing or interviewing people in the present, the historical researcher relies on historical documents and past written records. These might include diaries, letters, newspapers, articles, books, audio or videotapes, government or professional records, and archives. People might be interviewed, but it would be to elicit their recollections of a past event.

Historical research is not nearly as prevalent in the qualitative nursing research literature as some of the other classifications we have discussed. However, current examples can be found in an article by Neiderhauser (1999) entitled "Varicella: The Vaccine and the Public Health Debate" and an article by Shermer and Raines (1997) entitled "Positioning During the Second Stage of Labor: Moving Back to the Basics." The varicella study examines the historical development of the chicken pox vaccine and concludes that the vaccine should be administered as a part of a routine immunization schedule. The positioning study examines the upright position for labor looking at historical influences such as anesthesia and fetal monitoring. It concludes that the upright position is advantageous in labor and makes recommendations for facilitation of the upright position.

CASE STUDY

A **case study** is an in-depth examination of certain phenomena in an individual or in small numbers of individuals. It has also been used to examine the workings of a group, organization, or institution. It is a study of the particular. Nursing and medicine have long used this approach to detail what happens when a person has a certain disease. Medicine focuses on the disease and its processes, while nursing focuses on how the individual responds to the disease, the treatment, and the environment. Much of the early research reported in the nursing literature used a case study approach.

Many researchers would argue that a case study is not a qualitative research design at all, but a sampling choice (Denzin and Lincoln, 1994). Others see the case study method as using both qualitative and quantitative elements of research (Denzin and Lincoln, 1994). For example, if you study an ill individual, some characteristics can be quantified or measured (e.g., vital signs, frequency of signs and symptoms). Other characteristics are better qualified or described in narrative fashion (e.g., the feelings associated with illness).

The case study is used to examine one entity in depth and to study and analyze patterns occurring in that one case. When researchers study more than one unit (e.g., individual, group, or institution) they are really doing what is termed a **collective case study** or a series of case studies. This is done to see if patterns carry over from one case to the next. Case studies provide a way to study and analyze phenomena that are relatively rare in occurrence. Case studies are not seen as frequently in the nursing literature as they once were, but examples can still be spotted. One such example is the study by Boehm and coworkers (1995), which used two cases to examine behavioral analysis with dementia patients.

ADVENTURE
CD
6-3

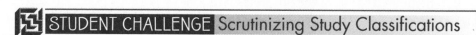

🔲 STUDENT CHALLENGE Scrutinizing Study Classifications

1. Go to the library and look up the research studies cited as examples in the previous paragraphs. Can you tell why they are classified as they are?

2. Now choose several other current qualitative nursing research articles. See if you can locate one study in each of the five qualitative research design categories. (Hint: Use the design category as your search term and limit the results to 1 or 2 years.)

3. Observe the general look and feel of the articles you've located. Note how they differ from quantitative reports. Note how they differ from one another.

4. If your library has copies, look at the case studies reported in the *American Journal of Nursing* in the 1920s and 1930s. Save your articles; you will be using them again.

What Is the Qualitative Research Process?

As you have already observed, qualitative and quantitative research look different in final written report format. You will discover that while many of the terms used in qualitative research look like the terms in quantitative research, they often have different meanings and are used differently. The process is also different. The process used in conducting qualitative research is not as well defined or segmented as the process used for quantitative research, and it varies across the different qualitative designs. As a whole, the processes used are much more fluid. Several phases of a given process frequently occur simultaneously or are revisited numerous times during the course of a study. Many of the decisions about various aspects of the process are made or altered as data are collected and certain trends or patterns are noted.

In quantitative research, the conception and design of the study form a detailed blueprint for conducting, analyzing, and interpreting the study. In qualitative research, conceptualization and design form only a broad umbrella-like structure for the study. Data collection and analysis dictate detailed study decisions. We can use the broad research phases identified in Chapter 5 as we discuss the qualitative research process. However, we must keep in mind that the phases are more fluid and less distinct for qualitative research and that the process varies for the different research classifications we have identified. We will see that there are common issues to be addressed for all classifications of qualitative research. This section discusses those common features using the phases of the research process identified in Chapter 5.

> The qualitative process is fluid and repetitive and is ruled by data collection and analysis.

Phase I: Conceive the Study

Just as with quantitative research, the first task that a qualitative researcher faces is to make a decision about what to study. The activities in this phase focus on identifying the phenomenon to be studied. This means an identification of some "whole" or "whole process" that the researcher is interested in studying. This differs from quantitative studies in which specific measurable concepts are identified. Table 6-2 presents specific examples by research design.

The initial identification of the phenomenon to be studied is done in the broadest sense. Phenomenology studies may simply identify some group of individuals to be interviewed. For example, parents of children in an intensive care

Table 6-2 Identification of Phenomenon

RESEARCH DESIGN	IDENTIFICATION OF PHENOMENON
Phenomenology	Lived experience
Ethnography	Issue(s) of interest within a defined culture
Grounded theory	Basic social process
Historical method	Past event
Case study	Broad area for case(s) selection

unit (ICU) or students in a university might be selected. The ethnographer may choose a group of people or a field setting with a broad statement of what is to be investigated. For example, health beliefs and practices of Vietnamese immigrants might be selected. Grounded theorists begin with a broad area of social interest with no specific problem in mind. For example, the area of interest might be hopefulness and cancer. Historical research begins with a broadly defined historical event such as the influence of World War II on nursing.

Since qualitative research does not begin with preconceived theoretical notions, no theoretical framework or hypothesis is proposed. The exception to this statement is historical research, which often states a particular philosophical or theoretical perspective and proposes broadly stated hypotheses about expected relationships among historical phenomena. Other qualitative researchers may state their preconceived notions or ideas about the study at the outset and then "bracket them" or set them aside during the actual investigation.

Most qualitative designs do a literature review at this point. The review serves various purposes depending on the study classification. For example, phenomenological researchers may do a cursory literature review to ensure that the area of interest (i.e., the lived experience) has not been previously researched and that there is a demonstrated need for such a study. Ethnographers may do a literature review to help identify a culture or to identify a particular aspect of a culture that has not been previously researched. When a culture has been selected, they may do an extensive literature review for any available information about that defined culture.

Literature review is an integral part of historical research and the selection of the event to be studied. Historical researchers often conduct extensive literature reviews to place limits on the final topic to be studied. In fact, the initial literature review and narrowing of the event and the historical time span considered often requires a large investment of time. Some case studies do an extensive literature review for all information available on the identified area of interest (e.g., a disease process). Others may review literature as data are collected. Grounded theory researchers make a point not to look at the literature before beginning the study. Literature review occurs after data collection and analysis has begun and theory has emerged from the data. Then the literature is reviewed and related to the developing theory. This is done to avoid contamination of the data with preconceived concepts and notions about what might be relevant.

Once the phenomenon of interest is selected, a research aim is formulated. This might be expressed in the form of a research question, purpose, or objective. It may not be readily identified in the report of the study. The aim is generally broad and serves as a general focus or guide for the study. More defined focal areas of the research often emerge as data are collected and analyzed. Table 6-3 presents sample research aims for each design using the previously cited articles in the discussion on design classification.

Take the following Student Challenge and see if you can identify the researcher's intent in sample studies.

STUDENT CHALLENGE Reading Research Aims

Use the studies that you found in the previous student challenge.

1. For the studies that were identified in this text, see if you can locate where I came up with the research aims listed in Table 6-3. You will notice that some of the studies specifically state the aim or purpose while others imply it.
2. Now look at the other studies you located. Can you determine the research aim for each of them?
3. Examine the literature review. Can you tell when it was done? Is the review more comprehensive in some studies than in others?

Phase 2: Design the Study

Once the phenomenon has been identified and the general aim of the study is determined, the next phase is to design the study. In qualitative research, the research design itself (i.e., phenomenology, ethnography, and so on) is often known before the phenomenon is identified, or it is chosen simultaneously with the iden-

Table 6-3 Sample Research Aims

RESEARCH DESIGN	SAMPLE PURPOSE
Phenomenology	To describe the mental and emotional impact of treatment for breast cancer with a focus on the ways the body is experienced
	To explore the meaning for oncology nurses of caring for cancer patients with side effects from chemotherapy
Ethnography	To examine the meaning of vigilance in families who remained at the bedside of a hospitalized family member
	To explore the experience of nursing home living
Grounded theory	To investigate the processes involved when midwives engage in facilitating informed choices for women
	To learn how chronically ill children who are repeatedly hospitalized cope and how they feel others could help them cope
Historical method	To examine the historical development of varicella vaccine to determine if need for the vaccine exists
	To examine the historical evolution of positioning during labor to determine the moves away from upright position
Case study	To examine the potential of behavioral analysis intervention in decreasing disruptive behaviors in persons with dementia

tification of what is to be studied. The chosen design dictates the general structure of the study and includes initial decisions about setting, sample selection, and data collection methods. Remember that the qualitative process is fluid, and sampling and data collection methods may evolve during the course of data collection.

SETTING

The setting in qualitative research is often referred to as the **field** because the study is set "in the field" (i.e., the natural setting where the phenomena under investigation occurs). Settings vary by type of research design. The selected setting assumes more importance in some research designs than in others. The type of data collection method may also influence the selected setting. Phenomenological research settings are usually chosen based on the convenience of the people who are

Table 6-4 Examples of Research Settings

RESEARCH DESIGN	SAMPLE SETTINGS
Phenomenology	Outpatient treatment area of a cancer treatment center
	Work, home, and social setting
Ethnography	Hospital
	Two 80-bed nursing homes
Grounded theory	Wherever the pregnant woman and midwife dyads interacted
	Hospital
Historical method	None listed
	None discussed
Case study	Mental institution

being studied. Since most of the data are collected through a series of interviews with individual participants, setting is secondary.

Ethnographical studies take place in a setting where the researcher can readily observe and interact with a grouping of people of a particular culture. If the culture of interest is Native Americans, the setting might be an Indian reservation. If the culture of interest is the critically ill, the setting might be an ICU. It is important that the setting in ethnographical research allow the researcher to see and interact with the people collectively.

Grounded theory research takes place in a setting that allows the researcher to observe the selected social processes in action. This means an ability to observe both the environment and the selected participants in the study. Case study settings allow the researcher to view and interact extensively with the chosen case. Historical studies have no real setting. Data are collected from records, relics, and artifacts that may be located in libraries, museums, personal collections, or boxes in storage. Table 6-4 lists the settings for the studies we've been following.

SAMPLES AND SAMPLING

The concepts of samples and sampling are viewed differently in qualitative research. In quantitative research, the key issue in sampling is to determine whether a representative sample was taken from the population to ensure that the study results from the sample could be applied back to the population.

Generalizability in this sense is not usually seen as an issue in qualitative research. Phenomenological and ethnographical research are more concerned with careful documentation and description of what is occurring in a given setting or with a given group of subjects. Further research over time will identify how the findings fit into the overall scheme of things. Grounded theory research is aimed at deriving broad statements about general social processes. The question for these researchers is not whether the findings are generalizable but to which other settings and people they are generalizable. This is addressed through the generation of theory that can then be tested in other settings.

Samples in qualitative research tend to be small and selected using purposive sampling techniques. The researcher is concerned that the selected sample be what is termed "information rich." This means that the selected sample provides a powerful picture of the phenomena under study. Several sampling techniques can be used to help provide an "information rich" sample. These include extreme, intensity, maximum variety, and critical case (Denzin and Lincoln, 1994). Box 6-2 discusses these techniques.

Grounded theory studies use a sampling technique called **theoretical sampling**. In theoretical sampling, the researcher begins by collecting and analyzing

Box 6-2 Qualitative Sampling Techniques

Extreme (deviant) sampling   Selection of subjects who exemplify the phenomena to be studied. (e.g., In a study about the "experience of pain", extreme sampling would chose those in extreme pain.)

Intensity sampling   Selection of subjects who are experiential experts or authorities about the selected phenomena. (e.g., In the pain study, intensity sampling might choose those who have chronic pain.)

Maximum variety sampling   The deliberate selection of subjects who are different, who come from different backgrounds, for the purpose of observing commonalties of experience. (This is particularly helpful when exploring abstract phenomena such as love, joy, or hope.)

Critical case sampling   Selection of subjects that have been identified as demonstrating what has been identified as a "critical incident" while collecting and analyzing data. (Once critical cases have been identified, additional purposive sampling is conducted to find cases that confirm or disconfirm the critical case.)

data on an initial sample. This sample is called an open sample because the sampling process was not guided by data analysis. As data are collected and analyzed (coded), concepts begin to emerge that will help form an evolving theory. These concepts are called categories and are identified by their repeated presence or absence in the data. The researcher then samples again looking for additional data to support identified categories. The researcher continues sampling, data collection, and analysis until all identified categories are fully explored or **saturated**.

Sample selection in historical research is unique because the sample is comprised of data sources rather than people. The sampling process occurs simultaneously with data collection and analysis and is ongoing as the researcher refines the study topic. As the topic becomes more clearly defined, the pertinent data sources become more readily identified. This sampling process can cover an extended period of time. Initially the needed data are known only generally. The researcher spends time collecting and reading data sources, which allows the researcher to add greater clarity and definition to the chosen historical topic, which in turn allows the researcher to more clearly identify needed data sources. Sampling and data collection cease when no new information is uncovered from several successive sources.

DATA COLLECTION METHODS

Data for qualitative studies are gathered chiefly by use of observation and interview. When a researcher desires to study behavior, activity, and sequences of interaction or the context or environment in which these behaviors and actions take place, observation is used. Observations may be classified by several features such as structure, participation of the researcher, and visibility of the researcher. Box 6-3 presents a fuller description of these classifications. Observations in quantitative research tend to be structured and nonparticipant. Qualitative research observations are unstructured. Ethnographical studies use an unstructured participant approach. Grounded theory uses a combination of observational approaches.

Interviews allow the researcher to tap into the opinions, attitudes, and belief systems of participants. Interviews can be placed on a continuum from structured to unstructured. Highly structured interviews are used primarily in quantitative research and were discussed in Chapter 5. Semistructured or unstructured interviews are generally used in qualitative research. Unstructured interviews are guided by a

Box 6-3 Classification of Observation Features

Structure

1. *Structured* Specified behaviors are predetermined and listed on a checklist to be counted or checked off during an observation period.
2. *Unstructured* Behaviors are described and recorded as or after they occur using a journal, diary, or field notes. A detailed descriptive picture is recorded.

Participation of the Researcher

1. *Participant* The researcher is an active part of the activities or behaviors engaged in by the participants being observed.
2. *Nonparticipant* The researcher is a bystander or passive participant in the activities being observed.

Visibility of the Researcher

1. *Concealed* The nonparticipant observer is hidden from view of those being observed. The activities might be recorded on videotape for later viewing and analysis, or activities might be viewed from a concealed space such as behind a two-way mirror.
2. *Nonconcealed* The observer is in full view of the participants. Participants are aware of being observed.

general aim of the research and are conducted in a conversational, story telling style. The researcher might begin with a very broad request such as "tell me about . . ." As the person being interviewed tells his or her story, the interviewer may ask additional questions that encourage elaboration on a certain part of the story. These questions are known as *probes*. Semistructured interviews may have a series of general questions and/or probes that were planned in advance of the interviewing process and are asked of all interview participants.

Most qualitative studies combine the use of observation and interviewing techniques to collect data. Some would say that the real instrument in a qualitative study is the researcher. This is because the amount, type, and quality of data retrieved are due in large part to the skills and abilities of the researcher. The researcher must be able to enter an environment and gain the trust of the people in that environment. Interviewing skills must be well-honed with a good feel for the ebb and flow of conversation and the ability to keep the interview flowing with a well-placed probe. Interviewing requires active listening and the ability to pick up and follow up on subtle leads or clues dropped in the course of the interview. The researcher must be able to put the participant at ease and know how to elicit information that participants may be reluctant to divulge. The researcher must have an eye for detail and be attuned to variations and changes when observing. The researcher needs to be able to capture in depth what has been seen and heard. Finally, the researcher must have a good grasp of self. He or she must be aware of and able to articulate feelings and biases that may influence data collection and analysis. In short, quality data collection in a qualitative study demands a skilled researcher.

> Quality data collection demands specialized skills on the part of the researcher.

Researchers use several tools to record their observations or interview results. These include the use of audio and video recordings and field notes. Audio and video recordings are later transcribed for closer analysis. **Field notes** are a written account of what the researcher sees, hears, experiences, and thinks during the course of data collection. Field notes can be classified into four basic types. The first is a brief description of what has occurred. These contain key phrases and major events and are often jotted down in the field. The second type of note is an expansion of the first set of notes. These are recorded immediately after a data collection session and expand on the brief notes, adding detail. A running journal is also kept by many researchers, describing personal thoughts and feelings that occur during the process of data collection. Finally, any insights, analysis of observations, judgments, and interpretations that are made in the field are recorded and kept.

The questions of reliability and validity have somewhat different meanings in qualitative research. Qualitative researchers are concerned with the accuracy and comprehensiveness of the data they collect. Data are considered **reliable** when what is recorded matches what actually occurred. The use of audio and video recordings and multiple samplings help ensure data are reliable. **Validity** in qualitative research examines whether or not the explanation or interpretation of data matches what has been described or recorded. Validity then is a question of **credibility.**

Validity is often examined and cross-checked through the use of two techniques: member checks and audit trails (Denzin and Lincoln, 1994). Member checks are made by having study participants review the material once it has been analyzed and interpreted. Audit trails (decision trails) ensure adequate documentation is available about the data collection and analysis processes. This includes the raw data and written evidence of each step of the analysis process (e.g., showing how data were collapsed, categorized, synthesized, or discarded).

STUDENT CHALLENGE Scrutinizing Phase 2

Look again at those qualitative nursing research studies that you examined for phase 1. Scan these studies and see if you can identify each of the elements we've discussed in phase 2.

1. Identify the settings.
2. Identify the sample and sample size.
3. Did any of the studies use extreme, intensity, maximum variety, critical sampling, or theoretical sampling techniques?
4. What data collection methods were used?
5. Did any of the studies address the issues of reliability and validity? (Hint: Look for key words such as accuracy, credibility, member checks, or audit trails.)

Phase 3: Conduct the Study

This phase receives a lot of time and attention in qualitative research. The conceptualization and planning stages are usually preliminary and loosely defined to lay a broad set of boundaries for data collection. As data collection begins, data analysis also occurs. Data collection and analysis lead to ongoing conceptualization and planning about further collection and analysis. So we again see the fluid and repetitive nature of the qualitative research process.

The issues of human subjects approval and informed consent as they apply to qualitative research differ from quantitative research. Most of the guidelines and procedures used by institutional review boards (IRBs) were designed for quantitative research methods. Qualitative studies do not involve invasive procedures and pose little threat to the participants. So, the review process is usually cursory and may be expedited.

Consent forms often do not contain a detailed description of the study or the risks and benefits because they aren't known at the time of data collection. Permission is obtained for interviews and for the use of audio and video recording equipment. Confidentiality is assured. Consent is often renegotiated with participants as data collection progresses and information emerges, which sends the collection process in a new direction.

Observations are often conducted without informed consent if the researcher can give assurances to the IRB that identifying information about participants will be kept confidential. Researchers opt not to use a consent form when the behavior being observed is likely to be altered if the subject is made aware of the study or its intent. For example, if a researcher were observing handwashing behaviors after use of a public toilet, subjects might alter their normal handwashing patterns if they knew they were being studied. Historical studies often use consent forms to get permission to use certain recorded information that is not in the pubic domain (e.g., privately held letters, diaries, photos).

Subjects of qualitative research studies are often called participants or informants rather than subjects. Many qualitative researchers see the term "subject" as too closely associated with the concept of experimentation and the connotation that people are being experimented on like laboratory animals. The term participant or informant is used to convey the sense of mutual participation and trust building that occurs between the researcher and the people being researched.

Data collection is a lengthy process in most qualitative studies. Whereas data collection in typical quantitative studies might take from several minutes to several weeks, data collection in qualitative studies may last for months or even years. The process of data collection is often described in more detail in qualitative studies because the collection process is often used to make decisions about the credibility of the data. Take the following challenge.

STUDENT CHALLENGE Study Conduct

Look again at those qualitative research studies you examined for phases 1 and 2. Look for evidence of the steps in phase 3.

1. Were the rights of human subjects protected in these studies? What evidence did you find to support this?
2. Is there evidence of IRB approval?
3. Was an informed consent obtained?
4. What information was provided about what occurred during data collection?

Phase 4: Analyze the Study

Analysis of data in qualitative studies involves examining words, descriptions, and processes rather than statistical analysis of numbers. The researcher reads and rereads field notes and transcripts, becoming familiar with the data. This is often called **data immersion** or dwelling with the data. It lets the researcher get in touch with not only the content but also the feeling, tone, and emphasis being communicated.

Initial analysis efforts are directed at setting up a system to make large volumes of data more manageable. A system is needed that allows the researcher to file, code, and easily retrieve needed data. Computer programs can assist in this management and analysis process. Raw data must be reduced and given some sense of meaning and order. This is done through several processes that simplify, focus, and transform the raw data. The researcher then searches for patterns and meaning of the data and arranges the data in some way that classifies or categorizes the data. This may be done by using an established classification scheme or by inventing a new scheme. This initial analysis may lead to additional observations or interviews to confirm patterns or find additional data to support the existence of an emerging pattern.

METHODS

Several specific formats and methods have been developed to analyze the data collected for various types of qualitative research. Common techniques used in phenomenological research include methods by Giorgi (1970); Spiegelberg (1976); Colaizzi (1978); Van Kaam (1984); and Parse, Coyne, and Smith (1985). All of these methods are similar, requiring qualitative researchers to immerse themselves in the data and use inductive reasoning to sort and make sense of the data and to extract and synthesize meaning from the data. Once it is more manageable, the researcher begins to refine categories and to assign meaning to the data. Data are compared and contrasted, similarities and differences are noted, and processes and relationships are defined. Finally, descriptions are constructed that represent the synthesis of material. These descriptions may take the form of a metaphor or an analogy or may be presented as a common theme.

Grounded theory has a very well-defined method of data collection and analysis described by Strauss (1987, 1990). The key is the use of techniques known as theoretical sampling and the constant comparative method. Theoretical sampling was discussed earlier in the sampling section. In the **constant comparative method** of analysis, the researcher categorizes units of meaning through a process that compares recorded incident to recorded incident until concepts and categories of concepts begin to emerge. As this occurs, theoretical constructs and relationships are developed and a theory emerges.

Ethnography uses several analytic methods such as ethnoscience, life history, network and event analysis, and the natural history method to examine conceptual and structural patterns in an identified culture. Ethnoscience techniques are designed to explore the "mental maps" that people use to navigate everyday life (Dobbert, 1984). Examination takes place at four levels. Data are described, classified, compared, and explained. Description occurs using a technique known as domain analysis; classifications are made through taxonomic analysis and comparisons through componential analysis. Explanation occurs by using the information from the first three analytic steps to make sense of the cultural patterns that emerge. (Spradley [1979, 1980] provides a good basic discussion of the four levels used in the ethnoscience approach.)

A life history gathers in-depth information about an informant's life and examines how similar or different individual patterns were from surrounding cultural patterns. Network and event analysis techniques are used to examine social structures. The natural history method provides a five-step method for organizing observational data to make sense of the process underlying the observations.

Historical studies use analytic techniques that examine the documents gathered to determine their importance and their reliability and validity. Initial importance is judged by a gross classification into three categories: clearly valuable, "mildly interesting," and not valuable. Valuable documents are included in the write-up. Interesting documents are rereviewed and nonvaluable documents are deleted from the study.

Validity is examined through a process of external criticism that seeks to authenticate the data source. Reliability is examined using a process known as internal criticism. Here the researcher must decide if the document is true to the language and customs of the historical time period in which it was written. The researcher must also decide whether the account of the event is from a first-hand or primary source or is a second- or third-hand account (secondary source). Material is then labeled as fact, probable, or possible, based on the type of source (primary versus secondary) and critical evaluation of those sources (Christy, 1975).

Case studies use a content analysis methodology that allows the researcher to search for patterns or themes in the data using a specific set of rules that govern coding and the formation of categories and category relationships.

FINDINGS

The findings in most qualitative studies are presented in a way that is more immediately understandable to the novice reader (you) than the results in most quantitative studies. This is because the language used is a descriptive narrative form. We are familiar with this form, and it doesn't require us to learn a new vocabulary. Frequently findings are illustrated by further examples or data highlights. A good qualitative presentation of findings leaves the reader with a clear cohesive picture of the phenomena that was the focus of the study.

STUDENT CHALLENGE Analysis and Results

Examine your chosen research studies for the analyses used and the results of the analyses.

1. Can you identify the specific analytic methods that were employed?
2. Were the results understandable? Did you get a sense of what had been uncovered in the study?
3. Did you find the results easier to decipher than in the quantitative studies you examined in Chapter 5?

Phase 5: Use the Study

Qualitative studies also make conclusions about their research findings. However, the conclusions may not draw inferences that are as easily applied to clinical practice. The reader is often left with the task of applying the results. Recommendations for further research are not usually a product of a qualitative study because definition and focus emerge with the collection and analysis of data and are not preconceived at the outset of the study.

The qualitative researcher is under the same obligation as the quantitative researcher to disseminate the results of the research study. The avenues for this dissemination are much the same and include journal articles and conference presentations. However, many qualitative studies may be found in monograph or book form because of the length of presentation. These formats allow fuller description and use of a greater number and variety of example illustrations obtained from data collection.

STUDENT CHALLENGE Entertaining the End

Examine your chosen research studies.
1. What did you glean from the studies' conclusions that might be helpful in the practice of nursing.
2. How would you compare your overall experience of reading qualitative research studies with reading quantitative research studies. Did you find one type easier to read and comprehend than the other?

Using Qualitative and Quantitative Research Approaches Together?

One question students frequently raise is whether quantitative and qualitative methods can be used together. Some researchers do combine the two methodologies to study certain phenomena. This approach is known as **triangulation**. Both methods may be used at the same time in one study (simultaneous triangulation), or one method at a time may be used in a series of studies (sequential triangulation).

When simultaneous triangulation is used, the researcher must use either a qualitative or quantitative approach as a foundation. The other approach then provides additional or complementary data. For example, a quantitative study might initially use unstructured interviews or observations to help develop more structured and hence measurable questions or behaviors. Qualitative research might use statistics to describe a sample of informants or to count frequencies of certain categorized events. A qualitative researcher might also use a quantitative scaled instrument to add an additional dimension to data on a particular concept.

However, use of both methods in a single study raises several issues because the philosophical approaches and assumptions underlying the study methodology are so different. Often a researcher who attempts simultaneous methods produces a finished product that fails to meet the criteria for good research in either approach.

Resource Kit

Want to Know More About Qualitative Research?

Try entering "qualitative research" as a search phrase using a search engine on the Internet. A variety of interesting websites are devoted to qualitative research.

 Visit the book's MERLIN website at
www.mosby.com/MERLIN/Langford/maze
for further information.

Check out the puzzles, mazes, and games on your **CD-ROM.**

References

Boehm S et al: Behavioral analysis and nursing interventions for reducing disruptive behaviors of patients with dementia, *Appl Nurs Res* 8(3):118, 1995.

Boyd JR, Hunsberger M: Chronically ill children coping with repeated hospitalizations: their perceptions and suggested interventions, *J Pediatr Nurs* 13(6):330, 1998.

Carr JM, Fogarty JP: Families at the bedside: an ethnographic study of vigilance, *J Fam Pract* 48(6):433, 1999.

Christy TE: The methodology of historical research: a brief introduction, *Image J Nurs Sch* 24(3):189, 1975.

Christy TE: The hope of history. In Fitzpatrick J, editor: *Historical studies in nursing,* New York, 1978, Teacher's College Press.

Cohen MZ, Kahn Dl, Steeves RH: Beyond body image: the experience of breast cancer, *Oncol Nurs Forum* 25(5):835, 1998.

Colaizzi P: Psychological research as a phenomenologist views it. In Vaille RS, King M, editors: *Existential phenomenological alternatives for psychology,* New York, 1978, Oxford University Press.

Denzin NS, Lincoln YS: *Handbook of qualitative research,* Thousand Oaks, Calif, 1994, Sage Publications.

Dobbert ML: *Ethnographic research: theory and application for modern schools and societies,* New York, 1984, Praeger Publishers.

Fall-Dickson JM, Rose L: Caring for patients who experience chemotherapy-induced side effects: the meaning for oncology nurses, *Oncol Nurs Forum* 26(5):901, 1999.

Fiveash B: The experience of nursing home life, *Int J Nurs Pract* 4(3):166, 1998.

Giorgi A: *Psychology as a human science: a phenomenologically based approach,* New York, 1970, Harper and Row.

Leininger MM: *Caring: an essential human need,* Thorofare, NJ, 1981, Charles B. Slack.

Levy V: Protective steering: a grounded theory study of the processes by which midwives facilitate informed choices during pregnancy, *J Adv Nurs* 29(1):104, 1999.

Neiderhauser VP: Varicella: the vaccine and the public health debate, *Nurs Pract* 24(3):74, 1999.

Parse RR, Coyne AB, Smith MJ: *Nursing research qualitative methods*, Bowie, Md, 1985, Brady.

Shermer RH, Raines DA: Positioning during the second stage of labor: moving back to the basics, *J Obstet Gynecol Neonatal Nurs* 26(6): 727, 1997.

Spiegelberg H: *The phenomenological movement*, The Hague, 1976, Martinus Nijhoff.

Spradley JP: *The ethnography interview*, New York, 1979, Holt, Rinehart and Winston.

Spradley JP: *Participant observation*, New York, 1980, Holt, Rinehart and Winston.

Strauss AL: *Qualitative analysis for social scientists*, New York, 1987, Cambridge University Press.

Strauss AL, Corbin J: *Basics of qualitative research: grounded theory procedures and techniques*, London, 1990, Sage Publications.

Van Kaam A: *Existential foundation of psychology*, New York, 1984, Doubleday.

Learning Objectives

1 Identify reputable research and clinical nursing journals with a research focus.

2 Describe the elements found in a standard research article format.

3 Discuss the relationship of a standard article format and the quantitative and qualitative research processes.

4 Describe a strategy that can be employed to more effectively read and comprehend research articles.

5 Apply the specified reading strategy to survey, examine, critically read, and evaluate a sample quantitative article and visualize practice applications.

6 Apply the specified reading strategy to survey, examine, critically read, and evaluate a sample qualitative article and visualize practice applications.

Chapter Outline

How Is Research Reported?
  Research and clinical journals
  Journal presentation format
    Title and abstract
    Introduction/background
    Methodology
    Results/findings
    Discussion/conclusions
    References

How to Read a Research Article
  Research reading strategy
  Using the reading strategy with sample research studies
    Quantitative research example
    Qualitative research example

Reading Research: Critical Approaches to Effective Understanding

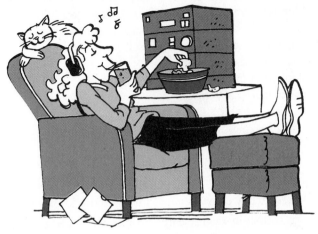

CHAPTER 7

Well the directions did say to "select a conducive environment!"

Student Quote *"I thought reading the article three times was going to be a colossal waste of time; but when I followed the strategy, I really did come away with a better understanding of what the researcher was doing."*

Abstract Research results are disseminated primarily through journal articles and are generally presented in a standard format that includes a title and abstract, introduction, methods, results, discussion, and references. These sections encompass the steps of the research process. A reading strategy can improve comprehension and use of research results. The described reading strategy consists of five phases. The article is read three times: once to survey the study, once to examine it for key ideas, and once to identify key elements of the research process. The study is then evaluated, and practice applications are visualized. Sample quantitative and qualitative articles are used to illustrate the use of the research reading strategy.

165

KEY TERMS
Reading Strategy Rhetoric

Abstract A clear concise summary of a study.

Critically read Step 3 of the research reading strategy; designed to focus on key steps in the research process.

Evaluate Step 4 in the research reading strategy; designed to judge the quality of the article.

Examine Step 2 of the research reading strategy; designed to identify key ideas and sort out the meaning of the article.

Research critique A detailed critical examination and evaluation of the theoretical and methodological merits of a given research study.

Research reading strategy A five-step process designed to increase comprehension and application of research studies. The steps are survey, examine, critically read, evaluate, and visualize.

Survey Step 1 of the research reading strategy; designed to provide a general overview and feel for the article.

Visualize Step 5 in the research reading strategy; designed to apply research results to practice.

Now that we have honed your library, Internet, and reading skills and introduced you to the world of research, we now begin to integrate this knowledge. This chapter helps you examine and critically read research articles. We look at the typical presentation format of research articles and introduce a set of criteria and a strategy to read by. We then dissect sample articles using the reading strategy and evaluation criteria.

How Is Research Reported?
Research and Clinical Journals

The most common way to disseminate research findings is by publication of a research article. We have already identified several journals that focus on nursing research. In addition, several clinical specialty journals devote at least half of their journal space to presentation of nursing research articles. There are also journals that review and critique the current state of nursing research. Box 7-1 lists some of the more common journals where research studies or discussions of studies can be located. As we discussed in Chapter 6, some qualitative studies are presented in monograph or book form because the presentation is lengthy and often not suited for an article format. Our focus is on research reports presented in article format.

STUDENT CHALLENGE Journal Set Ups

1. Peruse several of the research and clinical journals listed in Box 7-1. What do you see? What kinds of articles are present in addition to research articles?

2. Locate research articles in several different research and clinical journals. Compare the formats for presentation. Do you see similarities? Do the journals differ in emphases? What about the formats within a specified journal? Are they similar or different?

Box 7-1 Journals with a Research Focus

Nursing Research Journals

Nursing Research
Research in Nursing and Health
Western Journal of Nursing Research
Applied Nursing Research
Nursing Science Quarterly
Clinical Nursing Research
Image: Journal of Nursing Scholarship
Scholarly Inquiry for Nursing Practice

Clinical Nursing Journals (samples)

Cardiovascular Nursing
Heart and Lung: Journal of Critical Care
Issues in Comprehensive Pediatric Nursing
Issues in Mental Health Nursing
Journal of Community Health Nursing
Journal of Gerontological Nursing
MCN. The American Journal of Maternal Child Nursing
Oncology Nursing Forum
Public Health Nursing
Rehabilitation Nursing

Research Review Nursing Journals

Annual Review of Nursing Research
Online Journal of Knowledge Synthesis for Nursing
Research for Nursing Practice

As you probably just discovered, even research journals contain more material than just research studies. They may discuss statistical or methodological concerns, report on the development and testing of new research instruments, or discuss reliability or validity concerns of established instruments. They may even report on the reanalysis of old studies using a statistical technique known as *meta-analysis*. Clinical journals often contain anecdotal, clinical experience, and theoretical articles in addition to research articles.

Journal Presentation Format

You've probably also discovered that the format of a research article differs somewhat from the steps of the research process we discussed in Chapters 5 and 6. However, the format is very similar among the various journals. This format comes out of a quantitative research tradition and has six major sections: (1) title and abstract, (2) introduction or background, (3) methodology, (4) results or findings, (5) discussion, and (6) references. Slight variations may be seen in this format, but the sections are usually recognizable. Table 7-1 identifies the steps of the research process that are usually delineated under these section headings.

Table 7-1 Relationship Between the Research Process and the Format of Research Articles

ARTICLE SECTIONS	QUANTITATIVE PROCESS
Introduction/background	Problem statement/purpose
	Literature review
	Theoretical framework
	Hypotheses/research questions/objectives
Methods	Research design
	Sample and setting
	Data collection method
	Instrument quality
Results/Findings	Data analysis procedures
	Description of sample
	Presentation of results
Discussion/Conclusions	Interpretation of results
	Recommendations for research
	Implications for nursing
References	

Qualitative articles are often adapted to this format to provide a consistency in journal presentation. However, as qualitative research finds broader acceptance in nursing, we are beginning to see presentations that are much truer to the nature of the qualitative process. Thus, increasing numbers of qualitative articles are presented in a much looser narrative format tailored to the narrative presentation of the material discovered in the analysis process. The following discussion presents the typical quantitative presentation format and provides comments about qualitative studies when applicable.

TITLE AND ABSTRACT

The title of the study is the first thing you are likely to notice in any research article. It is set off in boldfaced large print and should capture the essence of the study. It typically states the variables or phenomena and population to be studied. The title section often lists the names and credentials of the researchers. Credentials may also be found at the end of an article.

Just below the title in italicized print is the abstract for the study. The **abstract** is a clear concise summary of the study. In about 100 to 300 words, the abstract describes the study purpose, research design, methodology, and findings. It serves as an overview of the article and should tell you what to expect in short.

INTRODUCTION/BACKGROUND

The introduction is the first section in the body of the article. It may or may not be labeled as such. The introductory section serves to acquaint you, the reader, with the research problem and its context. In a quantitative study, the following basic elements are included in the introduction:

- Research problem
- Research questions or hypotheses
- The need for the study
- Review of literature
- Theoretical framework

Remember that the problem statement may be in either interrogative or declarative form and may be couched as a statement of purpose. It is typically located at the beginning or the end of the introductory section. The problem may then be broken down into smaller research questions or hypotheses. In some studies, you may see these stated in the results section rather than the introductory section. The introduction often begins with a statement of need followed by a brief presentation of the current literature and identification of the theoretical framework. At times, the literature review and/or framework are set out under separate headings. Many studies may not articulate a theoretical framework. The reported review of literature may not be complete because of space constraints. Therefore, only the most critical and current studies are cited.

Qualitative studies use the introductory section to present a broad overview and context of the phenomena under study. Study objectives may be identified and pertinent literature cited. When you finish reading the introduction of a study, you should have a good feel for what is being studied and why such a study is important.

METHODOLOGY

The methods section describes how the researcher carried out the study. In a quantitative study, this section usually identifies the research design; describes the subjects, sampling techniques, and setting; and discusses instrumentation. This section may also contain a rationale for what was done, thus informing the reader why the selected approaches were used for the study. Research journals generally place a greater emphasis on this section than clinical journals do. Qualitative studies identify the research design and discuss interview or observation techniques. However, the focus centers on a detailed description of the analysis process.

RESULTS/FINDINGS

The results section presents the key research findings. In quantitative studies, the results section is fairly short. The data are presented in succinct form with little discussion. Studies often begin by describing sample characteristics here. In other studies, this description is included in the methods section. The focus is centered on answering the research questions or hypotheses. The statistical test(s) used are identified, and the value of the calculated statistic and the p value are reported. A brief narrative translation of these statistical results is included. Much of the statistical information may be displayed in table or graph form.

The results section in qualitative studies is generally longer because the results are presented in narrative form. In addition, the researcher often uses this section to describe the themes, processes, or structures that emerged from the analysis and to integrate them into the researcher's theoretical perspective. Pertinent literature review is often seen in this section. Grounded theory studies use this section to present the theory that has emerged from the data analysis.

DISCUSSION/CONCLUSIONS

The discussion section focuses on interpreting the results and is sometimes labeled "conclusions." The researcher explains what the results mean and how they fit back into the existing body of literature. In quantitative studies, if the results are unexpected (e.g., the hypotheses were not supported) the researcher may try to explain why things turned out the way they did. Quantitative studies also discuss limitations of the study methodology in this section. Implications for nursing practice are also stated here, as are recommendations for further research.

The discussion section in qualitative studies is often very short. This may stem in part from the belief that results stand on their own merits. Interpretation is often left to the reader. Implications may or may not be drawn for nursing practice. When they are drawn, they may be very general in scope.

REFERENCES

Journal articles conclude with a listing of references. This lists journal articles, books, and other sources cited in the text of the article. This reference section can be a very valuable tool to a reader who is interested in further information on a given area of study. It provides a starting point for a preliminary review of the literature on that topic.

STUDENT CHALLENGE Qualitative and Quantitative Comparisons

Choose a quantitative article and a qualitative article that use the general format previously described. Select an additional qualitative article that does not follow the prescribed format.

1. View each of the first two articles. Identify each of the major sections. Note how the information is presented under each section. Were the sections readily identifiable?
2. Did you notice the differences in the qualitative and quantitative approaches?
3. Now look at the two qualitative articles. Which approach seemed more readable to you? Which approach did you like better?

How to Read a Research Article

The primary reason we read research articles is to determine whether the findings will be helpful to our own professional practice. As we discuss effective ways to

Box 7-2   Research Reading Strategy

Get prepared. Select a conducive reading environment and a time when you are mentally alert. Have a glossary of research terms available for reference. Follow the steps listed below.

1. **Survey** the article to get a general feel for what is being studied and the overall outcomes.
   a. *Examine the title* to give you a good idea of the study area and to identify the major concepts or phenomena under investigation. Identify authors and author qualifications.
   b. *Pay careful attention to the abstract* to help you determine the type of study you're reading and whether this particular study is pertinent to you and your nursing practice. The abstract also provides a quick sketch of the research results.
   c. *Skim the major sections of the article* to pick up the general flow and article highlights. Try not to get bogged down by unfamiliar terms or statistical treatments.
   d. *Look at the reference list.* Do articles cited seem comprehensive, relevant to the topic, and current?

2. **Examine** the article. Go back and read the article more carefully. Proceed one section at a time. Draw out the key idea in each paragraph. Write down questions about terminology, concepts, or ideas that are puzzling. Consult needed resources to answer the questions you've raised.

3. **Critically read** the article. Using the criteria listed in Box 7-3 or 7-4 as a guide, read the article once more and locate the key elements of the study. Write them down as you find them.

4. **Evaluate** the article. Was the study a good one? Can results be applied to practice?

5. **Visualize** practice applications. Think about the results and how you might use them in your own nursing practice. Make written notes of your ideas.

read research articles, you may wish to quickly review Chapter 3. We introduce a reading strategy and a set of criteria to help you read research articles effectively and critically. The reading strategy as applied to research articles is outlined in Box 7-2. Criteria for increasing your comprehension of quantitative and qualitative studies are outlined in Boxes 7-3 and 7-4.

| Box 7-3 | Guidelines to Aid in the Comprehension of Quantitative Research Studies |

Introduction

Determine what is being studied:

 Locate a problem statement and/or statement of purpose.

 Locate hypotheses and/or research questions.

 Identify research variables and the population.

Determine why the study is important:

 Locate the rationale for the study.

Examine how the study contributes to existing knowledge:

 Look at literature review and the theoretical/conceptual framework.

Methods

Determine how the study was conducted:

 Identify the research design (e.g., Experimental or nonexperimental?
  Descriptive, exploratory, explanatory, or predictive?) Identify sampling
  issues (e.g., Probability or nonprobability? Number of subjects used?).

Identify study setting (i.e., Where did data collection occur?):

 Locate instruments used and reported reliability and validity measures.

Determine how study was analyzed:

 What statistical measures were used?

Results

Examine a description of the subjects (remember this may be in the methods
 section).

Determine the answers found by the study:

 Were statistical results significant or not? What does that mean?

Discussion

Determine implications for nursing practice:

 How were results related to practice?

 What limitations were placed on the study results?

 How were results tied back to existing knowledge?

ADVENTURE
CD
7-2

Box 7-4   Guidelines to Aid in the Comprehension of Qualitative Research Studies

Remember that many qualitative studies are not found in a set article format.

Introduction

Determine what phenomena are being studied:
   Look for a statement of purpose.
   Locate study questions or objectives.
Determine the context of the study:
   Read the literature review.
   Look for why the study was deemed important.

Methods

Determine how the study was conducted:
   Identify the research design (e.g., phenomenological, ethnographical, historical, grounded theory, or case study).
   Identify study setting, sampling techniques, data collection techniques, and reliability (accuracy) and validity (credibility) issues.
Determine how the study was analyzed:
   Look for descriptions of the analysis process. (e.g., How were data processed to establish themes, structures, or processes?)

Results

Examine a description of the subjects. (Remember, this may be the one place you see statistics used in a qualitative study.)
Determine the answers found by the study:
   What themes, metaphors, processes, or structures were identified to describe the data collected?

Discussion

Determine the implications for nursing practice:
   How were results related to practice?
   Were results tied back to existing knowledge?

Research Reading Strategy

As you can see by reviewing Box 7-2, which details the **research reading strategy,** you are going to read the article a minimum of three times. The first time you are skimming to detect the general purpose and direction of the study. The second time you are reading for understanding and to detect areas that may be confusing or present roadblocks to understanding. The third reading focuses in on specific pieces of the research process that need your attention. As you become more proficient at reading research articles, the middle reading step is often no longer necessary. This process will seem cumbersome and tedious at first. Stick with it, and ultimately you will be able to read research articles with greater ease and understanding.

Once you have surveyed, examined, and critically read the research article, the next step is to evaluate the study. This involves making judgments about the value of the study and deciding whether the study is a good one. You do not yet possess the knowledge or skills necessary to offer a critical evaluation of a reported research study. This process is commonly known as a **research critique**. It judges the theoretical and methodological merits of the study and addresses issues such as whether a study is theoretically sound, whether it was appropriately designed, and whether the methods or statistical analysis were correctly applied. These judgments require considerable knowledge of research and statistical methodologies. Your best bet is to stick to research reported in established professional journals and to rely on the editors and reviewers of the journal to make those evaluations.

However, you can ask yourself questions that have a bearing on the quality of the study. These include such queries as the following:
1. Were the key elements of the study clearly identified?
2. Could you readily follow the steps of the research process?
3. Were ideas concisely and comprehensively presented?
4. Were study findings clearly tied to existing knowledge?
5. Do the ideas make logical or intuitive sense?
   In qualitative studies, you want to ask the following questions:
1. Was the phenomena fully described?
2. Did the narrative paint a clear picture of the phenomena?
3. Were themes, structures, or processes clearly presented?

4. Did these themes, structures, or processes make sense?
5. Did they flow logically from the data?

When evaluating a study you are also concerned with whether the results can be applied to a particular practice setting. In a quantitative study, the question is: Are the results generalizable to subjects other than those in the study? If you remember from Chapter 5, results are generalizable to the population when the sample is a probability sample. If the sample is not a probability sample, then you must decide whether other studies have generated similar results. If more than one study is showing similar results, confidence in the results is increased. Use of a theoretical framework can also broaden the application of results to other groups of subjects. You want to ask questions such as what sampling technique was used? Is there a theoretical framework? Were results of similar studies reviewed in the article? How similar is my practice setting to the study setting?

Applicability of qualitative results is not concerned with generalizability. The question here is whether the results have any relevance to your particular practice. That is, does the interpretation of the data and the resulting themes, patterns, structures, or processes make sense in your practice? Do the ideas make sense? Are they useful?

The final step in the reading of a research article is to visualize how the study results might be helpful in your nursing practice. The study itself will suggest some ideas for application of the research results. You need to personalize the results; that is, think about them for your own practice. If you can visualize using the results, then you are more likely to incorporate them into your ongoing practice.

Using the Reading Strategy with Sample Research Studies

In this section, we use the research reading strategy and the comprehension guidelines to walk through two actual research articles step-by-step. The first article (Korniewicz et al, 1989) is a quantitative study and the second (Beck, 1992) is a qualitative study.

QUANTITATIVE RESEARCH EXAMPLE

If you are ready to get started, begin with the following Student Challenge.

STUDENT CHALLENGE Quantitative Surveying

1. Go to the CD-ROM and locate the Article Access exercise in Chapter 7. Print out the reading strategy, the guidelines for comprehending quantitative studies, and the quantitative research article entitled "Integrity of Vinyl and Latex Procedure Gloves."

   This article is not current. It was selected because it is short, appears in a standard format, involves few variables, and covers a basic topic that would be of interest to a wide variety of nurses.

2. Take your textbook; article, strategy, and guideline printouts; and notepad and pen, and find a conducive reading and study environment.

3. Note that each part of the article has been labeled with a letter and a number. The letter corresponds with the six sections of a standard research article. The numbers identify subsections of the specific section.

4. Now survey the article using Step 1 of the Research Reading Strategy found in Box 7-2. Print out. Make notes of what you gleaned from your survey. After you've finished, read the "Survey the Quantitative Article" section in this chapter and compare your notes with mine.

Survey the Quantitative Article.   The first stop on the survey is the title (labeled **A1**). This particular title informs us that the study examines the quality of two kinds of gloves used in doing procedures. This sounds like a study that could provide useful information about a product used daily in the clinical area. (Note: At the time this study was published, the use of universal precautions was just beginning to become a widespread and common practice).

Sections **A2** and **A5** (end of third page) identify four authors. All hold doctorates, three are nurses, two are postdoctoral students, and two are faculty members at a prestigious university. Infectious disease and infection prevention are identified specialty areas. This information gives us confidence that these researchers have enough expertise to conduct the study. Section **A4** gives us additional information about the study. It was published 7 to 8 months after acceptance by the journal. This means the material should still be relevant and timely at the time of publication. It was supported by an outside grant-funding source, and the results have been presented at an international conference, which lends further credence to the quality of the study.

ADVENTURE
CD
7-4

The abstract **(A3)** informs us that both types of gloves were tested using three different methods. From the description it sounds as if the gloves were tested for leaks of water, bacteria, and dye under simulated in-use conditions. It appears that the latex gloves performed better than the vinyl gloves across all tests. Twenty percent of the latex gloves and 34% of the vinyl gloves allowed penetration of bacteria; this raises some alarm. We need to read further to find out details about each of the testing methods and for a description of full results. After reading this far, I know this study has information that affects me personally in the clinical area.

As we skim the article, several things are readily apparent: Several pertinent articles are cited in the introduction, a purpose statement is clearly identified, the tests used seem well-described, results are straightforward, and the discussion has implications for practice. Articles included in the reference list are clearly related to the topic under study, include international sources and sources from various disciplines, and most were published in the 1980s.

STUDENT CHALLENGE Quantitative Examining

1. Now that you've surveyed the article and have a general idea of what it's about, go back and read the article paragraph by paragraph.
2. Jot down the key idea in each paragraph.
3. Make a note of anything you don't understand.
4. When you've finished, consult needed references to clarify those things that are unclear.
5. Now read the "Examine the Quantitative Article" section in this chapter for examples of abstractions of key ideas.

Examine the Quantitative Article.   The key ideas for each paragraph in the article are presented below and identified by their assigned code. See how they compare to your notes. Things that might raise questions about the research process are highlighted in bold.

B1   Fear of HIV exposure led to reevaluation of glove standards and practices that were designed to prevent the spread of hepatitis B virus (HBV).

B2   Several condom studies recommend latex condoms for protection against HBV and HIV, but we don't know if these results are applicable to gloves.

B3   Most of the studies on gloves have been done to test sterility during surgery.

B4   Data about protective abilities of latex and vinyl gloves are scarce. The purpose of the study is to examine the integrity of vinyl and latex gloves under in-use conditions.

C1   28 subjects

C2   Watertight method used to check for visible leaks in gloves. **Sensitivity of the watertight test was checked. Sensitivity is the ability of a test to adequately detect what it was designed to detect (i.e., how well the watertight test picked up leaks).**

C3   Three levels of hand manipulations (described in Table 1) were used to simulate hand activities during patient care.

C4   Each subject wore a vinyl glove on one hand and a latex glove on the other hand (Left hand versus right hand was randomly assigned). **Random assignment means that the hand wearing a certain glove type was chosen by chance.** Rubber bands were worn at wrists to prevent splashing and contamination. **This is a way to control extraneous variables.** Ninety manipulation tests were done for each glove type (30 each with no, partial, or full manipulation). Gloves were then tested for leaks using dye solution. Dye stains on hands were recorded by a person who was blind to (had no knowledge of) glove type. **This is a way to control bias in data recording.**

C5   *S. marcescens* cultures were used because it is not normally found on the skin. **This is another control placed over possible extraneous variables (e.g., contamination by bacteria already on a subject's skin).**

C6   Hands were washed and a baseline culture was done before testing.

C7   Subjects donned a vinyl and a latex glove, performed hand manipulations (no, partial, full), and then put hands into *S. marcescens* broth.

C8   Cultures taken from each glove. Cross-contamination controlled by frequent investigator glove changes. **This is another control over extraneous variable of cross-contamination.**

C9   Sensitivity of bacterial test examined. **(See sensitivity comment above.)**

D1   Visible defects were evident in 2.7% of latex and 4.1% of vinyl gloves ($\chi^2 = .58$, $\rho = .44$). χ^2 **stands for chi square; it is the statistical test used to determine whether any differences in defects were visible between latex and vinyl gloves. The ρ value of .44 tell us that differences in visible defects were not significant (see Chapter 5, page 130).**

D2   Watertight test not sensitive in the deliberately punctured latex gloves but was sensitive to vinyl.

D3   Fifty-three percent of vinyl and 3.3% of latex gloves leaked dye after full manipulation ($\rho = .0004$). The difference in performance of the two glove types after full manipulation was significant. Latex performed better. No difference in glove types was found for no or partial manipulation. Dye leaks occurred mainly on thumb and forefinger.

D4   All baseline cultures were negative. **This served as a pretest showing no *S. marcescens* on hands before the bacterial penetration test.** All deliberately punctured gloves were sensitive to bacterial test. Thirty-four percent of the vinyl and 20% of the latex gloves allowed bacterial penetration ($\chi^2 = 1.83$, $\rho = .18$). **The difference in the two glove types was not significant.** Brands of latex or vinyl gloves made no difference in the permeability.

E1   Concern over infection transmission and increased acceptance of universal precautions has increased glove use by health care workers.

E2   This study supports other evidence that shows that gloves are vulnerable to bacterial penetration.

E3   Glove testing protocols are under review by the Food and Drug Administration (FDA).

E4   Test sensitivity could be improved by use of a dye test that shows immediate results and the point of leakage with no risk of bacterial contamination to testers.

E5   Bacterial penetration tests are very sensitive but require too much time and delay test results. Contamination is a risk to testers.

E6   Both glove types provide some protection that decreases with use. Hands should be washed after patient care even if gloves are worn and gloves should not be reused or washed between patients.

STUDENT CHALLENGE Quantitative Critical Reading

1. Now that you've examined the article and summarized key ideas, go back and read the article a third time using the criteria outlined in the quantitative research guidelines.
2. Locate and record each key element of the research process.
3. Now review the section "Critically Read the Quantitative Article" in this chapter for confirmation of what you found.

Critically Read the Quantitative Article.   This section identifies the key elements of the research process used in our sample article. It follows the quantitative guidelines. The location of the identified elements in the article is indicated by the appropriate paragraph code.

Introduction
Determine what is being studied:
    The purpose is located in **B4** "The primary purpose of this study was . . ."
    No hypotheses or research questions are stated.
    Variables were not labeled, but can be identified.
    Independent variables: (1) type of glove (latex or vinyl), (2) in-use condition (none, partial, full)
    Dependent variable: glove integrity
    Extraneous variables that were identified and controlled for:
      Hand glove was worn on (left or right) hand **C4, C7**
      Dye splashing and contamination **C4, C7**
      Inspection bias **C4**
      Bacteria already on skin **C5, C6**
      Cross-contamination **C8**
    Population: procedure gloves
Determine why the study is important:
    The rationale is built in paragraphs **B1 to B4.** Perceived risk of exposure is increasing and insufficient data about barrier effectiveness of gloves.
Examine how the study contributes to nursing:
    No theoretical framework is identified.
    Brief literature review in **B1 to B4** supports need for additional testing.
    Nurses use gloves for barrier protection in the clinical area.

Methods

Determine how the study was conducted:

> Research design is experimental because the independent variable (in-use condition) was manipulated.
>
> The way the gloves were chosen (sampled) is not described beyond what appears in **D1.**
>
> We must assume that the sampling was convenience.
>
> Data collection sounds as if it were done in a lab, but this is not directly stated. One mention is made of a laminar flow cabinet in **C7.** Three biophysical tests were designed to measure glove integrity (watertight, dye, and bacterial penetration).
>
> Reliability and validity issues of tests were not discussed. This is not uncommon with biophysical measures.

Determine how the study was analyzed:

> Frequencies and percentages reported numbers of failed gloves. Differences between the vinyl and latex gloves were measured using chi square and Fishers exact tests. (These tests are designed to be used with nominal level data.) See **D1 to D4.**

Results

Examine description of subjects:

> This is confusing. A description of the people wearing the gloves is seen in **C1.** However, in this study, the gloves are the subjects. The only description of them is found in **D1.**

Determine the answers found in the study:

> The difference in the number of visible defects seen in latex versus vinyl gloves was not significant. Overall number of leaks seen was low (2.7 to 4.1%)—see **D1.** Latex gloves were significantly better than vinyl gloves at protecting against dye leaks after being fully manipulated (3.3% to 53%)—see **D3.** Differences between latex and vinyl gloves in the number of dye leaks under no or partial manipulation were not significant—see **D3.** One-fifth of latex and one-third of vinyl gloves were penetrated by bacteria. This difference was not significant—see **D4.** The difference in protection against bacterial penetration between the brands of latex gloves or between the brands of the vinyl gloves was not significant—see **D4.** The bottom line is that latex is generally better than vinyl in offering protection, particularly during use. However, neither performed well at keeping bacteria from penetrating.

Discussion

Determine implications for practice:

Practice implications are seen in **E6** where it stated that hands should be washed after patient care even if gloves are worn. Limits were discussed in **E5** where it was stated that bacterial test results occurred only under simulated conditions and risk of transmission was not studied. Study results were tied to the literature in **E2** and **E3.** The bottom line is gloves offer some barrier protection, and latex is generally better than vinyl. However, gloves should not be relied on for complete protection and should not replace handwashing.

STUDENT CHALLENGE Evaluation and Visualization

1. Now that you've read the article three times, it's time to do a general evaluation of the article and visualize practice applications.
2. Use the questions raised on page 175 of this chapter as you decide whether the study was a good one.
3. Then think about how these results might be applied to your own practice.
4. Now review the section "Evaluate and Visualize the Quantitative Article" in this chapter for a sample evaluation of the article and sample practice applications.

Evaluate and Visualize the Quantitative Article.   This section evaluates the quality of the sample article and then discusses how results might be used in clinical practice. Your evaluation may differ from mine, just as your level of comprehension and understanding differ from mine. Thus what seems clear cut to me may not seem so clear to you. Your ideas for application to your clinical practice may also differ. The applications stated here are general. Hopefully, yours is individualized to your personal situation.

This article is good. The key elements of the study are easy to identify, and the steps of the process generally are easy to follow. The ideas are presented clearly. The introductory argument clearly leads to the primary purpose of the article. Methods are described clearly. There is some confusion over the sample and sampling technique, but the procedure is discernible. Reliability and validity issues could have been directly addressed. Results are succinctly presented and logical. Study findings are easy to understand and are clearly tied to existing knowledge. Convenience sampling means results must be confined to the gloves tested. However, because these results are consistent with other study results, the findings can be applied to clinical situations with some degree of confidence.

As nurses, we should use gloves to provide some measure of barrier protection against disease. The choice of latex is better than vinyl. However, we should not rely on gloves to provide complete protection against bacteria. Good and frequent handwashing techniques are still much needed before and after patient contact, whether or not gloves are worn.

QUALITATIVE RESEARCH EXAMPLE

We have made it through the research reading strategy process using a quantitative article as an example. Now we are going to repeat the process using a qualitative article. So, if you are ready to move ahead, try the following Student Challenge.

STUDENT CHALLENGE Qualitative Survey and Examination

1. From the CD-ROM, print the qualitative research comprehension guidelines and the qualitative research article entitled "The Lived Experience of Postpartum Depression: A Phenomenological Study." This article was selected because it is relatively short, appears in the same format as the previous article, and is written for an audience who is not familiar with the phenomenological method.
2. Note that each part of the article has been labeled with a letter and a number (e.g., **A1**). The letter corresponds to the six sections of a standard research article. The numbers identify subsections of the specific section.
3. Now survey the article using Step 1 of your research reading strategy. Make notes of what you gleaned from your survey.
4. Now reread the article and jot down the key idea in each paragraph, making note of anything confusing. After you've finished, read the section "Survey and Examine the Qualitative Article" in this chapter.

Survey and Examine the Qualitative Article.   The title (**A1**) tells us that this study is a qualitative phenomenological study and that the phenomenon under investigation is postpartum depression. The author (**A2, A5**) holds a doctorate, is a certified nurse midwife, and a faculty member at a college of nursing. It was published 5 months after acceptance. The abstract (**A3**) succinctly identifies the study design, the purpose, the sample size, the method of analysis, and the results. An immediate picture is painted of postpartum depression as a horrifying experience. After I finished with the abstract, I was hooked and wanted to know the details of life for these women.

A quick survey of the article reveals a well-organized approach to presentation of the study. Elements of the research process are clearly labeled and well-defined. Each theme is identified discussed and illustrated with a concrete example from actual data. References cover the 1960s to the mid-1980s, are clearly related to the topic under study and include international sources and sources from various disciplines, as well as several references about the phenomenological research process.

At this point, you should be getting pretty good at pulling key ideas from a paragraph. So, the following includes selected examples pulled from identified paragraphs.

C1   Purposive sample of seven women from a postpartum support group for whom the researcher was a facilitator. Sample description: 22 to 38 years old, high school/college educated, primiparas/multiparas, vaginal/C-section, all but one under psychiatric care.

C7   Data analysis—interview transcripts analyzed using Colaizze's 6-step method **(specific method used in phenomenological analysis)**: (1) read, (2) extract phrases directly related to postpartum depression, (3) formulate meaning, (4) organize into themes, (5) integrate data analysis, (6) return to participants to validate.

C8, C9   Credibility, auditability, and fittingness were addressed using member checks and audit trails. **(These are specific terms used by phenomenologists to look at confirmability of results. Confirmability is a concept parallel to the concepts of credibility [validity] and accuracy [reliability] that were discussed in Chapter 6. Fittingness is a somewhat vague concept that refers to whether study results fit the data and are understood by the reader.)**

D2   Theme 1: Loneliness

D3   Loneliness because women felt no one understood, pleas for understanding ignored, so began to isolate selves.

D4   Theme 2: Death seen as hope.

D5   Death seen as a way out of living hell.

D6   Theme 3: Consumed by obsessive thoughts of experience and being a bad mother.

D7   Obsessive thinking left them mentally and physically exhausted, but sleep is not possible because of racing thoughts.

STUDENT CHALLENGE Qualitative Critical Reading

1. Now that you've examined the article and summarized the key ideas, go back and read the article a third time using the qualitative research comprehension guidelines.

2. Locate and record each key element of the research process.

3. Now review the section "Critically Read the Qualitative Article" in this chapter for confirmation of what you found.

Critically Read the Qualitative Article.   This section identifies the key elements of the research process used in our sample article. It follows the qualitative guidelines. The location of the identified elements in the article is indicated by the appropriate paragraph code.

Introduction

Determine what phenomena are being studied:

> The purpose of the study is stated in the abstract **(A3)** and in the introduction at the end of the paragraph **B3**. A research question is also present in **B3** and stated as "What is the essential structure of the lived experience postpartum depression?" The phenomenon is postpartum depression.

Determine the context of the study:

> Literature review is used to establish a need and clarify terms **(B1 to B4)**. Study importance is developed in paragraphs **B1, B3,** and **B4**. Depression occurs in 10% to 26% of mothers **(B1)**. No qualitative research is available on the experience **(B3)**. Results could be used to enhance content validity of quantitative instruments **(B4)**

Methods

Determine how the study was conducted:

> Phenomenological research design was used **(A1, A3, C2)**. A description of phenomenology as a philosophy is described in **C2**, and phenomenology as a research design is described in **C3**.
>
> Sampling is purposive **(C1)**; sample was taken from a postpartum support group **(C1, C4)**.
>
> Data were collected using interviews **(C4)** and bracketing **(C5)**.
>
> Interviews were taped and transcribed **(C6)**.
>
> Collection continued until repetition occurred with no new themes **(C6)**.
>   Setting was private home or private interview in psychiatric clinic **(C6)**.
>
> Reliability and validity issues are covered in **C8**.
>
> Credibility was examined using a member check and auditability **(audit trail)**.
>
> Accuracy was examined by using tape recordings, verbatim transcriptions, use of an independent judge experienced in phenomenological analysis to check each stage of analysis.

Determine how study was analyzed:

> Analysis used Colaizzi's method **(C7)**. Significant statements are presented in Table 1 and decision trail examples are in Table 2.

Results

Examine a description of the subjects:

> Description is found in **C1.** Mothers who were in a support group, 22 to 38 years of age, high school or college educated, both primiparas and multiparas, both vaginal and C-section deliveries. Six were under psychiatric care.

Determine the answers found by the study:

> Results were discussed as identified themes. Themes can be found in **D2 to D26.** Eleven themes are identified and discussed. Specific examples are quoted. The eleven themes are loneliness, suicidal thoughts, obsessive thoughts, grieving over loss of normalcy, emptiness of life, guilt and fear, inability to concentrate, going through the motions, uncontrollable anxiety, loss of emotional control, and need to be mothered.

Discussion

Determine the implications for nursing practice:

> A direct relationship to practice is not discussed. The focus is on using results to improve quantitative instruments **(E1 to E3).** Results are related to existing tools.

STUDENT CHALLENGE Evaluation and Visualization

1. Now that you've read the article three times, it's time to do a general evaluation of the article and visualize practice applications.
2. Use the questions raised on pages 175 and 176 of this chapter as you decide if the study was a good one.
3. Then think about how these results might be applied to your clinical practice.
4. Now review the section "Evaluate and Visualize the Qualitative Article" in this chapter for a sample evaluation of the article and sample practice applications.

Evaluate and Visualize the Qualitative Article.   This study is easy to follow. The steps of the process are identified easily and described clearly. After reading the results, a picture emerges as to what it might be like to suffer from postpartum depression. Included data support the identified themes. It would have been helpful if the discussion included uses of the results in clinical practice.

The themes are relevant to clinical practice. The picture painted of postpartum depression enhances the nurse's ability to identify and more adequately assess signs and symptoms of potential postpartum depression. It allows for greater identification, understanding, and empathy with a client who has postpartum depression. The themes can lend direction to interventions, including such actions as referral for support or counseling and suicide precautions. If I were a psychiatric or maternal-child nurse who participated in individual or group support sessions, this information might help facilitate such sessions.

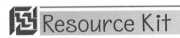 Resource Kit

 Visit the book's MERLIN website at **www.mosby.com/MERLIN/Langford/maze** for further information.

 Check out the puzzles, mazes, and games on your **CD-ROM**.

References

Beck CT: The lived experiences of postpartum depression: a phenomenological study, *Nurs Res* 41(3):166, 1992.

Korniewicz DM et al: Integrity of vinyl and latex procedure gloves, *Nurs Res* 38(3):144, 1989.

Three

WALKING THE WALK

Applying Research Results in a Variety of Clinical Practice Situations

... Practice, Practice, Practice

The ability to consistently read and apply nursing research requires that we become comfortable with our new found strategic skills. This means practicing these skills with research articles from various sources across a wide range of clinical practice situations. This allows us to become more proficient at using the strategic reading strategy and to discover a wide range of uses for research results. This section is designed to let you practice and develop your skills as a research consumer, by examining and applying example research results across the lifespan. Finally, the concept of research utilization is explored, and you are provided with approaches, criteria, and strategies to enhance your research utilization capabilities.

Learning Objectives

1 Identify maternal-infant clinical nursing journals that publish research articles.

2 Discuss clinical and research priorities in the practice of maternal-infant nursing.

3 Use research literature to clarify identified maternal-infant practice problems.

4 Explore examples of research that have been conducted in various areas of maternal-infant clinical practice.

5 Discuss application of sample research results in clinical practice.

6 Apply the reading strategy to survey, examine, critically read, and evaluate sample research articles on maternal-infant care.

Chapter Outline

What Research Resources Are Available for Mothers and Infants?
What Approaches Can Be Used for Review of the Research Literature?
  Addressing clinical and research priorities
  Using issues that arise from clinical practice
  Scanning available resources

What Current Research Is Available?
  Nursing research journals
  Clinical nursing journals
  Other journals
  Summarizing and using scanning results
How to Read and Evaluate a Research Article on Maternal-Infant Care

Reading and Using Research in Maternal-Infant Care

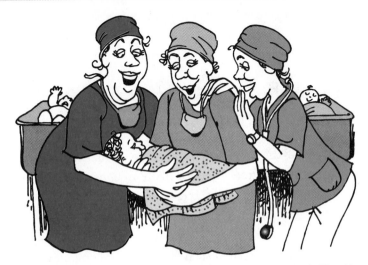

I know the study said we needed to improve patient-staff ratios, but we seem to be taking it just a bit too far.

Student Quote   *"In clinical conference, we discussed a research article that I had found on how to improve feeding patterns in a premie. I really felt like I was contributing to better care."*

Abstract   Several research sources publish articles pertinent to maternal-infant care. These sources can be used to view the latest research on maternal-infant care and research priorities, address identified problems and questions uncovered in clinical practice, or provide a broad view of currently available maternal-infant research. An abundant number of current research studies are available for use in the clinical practice of maternal-infant care. Samples of current studies are reported, and clinical applications are discussed. The use of the research reading strategy is illustrated with one maternal-infant research article.

You now have a reading strategy, and we have tentatively tested that strategy on two sample articles. The next four chapters are designed to allow you the opportunity to develop and hone your abilities to find, read, interpret, and apply research findings in specified clinical situations and settings. The chapters are divided using a lifespan schema. Chapter 8 covers maternal-infant care, Chapter 9 looks at children and adolescents, Chapter 10 discusses adults, and Chapter 11 addresses older adults.

In this chapter, we identify additional publications that contain nursing research on maternal-infant care, explore strategies to simplify the search process and target relevant research articles, and preview sample selections of currently published research. Finally we dissect a sample article using the reading strategy and evaluation criteria presented in Chapter 7.

What Research Resources Are Available for Mothers and Infants?

To effectively view the current research in maternal-infant care, it is helpful to be able to identify resources that are likely to contain research articles on the maternal-infant experience. All the research journals we have discussed in previous chapters contain articles on maternal-infant care. Several clinical specialty journals also regularly publish research articles for maternal-infant care. Clinical journals in other specialty areas such as pediatrics, community health, or mental health nursing also occasionally contain research articles relevant to maternal-infant care. Box 8-1 contains a list of journals most likely to contain research relevant to the practice of maternal-infant care.

STUDENT CHALLENGE Perusing Specialty Journals

1. If some of the journals listed in Box 8-1 are unfamiliar to you, take time to locate those available in your library. Scan two or three issues of each journal.
2. Note how they are organized. What types of articles are prevalent? Can you readily distinguish research articles from other featured articles? Do you notice a difference in the focus of the various journals?
3. Where might you locate a description of the journal's focus or purpose? (Locate one electronic and one print source.)

STUDENT CHALLENGE Perusing Specialty Journals—cont'd

4. Do you see any differences between articles in research journals and research articles in clinical journals? Can you detect differences in presentation and article selection among the various research journals? What about differences in the content style of research articles in the various clinical journals? Are some journals more readable than others? More helpful?

Box 8-1 Journals Containing Maternal-Infant Nursing Research

Nursing Research Journals
Nursing Research
Research in Nursing and Health
Western Journal of Nursing Research
Applied Nursing Research
Clinical Nursing Research
Nursing Science Quarterly
Image: Journal of Nursing Scholarship
Scholarly Inquiry for Nursing Practice

Clinical Journals that Regularly Contain Research Articles About Maternal-Infant Care
MCN: The American Journal of Maternal Child Nursing
Journal of Obstetric, Gynecologic and Neonatal Nursing
Neonatal Network-Journal of Neonatal Nursing
Pediatric Nursing

As you become more familiar with the various clinical and research journals you should begin to note which provide the most useful information for improving maternal-infant care. You should also discover that journals have varying foci and purposes, as well as differing formats and reading levels. Discover which journals are most helpful to you.

What Approaches Can Be Used for Review of the Research Literature?

There are three major ways that we might approach the current research literature to help guide and enhance our clinical practice for mothers and infants. One is dictated by the clinical and research priorities that have been identified in the area of maternal-infant health care. A second is dictated by problems you routinely encounter in your day-to-day clinical practice with mothers and their infants. A third approach is to regularly scan the readily available published resources.

Addressing Clinical and Research Priorities

Keeping informed of the current clinical and research priorities in a given area can help direct and guide your practice with whatever target population you choose to work. Let's use mothers and infants as an example. The overall goal in maternal-infant care is focused on improving outcomes for mothers and children. Priority issues in maternal-infant care and research can be drawn from several sources.

Healthy People is a far-ranging government effort to address the illness prevention, health maintenance, and health promotion needs of the people in the United States. *Healthy People 2000* was the public policy statement that resulted from the initial effort. It details 22 priority areas and numerous objectives for illness prevention, health promotion, and health protection across four age groups. The second major effort resulted in *Healthy People 2010*. This document builds on *Healthy People 2000* and details 28 priority areas with corresponding objectives. Several of the *Healthy People* objectives are pertinent to maternal-infant care. Pertinent objectives from *Healthy People 2000* are summarized in Box 8-2. We address *Healthy People 2010* objectives in the next Student Challenge.

The research priorities of the National Institute for Nursing Research (NINR) that were identified in Chapter 4 also included issues related to maternal-infant care (e.g., the prevention and care of low-birth-weight infants). In 1998, the area concerning low-birth-weight infants was narrowed to focus particularly on minority populations. As you can see, these priorities may assist you in identifying areas of concern in your own maternal-infant practice. They also let you know what areas of care receive funding priority for research.

Professional and volunteer associations often promote certain research priorities. The American Association of Women's Health, Obstetrical, and Neonatal Nurses (AWHONN), for example, has generated a list of clinically relevant areas that are viewed as research priorities. These include research on breastfeeding, childbearing, early parenting, infertility, low-birth-weight infants, and pregnancy. The March of Dimes has targeted issues such as immunizations and birth defects as research and funding priorities.

Box 8-2   *Healthy People 2000* Objectives Related to Maternal-Infant Care

Reduce fetal, infant, and maternal mortality
Reduce fetal alcohol syndrome
Reduce low birth weight in infants
Increase weight gain during pregnancy
Reduce severe complications of pregnancy
Reduce Cesarean deliveries
Increase breastfeeding
Increase abstinence from tobacco, alcohol, cocaine, and marijuana during
    pregnancy
Increase first trimester prenatal care
Increase age-appropriate counseling
Increase screening and counseling on detection of fetal abnormalities
Improve risk-appropriate care
Increase screening and treatment for genetic disorders
Improve primary care for babies
Reduce the incidence of spina bifida and other neural tube defects

From U.S. Department of Health and Human Services, Public Health Service: *Healthy People 2000: national health promotion and disease prevention objectives*, Washington, DC, 1991, Author.

You can view the *Healthy People 2000* and *2010* goals and objectives, the NINR priorities, the AWHONN areas, the March of Dime areas, and other maternal-infant resources on the web. They can be accessed through the book's MERLIN website. See the Resource Kit listing at the end of this chapter.

Activity

13

🔲 STUDENT CHALLENGE Checking Maternal-Infant
                                     Priorities

1. Check the *Healthy People 2010* goals and objectives presented on the *Healthy People 2010* website. Locate the objectives relevant to maternal-infant care. Compare them to the objectives in Box 8-2. Note similarities and differences.
2. Check the NINR research priorities. Have any new areas been added that affect maternal-infant care?

Continued

STUDENT CHALLENGE Checking Maternal-Infant
Priorities—cont'd

3. Can you locate any other sources that list or discuss priorities in maternal-infant care or research?
4. Choose one of the priority areas that have been listed or that you have discovered. Run a literature search for the years 2000 to the present and see what, if any, nursing research has been conducted in your selected area. Did you find anything that might be applicable to the clinical area of maternal-infant care?

Using Issues that Arise from Clinical Practice

When you practice in a particular clinical setting and interact on a regular basis with mothers and their infants, certain questions and problems routinely arise in the course of providing care. Answers to some of these identified problems may be found in the research literature. When a problem surfaces you may wish to define that problem by certain parameters before going to the literature. If you have a clear frame of reference from which to think about nursing care, it makes the search and use of research materials much easier. You need to ask yourself questions such as who is the target of care—the mother, the infant, or the mother-infant dyad? You might clarify what phase of care is involved (e.g., antepartum, intrapartum, or postpartum for the mother; fetus, newborn, or neonate for the infant)? What level of care is involved? Is the problem one of prevention, acute care, or chronic care? The aspect of care is also important. Are you concerned with physical, psychological, sociocultural, or spiritual needs? Finally what care setting did the problem arise in—a clinic, physician's office, home, or the hospital?

For example, I may be a staff nurse working in labor and delivery in a hospital. I notice that many of my patients are exhausted by labor, and I wonder if there is anything I can do to lessen the fatigue. The target of concern is mothers. The phase of care is intrapartum. The level of care is acute. The care aspect might be the physical and/or psychological components of fatigue. The care setting is hospital labor and delivery or birthing centers. If I do a MEDLINE search using the key words "maternal," "fatigue," and "labor" for the past 3 years, I find no research. I do find one article (Gennaro et al, 1999) that identifies potential effects from the fatigue associated with second stage labor and makes practice recommendations.

The article also discusses research that needs to be done on this problem. This article does contain more information than what is available in my maternal-child nursing text. If I look at the related literature available in the MEDLINE citation, I find 20 articles stretching back over 30 years that discuss labor and delivery practices or maternal fatigue in the postpartum period. None shed much relevance on my problem.

Maybe I work as a nurse in a neonatal intensive care unit and am concerned about the fact that many of the premature infants in my care seem to have patches of skin loss as a result of various treatments and procedures. I wonder if there are things I can do to decrease this problem. There is no skin protocol in this unit. A MEDLINE search for 3 years using the keywords "premature", "infant," and "skin" yielded a total of five articles. Two were research articles (Maguire, 1999; Munson et al, 1999). One discussed skin care protocols or management in infants (Lund, 1999), another reviewed the existing literature on neonatal skin care from 1993 to 1999 (Lund et al, 1999), and the final one discussed the thermoregulation and fluid maintenance problems associated with the congenital absence of skin in some preterm infants. This last article was deemed irrelevant. The third and fourth articles served to provide baseline data from which to better read the two research articles.

The first research article (Maguire, 1999) was a quantitative descriptive survey of 215 different neonatal intensive care units (NICUs) nationwide with one registered nurse with 2 or more years of NICU experience from each institution. The nurses were asked questions to describe and measure the incidence of skin breakdown in low-birth-weight infants in their units and to describe interventions to treat or prevent breakdown. Findings determined that about 20% of low-birth-weight infants suffered from skin breakdown across the 215 units. Those nurses reporting the least breakdown followed skin care protocols that limited use of tape and made liberal use of Aquaphor as a skin barrier. Recommendations included further study of the effectiveness of various products used to treat breakdown. This study might lead the way for me as a staff nurse to propose to the unit coordinator that the unit adopt a standard skin care protocol and perhaps try Aquaphor as a skin breakdown prevention measure.

The second research article (Munson et al, 1999) was a descriptive survey of 104 hospitals that delivered at least 2,500 babies a year and had a level III NICU with at least 20 beds. The purpose of the survey was to ascertain current skin care practices and protocols. This study was not helpful in solving my problem, but it did reinforce the fact that 25% of the surveyed hospitals had no standard protocols, and the others surveyed showed a wide variation in their approach to skin care.

The identification of a specific clinical problem often sheds more light on the research that still needs to be conducted rather than the research that is available. Literature searches targeted at specifically identified clinical problems can still prove worthwhile and may provide much needed help for a vexing clinical situation.

STUDENT CHALLENGE Chasing Maternal-Infant Challenges

1. Review your experiences in maternal-infant nursing and think about a situation that you wish to explore in the current research literature.

2. Identify appropriate search parameters for the subject material and conduct a library search for the year 2000 to the present. What did you find? (Hint: If your search yielded too many entries, try one of the following ideas. If you conducted an electronic MEDLINE search, try creating a specialized journal list. List only those journals found in Box 8-1. Then perform your search. The search mechanism will be confined to those selected journals. If you are conducting an electronic CINAHL search, try limiting results to research by checking that option on the search page. If you had too few entries, broaden your search parameters or check the related reference option available on MEDLINE.)

3. If your search was fruitful, retrieve one or two promising articles. (Remember, abstracts are very helpful in deciding if an article is worth retrieving).

4. Review the article. How might the results of the study be helpful in clinical practice?

Scanning Available Resources

As we have just seen, your clinical practice and the concerns that arise from day-to-day experience often lead to a search for research literature that may prove helpful and be of interest. However, many students say to me such things as, "I don't know enough yet to identify areas of concern in practice," or "I can identify things that need attention, but I'm not sure what the standard of care is let alone the new or changing care." One way to get connected to the research literature in a particular area such as maternal-infant nursing is to regularly scan the table of contents and the abstracts of the research and clinical specialty journals listed in Box 8-1. Look at what is available. Ask yourself if any of the articles seem relevant to what you are currently learning or practicing in the clinical area. If so, check out the full article. Use research results that you have found in your clinical care plans and in clinical conferences. Believe me, you will impress your instructor and amaze your classmates.

STUDENT CHALLENGE Scanning Maternal-Infant Journals

Select one research journal and one clinical journal from those listed in Box 8-1 that are available in your library.
1. Scan the year 2000 table of contents for each of these journals and note those articles that seem relevant to maternal-infant care.
2. Read the abstracts for the selected articles. Weed out any articles that are not clinically relevant. How long did this take you? Did you use electronic resources or the actual journal?

Save these articles. We will use them again in the next exercise.

You have just finished looking at two journals for a period of 1 year. However, an effective scan must take into account several journals that are likely to contain maternal-infant research. You can conduct a fairly rapid scan of several journals through the use of the Internet and your electronic library resources. Several publishing websites on the Internet allow you to peruse the table of contents and abstracts for various journals. Your library may also permit you access to the current abstracts of several journals. Some of these journals even have the entire article available on-line for reading and/or downloading. The publishing company websites usually charge a fee for these services, but they are often free through your library if you are a cardholder. Check out the Resource Kit at the end of this chapter for a listing of helpful publishing company journal sites, and then use the book's MERLIN website to get a link to one of these journals.

Armed with these tools plus MEDLINE and CINAHL search capabilities, it is possible to do a periodic journal scan from the comfort of your own home. You need only go to the library once you have pinpointed articles that seem relevant to your practice. Some libraries will even allow you to pay a fee for delivery of articles to your doorstep. I suggest conducting a scan about once every 6 months. When

MERLIN
Activity
14

you get proficient, you can conduct a scan of all of the journals listed in Box 8-1 in about 2 hours.

What Current Research Is Available?

The following are specific examples of pertinent maternal-infant research articles that I found by simply scanning the 1999 table of contents of the research and clinical journals listed in Box 8-1. Selected articles are briefly summarized and clinical implications are discussed. The articles are arranged by journal. This allows you to see which of the journals might provide you with the most insight about various maternal-infant clinical topics.

Nursing Research Journals

The articles found by scanning the tables of contents of the various research journals yielded the list of possibly relevant maternal-infant articles shown in Box 8-3.

Box 8-3 Relevant Maternal-Infant Article Titles in Research Journals

Nursing Research

Physiological Responses of Preterm Infants to Breastfeeding and Bottle-Feeding with the Orthodontic Nipple (Dowling, 1999)

Mother-Infant: Achieving Synchrony (Leitch, 1999)

Distress and Growth Outcomes in Mothers of Medically Fragile Infants (Miles-Shandor et al, 1999)

The Effects of Prescribed Versus Ad Libitum Feedings and Formula Caloric Density on Premature Infant Dietary Intake and Weight Gain (Pridham et al, 1999)

The Efficacy of Developmentally Sensitive Interventions and Sucrose for Relieving Procedural Pain in Very Low Birth Weight Neonates (Stevens et al, 1999)

Effects of Caring, Measurement and Time on Miscarriage Impact and Women's Well-Being (Swanson, 1999)

Research in Nursing and Health

Nursing Care and the Development of Sleeping and Waking Behaviors in Preterm Infants (Brandon, Holditch-Davis, and Beylea, 1999)

Preterm Infant Behavioral and Heart Rate Responses to Antenatal Phenobarbital (McCain, Donovan, and Gartside, 1999)

Testing an Intervention to Prevent Further Abuse to Pregnant Women (Parker et al, 1999)

The Adaptiveness of Mothers Working Models of Caregiving Through the First Year: Infant and Mother Contributions (Pridham, Schroeder, and Brown, 1999)

Developmental Intervention for Preterm Infants Diagnosed with Eriventricular Leukomalacia (White-Traut et al, 1999)

Western Journal of Nursing Research

Perceived Impediments to Prenatal Care Among Low Income Women (Mikhail, 1999)

Applied Nursing Research

Nutrition and Exercise in Overweight and Obese Postpartum Women (Morin, Gennaro, and Fehder, 1999)

Fatigue in Mothers of Infants Discharged to Home on Apnea Monitors (Williams et al, 1999)

Clinical Nursing Research

Testing a Model of the Nursing Assessment of Infant Pain (Fuller et al, 1999)

Skin Protection and Breakdown in ELBW Infant: A National Survey (Maguire, 1999)

Behavioral Responses of Newborns of Insulin-Dependent and Nondiabetic Healthy Mothers (Pressler et al, 1999)

A Comparison of Fatigue and Energy Levels at Six Weeks and 14 to 19 Months Postpartum (Troy, 1999)

The Relationship Between Method of Pain Management During Labor and Birth Outcomes (Walker and O'Brien, 1999)

Nursing Science Quarterly

The Construct of Thriving in Pregnancy and Postpartum (Walker and Grobe, 1999)

Image: Journal of Nursing Scholarship

No relevant articles

Scholarly Inquiry for Nursing Practice

No relevant articles

A scan of the 1999 issues of *Nursing Research* reveals six potentially relevant articles. An examination of the titles quickly reveals two studies that focus on women and the measurement of psychological adjustment after certain pregnancy outcomes (i.e., adjustment to miscarriage, adjustment to the birth of a medically fragile infant). Three studies focus on preterm and or low-birth-weight infants and examine the effectiveness of various interventions such as differing feeding schedules, differing pain relief measures, and the use of an orthodontic nipple. A final study examines mother-infant dyads. Further examination of article abstracts shows that all six articles might provide relevant information for varying clinical situations. Further selection would need to be based on your own clinical position, setting, and interests.

Research in Nursing and Health contained 5 articles related to maternal-infant concerns. Three studied preterm infants and one studied pregnant women, and the last looked at maternal-infant dyads.

The *Western Journal of Nursing Research* devoted a partial issue to maternal-infant concerns. Three of the five articles looked promising. A scan of the abstracts quickly revealed that one article was a historical study centering on maternal care after World War II and another was studying patient satisfaction with prenatal clinics in Russia. The findings were not relevant for practice. The remaining article surveyed impediments to prenatal care.

Applied Nursing Research had two articles both related to maternal postpartum issues, and *Clinical Nursing Research* had five relevant articles: three about infants and two about mothers. *Nursing Science Quarterly* had one relevant article that examined the specific concept of "thriving" in the mother. No relevant articles were found in *Image: Journal of Nursing Scholarship* or *Scholarly Inquiry for Nursing Practice*.

Examining the titles of the articles across all the research journals reveals a total of 20 articles (9 on mothers, 9 on infants, and 2 on maternal-infant dyads). Three of the maternal articles addressed prenatal issues, 1 addressed intrapartum issues, and 6 addressed postpartum issues. The infant articles were predominantly about preterm babies (7 articles) and examined such areas as feeding, pain, sleeping, skin care, and behavior. There was 1 qualitative study that viewed maternal-infant dyads for synchrony. Nursing interventions were tested in 6 studies (nipple use, feeding schedules, pain treatments, pain assessment, abuse intervention, developmental intervention). Studies on fatigue, pain, and feeding occurred more than one time.

Clinical Nursing Journals

The articles found by scanning the tables of contents of the clinical journals yielded the list of possibly relevant maternal-infant research articles shown in Box 8-4.

Box 8-4 Relevant Maternal-Infant Research Article Titles in Clinical Journals

MCN: The American Journal of Maternal Child Nursing

Pregnancy Wantedness in Adolescents Presenting for Pregnancy Testing (Bloom and Hall, 1999)

Comparison of a Rocking Bed and a Standard Bed Decreasing Withdrawal Symptoms in Drug Exposed Infants (Dapolito, 1999)

Living with Postpartum Depression: The Father's Experience (Davis et al, 1999)

Infant Sleep Position: Nursing Practice and Knowledge (Peeke et al, 1999)

Kangaroo Care for a Restless Infant with Gastric Reflux: One Nurse Midwife's Personal Experience (Roller, 1999)

Birth Kangaroo Care and Breastfeeding: A Eclamptic Woman's Story (Roller, Meyer, and Cranston-Anderson, 1999)

Fantasies of the Unborn Among Pregnant Women (Sorenson and Schuelke, 1999)

The Essential Forces of Labor Revisited: 13 Ps Reported in Womens' Stories (VandeVusse,1999)

Journal of Obstetric, Gynecologic, and Neonatal Nursing

Neonatal Axillary Temperature Measurements: A Comparison of Electronic Thermometer Predictive and Monitor Modes (Christiani and Fallis, 1999)

Psychological and Demographic Factors Related to Health Behaviors in the First Trimester (Cooney, Riggs, and Walker, 1999)

Impact of Perinatal Loss on Subsequent Pregnancy and Self: Women's Experiences (Cote-Arsenault and Mahlangu, 1999)

Maternal Perceptions of Newborn Umbilical Cord Treatments and Healing (Ford and Ritchie, 1999)

One-to-One Nurse Labor Support of Nulliparous Women Stimulated with Oxytocin (Gagnon and Waghorn, 1999)

Maternal Fatigue: Implications of Second Stage Labor Nursing Care (Gennaro et al, 1999)

Continued

| Box 8-4 | Relevant Maternal-Infant Research Article Titles in Clinical Journals—cont'd |

Mother's Perceptions of Postpartum Stress and Satisfaction (Horowitz and Damato, 1999)

The Effect of Relaxation Therapy on Preterm Labor Outcomes (Janke, 1999)

Factors Explaining the Lack of Response to Heel Stick in Preterm Newborns (Johnson et al, 1999)

Transitioning Preterm Infants with Nasogastric Tube Supplementation: Increased Likelihood of Breastfeeding (Kliethermes et al, 1999)

Clinical Issues Longitudinal Changes in Fatigue and Energy During Pregnancy and the Postpartum Period (Lee and Zaffke, 1999)

Birth-Related Fatigue in 34-36 Week Preterm Infants: Rapid Recovery with Very Early Kangaroo Care (Ludington-Hoe et al, 1999)

Parents' Perception of Skin to Skin Care with Their Preterm Infants Requiring Assisted Ventilation (Neu, 1999)

What Happens When Fatigue Lingers for 18 Months After Delivery? (Parks et al, 1999)

Physical Abuse, Social Support, Self Care and Pregnancy Outcomes of Older Adolescents (Renker, 1999)

Neonatal Network—Journal of Neonatal Nursing

Neonatal Thermoregulation: Bed Surface Transfers (Altimier et al, 1999)

The Influence of Equipment Weights on Neonatal Daily Weight (Hermansen and Hermansen, 1999)

Neonatal Skin Care: The Scientific Basis for Practice (Lund et al, 1999)

A Survey of Skin Practices for Premature Low Birth Weight Infants (Munson et al, 1999)

Suspended Mothering: Women's Experiences Mothering an Infant with a Genetic Anomaly Identified at Birth (Raines, 1999)

Pediatric Nursing

Neonatal Drug Exposure: Assessing a Specific Population and Services Provided by Visiting Nurses (Mahony and Murphy, 1999)

Weight Change of Infants, Age Birth to 12 Months, Born to Abused Women (McFarlane and Soeken, 1999)

Infant Nasal-Pharyngeal Suctioning: Is it Beneficial? (Czarnecki and Kaucic, 1999)

Reliability of Three Length Measurement Techniques in Term Infants (Johnson et al, 1999)

The scan netted 8 relevant research articles from MCN: *The American Journal of Maternal Child Nursing*, 15 articles from *Journal of Obstetric, Gynecologic and Neonatal Nursing*, 5 articles from *Neonatal Network-Journal of Neonatal Nursing*, and 4 articles from *Pediatric Nursing*.

A survey of the titles revealed 15 studies about infants, 16 on mothers or potential mothers, and 1 on fathers. The infant studies examined preterm infants 4 times and normal neonates 8 times. Two studies addressed infant complications, while prenatal care was the focus in 3 articles, labor the focus in 2 articles, and postpartum experiences the focus in 5 articles. A mix of physical, psychological, and social issues was studied. There were 6 qualitative studies, including 2 case studies. Six quantitative studies examined the effectiveness of specific nursing interventions (rocking bed, relaxation therapy, NG tube supplementation, bed surface transfers, nasal-pharyngeal suctioning, length measurement techniques). Two others examined the effectiveness of certain types of equipment used in practice (electronic thermometers, weight scales). Others examined the state of current nursing knowledge and practice (infant positioning and infant skin care). Fatigue was a favorite topic with 5 studies, and Kangaroo (skin-to-skin) care was featured in 4 studies.

Other Journals

A scattering of nine research studies pertinent to maternal-infant care were also found across various other journals. The results are listed in Box 8-5.

Some of the results are expected. Studies on infants or adolescent mothers were found in pediatric journals; mental health issues for mothers were found in *Issues in Mental Health Nursing*; an article on adolescent motherhood was discovered in the *Journal of School Nursing*; a study on care at home was located in the *Journal of Community Health Nursing*. Five of these studies used a qualitative approach, which may indicate that researchers go outside traditional research journal sources to publish the results of qualitative studies. So remember these likely ancillary sources when scanning for current maternal-infant research literature.

Summarizing and Using Scanning Results

Several of the identified research articles have been selected to serve as examples for how research articles might be summarized and how the findings could be used in clinical practice. Their reviews follow.

Box 8-5 Relevant Maternal-Infant Research Article Titles from Miscellaneous Nursing Journals

Journal of Pediatric Health Care

Do Apnea Monitors Decrease Emotional Distress in Parents of Infants at High Risk for Cardiopulmonary Arrest? (Abendroth et al, 1999)

Journal for Society of Pediatric Nurses

Conflicting Responses: The Experiences of Fathers of Infants Diagnosed with Severe Congenital Heart Disease (Clark and Miles, 1999)

Broken Past, Fragile Future: Personal Stories of High Risk Adolescent Mothers (Williams and Vines, 1999)

Journal of School Nursing

Giving Voice to Child Bearing Teens: Views on Sexuality and the Reality of Being a Young Parent (Clifford and Brykczynski, 1999)

Journal of Community Health Nursing

Postpartum Home Visits: Infant Outcomes (Frank-Hanssen, Hanson, and Anderson, 1999)

Issues in Mental Health Nursing

Depressed Adolescent Mothers' Perceptions of Their Own Maternal Role (Lesser, Koniak-Griffin, and Anderson, 1999)

Issues in Mental Health Nursing

Battering in Pregnant Latinas (Mattson and Rodriguez, 1999)

Journal of Nurse Midwifery

Spontaneous Pushing During Birth: Relationship to Perineal Outcomes (Sampselle and Hines, 1999)

Journal of Transcultural Nursing

Engaged Mothering: The Transition to Motherhood for a Group of African American Women (Sawyer, 1999)

Several articles tested nursing interventions for effectiveness. They provide concrete data about the effectiveness of certain nursing interventions used in the care of mothers and infants. One article is a pain relief study that employed a quantitative, experimental approach using 122 very low-birth-weight infants in an NICU (Stevens et al, 1999). Four different pain interventions were used on all infants after heel-stick procedures. Findings showed that pacifiers with sucrose and pacifiers with sterile water were both effective in reducing pain after a single heel stick. Prone positioning did not decrease pain. Pain was greater when infants were subjected to multiple repeated procedures. The effectiveness of the interventions after multiple repeated heel sticks was unclear and is in need of further study. Nurses working with low-birth-weight babies in an NICU might want to try the use of a pacifier to help reduce pain during and after a painful procedure. This re-search study examines several standard pain relief measures to determine which were most effective. This study gives the practicing nurse additional information about the specific effectiveness of accepted pain relief measures for low-birth-weight babies.

A second article (Fuller BF et al, 1999) also looked at infant pain and tested a specific model used in the nursing assessment of infant pain to see if nurses using it obtained an accurate assessment of infant pain. Results indicated that the nurses did use the infant pain assessment model to accurately reflect likelihood of infant pain. Nurses might use these findings in decisions about what tools to use to assess the likelihood of infant pain.

Another article examined the use of a rocking bed with maternal intrauterine sounds to decrease withdrawal symptoms and promote adaptation in infants ex-posed to drugs in utero (Dapolito, 1999). The 14 infants were kept on a rocking bed and a standard bed during withdrawal. There was a significant increase in with-drawal symptoms and sleep deprivation when the infants were on the rocking bed. This suggests that the rocking bed provides too much stimulus. This article shows that the rocking bed while useful for other infants is not helpful in decreasing with-drawal symptoms in drug-affected infants.

A fourth article that tested nursing interventions examined the effects of re-laxation therapy on preterm labor outcomes (Janke, 1999). One hundred seven women who experienced preterm labor were randomly assigned to a control group or a group receiving relaxation therapy. The results showed that women who prac-ticed relaxation had larger newborns and longer periods of pregnancy prolonga-tion. This nursing intervention is an effective and cost efficient mechanism to en-able women in preterm labor to postpone delivery.

Several articles also examined common maternal or infant problems. Postpar-tum fatigue was addressed frequently. The first article (Williams et al, 1999) was a quantitative comparative study that examined the fatigue levels of mothers with preterm infants sent home on apnea monitors. These were compared to fatigue levels of mothers with preterm infants not on monitors. Measurements were made at discharge, at 1 week, and at 1 month. The two groups had the same levels of fatigue on discharge. However as time passed the group with babies on monitors were significantly more fatigued, and the fatigue increased with time. This study shows that fatigue is a special consideration for mothers of infants on apnea monitors and that increased diligence is needed in the assessment, monitoring, and alleviation of fatigue. This data could be particularly useful for nurses who do discharge planning for mothers going home with infants on apnea monitors and for nurses in clinics, physicians offices, home care, or public health who have contact with these mothers.

A second article (Troy, 1999) examined postpartum fatigue of first time mothers in a longitudinal quantitative study that spanned a period of 19 months after birth. The study found that contrary to conventional wisdom, women do not recover from pregnancy and childbirth within 6 weeks. In fact, women in this study were more fatigued and less energetic at 14 to 19 months postpartum than they had been at 6 weeks. Quality of sleep was not related to fatigue levels. This information can be used to revamp expectations about postpartum fatigue and to extend efforts at fatigue relief.

Persistent maternal fatigue was the subject of a longitudinal quantitative study in which fatigue was measured a total of 5 times in 229 mothers for 18 months after the birth of their babies (Parks et al, 1999). Those who reported persistent fatigue also reported more health problems and slowed infant development problems. Findings indicate that fatigue can have a negative effect on maternal health and infant performance outcomes. Therefore assessment for maternal fatigue is an important part of each postpartum nursing contact, as is assisting mothers to find strategies to conserve energy and get rest.

Now you have seen several examples of how studies might be applied in maternal-infant care across various settings. Practice with some articles of your own by completing the following Student Challenge.

STUDENT CHALLENGE Using Data from Journal Scans

Use the articles that resulted from your journal scan.

1. Read the articles to determine what and who was studied and what the study results were. Write a brief summary of each article. Use the articles cited in the previous section as examples.

> **STUDENT CHALLENGE** Using Data from Journal Scans—
> cont'd
>
> 2. Read the discussion sections of articles and make a quick determination about how the results might be used in a clinical practice setting. Write out how the findings might be used and by whom.

How to Read and Evaluate a Research Article on Maternal-Infant Care

Now that you have warmed up, we are going to examine one research article on maternal-infant care in more depth. We use the research reading strategy and the research study comprehension guidelines introduced in Chapter 7.

> **STUDENT CHALLENGE** Surveying and Examining a
> Maternal-Infant Research Study
>
> 1. Log onto your CD-ROM and look for the Survey, Examine, and Critically Read exercise in Chapter 8. Print out the reading strategy and the research article entitled "Testing an Intervention to Prevent Further Abuse in Pregnant Women."
> 2. Take your text, the article, the strategy, and a notepad and pen (or your computer) and find a conducive reading and study environment.
> 3. Survey the article using the strategy guidelines. Make notes of what you gleaned from your survey.
> 4. Now go back and read the article paragraph by paragraph and jot down the key idea in each paragraph. Be sure to note anything that you don't understand. (I know this takes time and may be tedious, but trust me, it helps in the long run.)
> 5. When you have finished, consult needed references to clarify those things that are unclear.
> 6. When you have completed these steps, go back to the CD-ROM and complete the Survey, Examine, and Critically Read exercise, the Study Evaluation exercise, and the Application Visualization exercise for Chapter 8.

ADVENTURE
CD
8-1

ADVENTURE
CD
8-2

ADVENTURE
CD
8-3

The CD-ROM exercises guide you through the critical reading, evaluation, and visualization of the selected research article. When you finish you will be able to print your answers and my responses to the exercises. You should be feeling more confident about reading a research article and pulling out the key ideas.

 ## Resource Kit

Web Sources for Maternal-Infant Research Priorities
  Healthy People 2000/2010
  National Institute for Nursing Research priorities
  American Association of Women's Health, Obstetrical, and Neonatal Nurses (AWHONN) priority areas
  March of Dimes
  National Maternal and Child Health Clearinghouse

Web Sources for Relevant Journal Table of Contents and Abstracts
  Nursing Research
  Research in Nursing and Health
  Journal of Obstetric, Gynecologic, and Neonatal Nursing (JOGNN)
  MCN: The American Journal of Maternal Child Nursing

  Visit the book's MERLIN website at
  www.mosby.com/MERLIN/Langford/maze
  for further information.

References

Abendroth D et al: Do apnea monitors decrease emotional distress in parents of infants at high risk for cardiopulmonary arrest? *J Pediatr Health Care* 13(2):13, 1999.

Altimier L et al: Neonatal thermoregulation: bed surface transfers, *Neonatal Netw* 18(4):55, 1999.

AWHONN: AWHONN's Research and Grant Priorities, online at www.awhonn.org/resour/RGPPriorities.htm, April 7, 2000.

Bloom KC, Hall DS: Pregnancy wantedness in adolescents presenting for pregnancy testing, *MCN Am J Matern Child Nurs* 24(6):296, 1999.

Brandon DH, Holditch-Davis D, Beylea M: Nursing care and the development of sleeping and waking behaviors in preterm infants, *Res Nurs Health* 221(3):217, 1999.

Christiani P, Fallis WM: Neonatal axillary temperature measurements: a comparison of electronic thermometer predictive and monitor modes, *J Obstet Gynecol Neonatal Nurs* 28(4):389, 1999.

Clark SM, Miles MS: Conflicting responses: the experiences of fathers of infants diagnosed with severe congenital heart disease, *J Soc Pediatr Nurses* 4(1):7, 1999.

Clifford J, Brykczynski K: Giving voice to child bearing teens: views on sexuality and the reality of being a young parent, *J Sch Nurs* 15(1):4, 1999.

Cooney AT, Riggs MW, Walker LO: Psychological and demographic factors related to health behaviors in the first trimester, *J Obstet Gynecol Neonatal Nurs* 28(6):606, 1999.

Cote-Arsenault D, Mahlangu N: Impact of perinatal loss on subsequent pregnancy and self: women's experiences, *J Obstet Gynecol Neonatal Nurs* 28(3):274, 1999.

Czarnecki KL, Kaucic CL: Infant nasal-pharyngeal suctioning: is it beneficial? *Pediatr Nurs* 25(2):193, 1999.

Dapolito K: Comparison of a rocking bed and a standard bed decreasing withdrawal symptoms in drug exposed infants, *MCN Am J Matern Child Nurs* 24(3):138, 1999.

Davis MW et al: Living with postpartum depression: the father's experience, *MCN Am J Matern Child Nurs* 24(4):202, 1999.

Dowling DA: Physiological responses of preterm infants to breast-feeding and bottle-feeding with the orthodontic nipple, *Nurs Res* 48(2):78, 1999.

Ford LA, Ritchie JA: Maternal perceptions of newborn umbilical cord treatments and healing, *J Obstet Gynecol Neonatal Nurs* 28(5):501, 1999.

Frank-Hanssen MA, Hanson KS, Anderson MA: Postpartum home visits: infant outcomes, *J Community Health Nurs* 16(1):17, 1999.

Fuller BF et al: Testing a model of the nursing assessment of infant pain, *Clin Nurs Res* 8(1):69, 1999.

Gagnon AJ, Waghorn K: One-to-one nurse labor support of nulliparous women stimulated with oxytocin, *J Obstet Gynecol Neonatal Nurs* 28(4):371, 1999.

Gennaro S et al: Maternal fatigue: implications of second stage labor nursing care, *J Obstet Gynecol Neonatal Nurs* 28(2):175, 1999.

Hermansen MG, Hermansen MC: The influence of equipment weights on neonatal daily weight, *Neonatal Netw* 18(1):33, 1999.

Horowitz JA, Damato EG: Mother's perceptions of postpartum stress and satisfaction, *J Obstet Gynecol Neonatal Nurs* 28(6):595, 1999.

Janke J: The effect of relaxation therapy on preterm labor outcomes, *J Obstet Gynecol Neonatal Nurs* 28(3):155, 1999.

Johnson CC et al: Factors explaining the lack of response to heel stick in preterm newborns, *J Obstet Gynecol Neonatal Nurs* 28(6):587, 1999.

Johnson TS et al: Reliability of three length measurement techniques in term infants, *Pediatr Nurs* 25(1):13, 1999.

Kliethermes PA et al: Transitioning preterm infants with nasogastric tube supplementation: increased likelihood of breastfeeding, *J Obstet Gynecol Neonatal Nurs* 28(3):264, 1999.

Lee KA, Zaffke ME: Clinical issues longitudinal changes in fatigue and energy during pregnancy and the postpartum period, *J Obstet Gynecol Neonatal Nurs* 28(2):143, 1999.

Leitch DB: Mother-infant: achieving synchrony, *Nurs Res* 48(1):55, 1999.

Lesser J, Koniak-Griffin D, Anderson NLR: Depressed adolescent mothers' perceptions of their own maternal role, *Issues Mental Health Nurs* 20(2):131, 1999.

Ludington-Hoe SM et al: Birth-related fatigue in 34-36 week preterm infants: rapid recovery with very early kangaroo care, *J Obstet Gynecol Neonatal Nurs* 28(1):94, 1999.

Lund C: Prevention and management of infant skin breakdown, *Nurs Clin North Am* 34(4): 907, 1999.

Lund C et al: Neonatal skin care: the scientific basis for practice, *Neonatal Netw* 18(4):15, 1999.

Maguire DP: Skin Protection and breakdown in ELBW infant: a national survey, *Clin Nurs Res* 8(3):222, 1999.

Mahony DL, Murphy JM: Neonatal drug exposure: assessing a specific population and services provided by visiting nurses, *Pediatr Nurs* 25(1):27, 1999.

March of Dimes: FY 2000 Federal Funding Priorities, online at www.modimes.org/Public Affairs2/AdvocacyUpdate/adup0499.htm

Mattson S, Rodriguez: Battering in pregnant Latinas, *Issues Mental Health Nurs* 20(4):405, 1999.

McCain GC, Donovan E, Gartside P: Preterm infant behavioral and heart rate responses to antenatal phenobarbital, *Res Nurs Health* 221(6):461, 1999.

McFarlane J, Soeken K: Weight change of infants, age birth to 12 months, born to abused women, *Pediatr Nurs* 25(1):19, 1999.

Mikhail BI: Perceived impediments to prenatal care among low income women, *Western J Nurs Res* 21(3):335, 1999.

Miles-Shandor M et al: Distress and growth outcomes in mothers of medically fragile infants, *Nurs Res* 48(3):129, 1999.

Morin K, Gennaro S, Fehder W: Nutrition and exercise in overweight and obese postpartum women, *Appl Nurs Res* 12(1):13, 1999.

Munson KA et al: A survey of skin practices for premature low birth weight infants, *Neonatal Netw* 18(3):25, 1999.

Neu M: Parents' perception of skin to skin care with their preterm infants requiring assisted ventilation, *J Obstet Gynecol Neonatal Nurs* 28(2):157, 1999.

Parker B et al: Testing an intervention to prevent further abuse to pregnant women, *Res Nurs Health* 221(1):59, 1999.

Parks PL et al: What happens when fatigue lingers for 18 months after delivery? *J Obstet Gynecol Neonatal Nurs* 28(1):87, 1999.

Peeke K et al: Infant sleep position: nursing practice and knowledge, *MCN Am J Matern Child Nurs* 24(6):301, 1999.

Pressler JL et al: Behavioral responses of newborns of insulin-dependent and nondiabetic healthy mothers, *Clin Nurs Res* 8(2):103, 1999.

Pridham K et al: The effects of prescribed versus ad libitum feedings and formula caloric density on premature infant dietary intake and weight gain, *Nurs Res* 48(2):86, 1999.

Pridham KF, Schroeder M, Brown R: The adaptiveness of mothers working models of caregiving through the first year: infant and mother contributions, *Res Nurs Health* 221(1):471, 1999.

Raines DA: Suspended mothering: women's experiences mothering an infant with a genetic anomaly identified at birth, *Neonatal Netw* 18(5):55, 1999.

Renker PR: Physical abuse, social support, self care and pregnancy outcomes of older adolescents, *J Obstet Gynecol Neonatal Nurs* 28(4):377, 1999.

Roller CG: Kangaroo care for a restless infant with gastric reflux: one nurse midwife's personal experience, *MCN Am J Matern Child Nurs* 24(5):244, 1999.

Roller CG, Meyer K, Cranston-Anderson G: Birth kangaroo care and breastfeeding: a eclamptic woman's story, *MCN Am J Matern Child Nurs* 24(6):294, 1999.

Sampselle CM, Hines S: Research exchange: Spontaneous pushing during birth: relationship to perineal outcomes, *J Nurse Midwifery* 44(1):36, 1999.

Sawyer LM: Engaged mothering: the transition to motherhood for a group of African American women, *J Transcult Nurs* 10(1):14, 1999.

Sorenson DS, Schuelke P: Fantasies of the unborn among pregnant women, *MCN Am J Matern Child Nurs* 24(2):92, 1999.

Stevens B et al: The efficacy of developmentally sensitive interventions and sucrose for relieving procedural pain in very low birth weight neonates, *Nurs Res* 48(1):35, 1999.

Swanson KM: Effects of caring, measurement and time on miscarriage impact and women's well-being, *Nurs Res* 48(6):288, 1999.

Troy NW: A comparison of fatigue and energy levels at six weeks and 14 to 19 months postpartum, *Clin Nurs Res* 8(2):135, 1999.

U.S. Department of Health and Human Services, Public Health Service: *Healthy People 2000: national health promotion and disease prevention objectives*, Washington, DC, 1991, Author.

U.S. Department of Health and Human Services, Public Health Service: *Healthy People 2000*, online at www.odphp.osophs.dhhs.gov/pubs/hp2000, October 2, 1999.

U.S. Department of Health and Human Services, Public Health Service: *Healthy People 2010*, online at www.health.gov/healthypeople April 7, 2000.

VandeVusse L: The essential forces of labor revisited: 13 Ps reported in womens' stories, *MCN Am J Matern Child Nurs* 24(2):176, 1999.

Walker LO, Grobe JJ: The construct of thriving in pregnancy and postpartum, *Nurs Sci Q*, 12(2):151, 1999.

Walker NC, O'Brien B: The relationship between method of pain management during labor and birth outcomes, *Clin Nurs Res* 8(2):119, 1999.

White-Traut RC et al: Developmental intervention for preterm infants diagnosed with periventricular leukomalacia, *Res Nurs Health* 221(2):131, 1999.

Williams C, Vines SW: Broken past, fragile future: personal stories of high risk adolescent mothers, *J Soc Pediatr Nurses* 4(1):15, 1999.

Williams PD et al: Fatigue in mothers of infants discharged to home on apnea monitors, *Appl Nurs Res* 12(2):69, 1999.

Learning Objectives

1 Identify clinical nursing journals that publish research articles relevant to children and adolescents.

2 Discuss clinical and research priorities in the care of children and adolescents.

3 Use research literature to clarify identified clinical practice problems about children and adolescents.

4 Explore examples of research that has been conducted in various areas of clinical practice with children and adolescents.

5 Discuss application of sample research results in clinical practice.

6 Apply the reading strategy to survey, examine, critically read, and evaluate sample research articles on care of children and adolescents.

Chapter Outline

What Research Resources Are Available for Children and Adolescents?
What Approaches Can Be Used for Review of the Research Literature?
  Addressing clinical and research priorities
  Using issues that arise from clinical practice
  Scanning available resources

What Current Research Is Available?
  Nursing research journals
  Clinical nursing journals
  Other journals
  Summarizing and using scanning results
How to Read and Evaluate a Research Article on Children

Reading and Using Research in the Care of Children and Adolescents

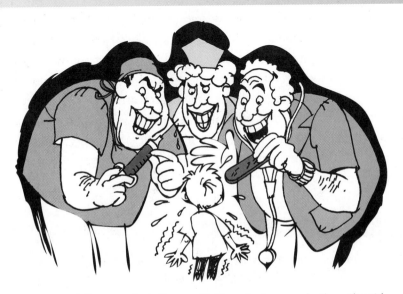

I wonder if this is what the qualitative study meant when it said that it collected the data from a child's point of view?

Student Quote   *"I read a research article about letting kids blow on a pinwheel to make getting a shot less of a big deal . . . and I tried it and it worked!"*

Abstract   Several research sources publish articles pertinent to the care of children and adolescents. These sources can be used to view identified priorities in the care and research of child and adolescent problems, address identified problems and questions uncovered in clinical practice, or to provide a broad view of currently available research about children and adolescents. An abundance of current research studies are available for use in clinical practice with children and adolescents. Samples of current studies are reported, and clinical applications are discussed. The use of the research reading strategy is presented with one research article on children.

215

In this chapter, we identify publications that contain nursing research on care of children and adolescents, explore strategies to simplify the search process and target relevant research articles, and preview sample selections of currently published research. Finally we dissect a sample article using the reading strategy and evaluation guidelines.

What Research Resources Are Available for Children and Adolescents?

To effectively view the current research in care for children and adolescents, it is helpful to be able to identify resources that are likely to contain research articles on the child and/or adolescent experience. All the research journals discussed in previous chapters contain articles on care of adolescents and children. Many clinical specialty journals also regularly publish research articles for care affecting children and adolescents. Clinical journals in other specialty areas also occasionally contain research articles relevant to children and adolescents. Box 9-1 contains a list of journals most likely to contain research relevant to the practice of nursing care for children and adolescents.

STUDENT CHALLENGE Perusing Specialty Journals

1. If any journals on the list in Box 9-1 are unfamiliar to you, take time to locate those that are available in your library. Scan two or three issues of each journal.
2. Note how they are organized. What types of articles are prevalent? Can you readily distinguish research articles from other featured articles? Do you notice a difference in the focus of the various journals?
3. Check out descriptions of the focus or purpose of any unknown journals.
4. Are some journals more readable than others? More helpful? More practical?

As you become more familiar with the various clinical and research journals, note which might provide the most useful information for improving your care to children and adolescents in various clinical settings. For example, if you are a school nurse, the *Journal of School Nursing* might be particularly helpful.

| Box 9-1 | Journals Containing Nursing Research Relevant to Care of Children and Adolescents |

Nursing Research Journals
Nursing Research
Research in Nursing and Health
Western Journal of Nursing Research
Applied Nursing Research
Clinical Nursing Research
Nursing Science Quarterly
Image: Journal of Nursing Scholarship
Scholarly Inquiry for Nursing Practice

Clinical Journals that Regularly Contain Research Articles About Care of Children and Adolescents
Issues in Comprehensive Pediatric Nursing
Journal of Child and Adolescent Psychiatric Nursing
Journal of Pediatric Health Care
Journal of Pediatric Nursing: Nursing Care of Children and Families
Journal of Pediatric Oncology Nursing
Journal of School Nursing
Journal of the Society of Pediatric Nurses
MCN: The American Journal of Maternal-Child Nursing
Pediatric Nursing

What Approaches Can Be Used for Review of the Research Literature?

In Chapter 8, we discussed three approaches to guide our use of the current research literature and help us enhance our clinical practice. These three approaches also work when searching for literature about children and adolescents. We explore the clinical and research priorities that have been identified in the care of children and adolescents; identify some example problems or questions that might arise from your routine practice with children and adolescents; and, finally, we scan the research literature and view what is available to enhance clinical practice.

Addressing Clinical and Research Priorities

Keeping informed about the current clinical and research priorities in a given area can help direct and guide your practice with whatever target population you choose to practice. Let's look at the care and research priorities for the care of children and adolescents. Health maintenance and promotion and health restoration are important goals in the care of children and adolescents. Children under the age of 5 use the health care system more than any other age group except for those 65 years of age and older.

Healthy People 2000 details several health care goals and objectives pertinent to children and adolescents. These objectives are geared toward health care prevention. Pertinent *Healthy People 2000* objectives are listed in Box 9-2.

Box 9-2 *Healthy People 2000* Objectives Related to Child and Adolescent Care

- Reduce number of overweight adolescents
- Increase exercise and leisure activities in children and adolescents
- Improve dietary intake for children and adolescents
- Reduce iron deficiency in children
- Reduce initiation and use of tobacco, alcohol, and drugs among adolescents
- Reduce child exposure to tobacco smoke in home
- Reduce steroid use among adolescent males
- Reduce sexual activity among adolescents
- Reduce suicide attempts among adolescents
- Reduce mental disorders among children and adolescents
- Reduce violent and abusive behavior toward children and adolescents
- Reduce violent behavior by adolescents
- Reduce deaths related to injury among children and adolescents
- Increase use of child safety seats, seat belts, and bicycle helmets.
- Reduce prevalence of mental retardation among children
- Reduce prevalence of lead poisoning among children
- Reduce childhood dental caries
- Reduce infectious diarrhea among children
- Reduce middle ear infections among children
- Increase immunization levels

From U.S. Department of Health and Human Services, Public Health Service: *Healthy People 2000: national health promotion and disease prevention objectives*, Washington, DC, 1991, Author.

The research priorities of the National Institute for Nursing Research (NINR) identified in Chapter 4 also included issues related to care of children and adolescents, such as health promotion. In the year 2000, the NINR identified two priorities that were directly targeted at children. The first was managing asthma symptoms in children, and the second was acute care of children with posttraumatic brain injury.

Other issues viewed as high priority in the provision of care to children and adolescents include immunization, nutrition, substance use, safety (injuries are the leading cause of disability and death for children and adolescents), child abuse and neglect, and sexuality. As you can see, these priorities may assist you in identifying areas of concern in your own nursing practice with children.

STUDENT CHALLENGE Checking Child and Adolescent Care Priorities

Activity
15

1. Check the *Healthy People 2010* goals and objectives that are presented on the *Healthy People 2010* website. (Refer to the Resource Kit at the end of this chapter to access this website.) Locate the objectives relevant to maternal infant care. Compare them to the objectives in Box 8-2. Note similarities and differences.
2. Check the NINR research priorities for 2000 to the present from the NINR website. (Refer to the Resource Kit to access this website.) Have any new areas been added that affect care for children or adolescents?
3. Can you locate any other sources that list or discuss priorities in care or research of children or adolescents?
4. Choose one of the priority areas listed or that you have discovered. Run a literature search for the years 2000 to present and see what if any nursing research has been conducted in your selected area. Did you find anything that might be applicable to the care of children and adolescents?

Using Issues that Arise from Clinical Practice

We look at two examples of clinical questions or problems that might arise during routine clinical practice and review the current research literature that might be helpful in addressing the identified problem. As a problem surfaces, you first need to define it by certain parameters to provide a clear frame of reference from which to think about nursing care. It can make the search and use of research materials much easier. Ask yourself the following questions: Who is the target of care—a toddler, preschooler, school-aged child, or adolescent; parents, siblings, or family? What level of care is involved (i.e., does the problem require health maintenance or prevention, acute care, or chronic care)? The aspect of care is also important. Are you concerned with physical, psychological, sociocultural, or spiritual needs? How do developmental and maturational issues come into play? Finally what care setting did the problem arise in—a clinic, physician's office, home, school, or hospital?

For example, I may be a nurse in a pediatric clinic where many children with asthma are treated. I notice that many of the children and their families have trouble keeping their asthma under control. I wonder if any research is available that would shed light on how to assist children to more successfully follow their treatment protocols. I am interested in toddlers through adolescents. This is a health maintenance/illness prevention problem. Developmental issues might have an effect on interventions.

I do a CINAHL search using the key words "asthma" and "children." I limit the search to the years 1997 to 1999 and to research. I get 11 citations. Only one was from a nursing journal, and it examined mothers' uncertainty of care in asthmatic children prior to diagnosis. The other 10 studies detailed various medical treatments. I drop the research limitation and get an additional seven studies. Three of these were pertinent to nurse interventions in asthma management. Two of these discussed current general management strategies for asthma, and one discussed emergency management measures during an acute attack. No information was obtained on successful maintenance of treatment protocols. Perhaps this is why this topic is on the NINR research priority list.

I work as a pediatric rehabilitation nurse in an acute rehabilitation center and want to update my knowledge on nursing care for children with head trauma. I am interested in all ages of children and adolescents and am looking for research that addresses all care aspects (physical, psychological, sociocultural, developmental, or spiritual). A CINAHL search using the keywords "head injury" and "children" with a 3-year limit yielded a total of seven related nursing articles. None were reports of research studies. Four studies spoke to the acute management of children with head injury. None of the studies shed any new light on nursing rehabilitation interventions. A review of nursing responsibilities serves to reassure me that my clinical practices are current.

As with the maternal-infant examples, identification of clinical problems in child health often sheds more light on the research that still needs to be conducted rather than the research that is available. Literature searches targeted at specifically identified clinical problems can still prove worthwhile and may provide much needed help for a vexing clinical situation.

STUDENT CHALLENGE Chasing Pediatric Challenges

1. Review your experiences in caring for children and think about a situation that you wish to explore in the current research literature.
2. Identify appropriate search parameters for the subject material and conduct a library search for the year 2000 to present. What did you find?
3. If your search was fruitful, retrieve one or two promising articles.
4. Review the articles. How might the results of the studies be helpful in clinical practice?

Scanning Available Resources

Let's explore what is available in the pediatric research literature when we use our third strategy and scan the table of contents and the abstracts of the research and clinical specialty journals listed in Box 9-1. Do the following Student Challenge to explore a sample of what is currently available. Then continue reading to see what a scan of articles in the year 1999 reveals. Check out the Resource Kit at the end of this chapter to find websites that allow you to see the tables of contents and abstracts for relevant journals.

Merlin
Activity
16

STUDENT CHALLENGE Scanning Pediatric Journals

Select one research journal and one clinical journal from those listed in Box 9-1 that are available in your library.

1. Scan the 2000 table of contents for each of these journals and note those articles that seem relevant to maternal care of children and adolescents.
2. Read the abstracts for the selected articles. Weed out any articles that are not clinically relevant. How long did this take you? Was the task easier this time than when you tried it for Chapter 8? Save these articles. We will use them again in the next exercise.

What Current Research Is Available?

The following are specific examples of pertinent research articles on the care of children and adolescents that I found by scanning the 1999 tables of contents of the research and clinical journals listed in Box 9-1. Selected articles are briefly summarized and clinical implications are discussed. The articles are arranged by journal. This allows you to see which of the journals might provide you with the most insight about various pediatric clinical topics.

Nursing Research Journals

The articles found by scanning the tables of contents of the various research journals yielded the pediatric article titles listed in Box 9-3.

Box 9-3 **Relevant Pediatric Article Titles in Research Journals**

Nursing Research

Alternate Child Care, History of Hospitalization and Preschool Child Behavior (Brooten and Youngblut, 1999)

Effects of Distraction on Children's Pain and Distress During Medical Procedures: A Meta-Analysis (Kleiber and Harper, 1999)

Diagnosis Disclosure by Family Caregivers to Children Who Have Perinatally Acquired HIV Disease: When the Time Comes (Ledlie, 1999)

Symptom Perception and Evaluation in Childhood Asthma (McMullen and Yoos, 1999)

An Empirical Test of Alternate Theories of Anger in Early Adolescents (Yarcheski, Mahon, and Yarcheski, 1999)

Research in Nursing and Health

Behavior Problems Among Young Children in Low-Income Urban Day Care Centers (Gross, Sambrook, and Fogg, 1999)

Medical and Ecological Factors in Estimating Motor Outcomes of Preschool Children (McGrath and Sullivan, 1999)

Maternal Perceptions of Family Provider Relationships and Well-Being in Families of Children with Down Syndrome (Van Riper, 1999)

Western Journal of Nursing Research

Parent-Teen Worry About Teens Contracting AIDS (Carroll et al, 1999)

Parent Child Interactions and Development of Toddlers Born Preterm (Magill-Evans and Harrison, 1999)

| Box 9-3 | Relevant Pediatric Article Titles in Research Journals—cont'd |

Parents Call for Concerned and Collaborative Care (Stubblefield and Murray, 1999)

Proximal and Distal Correlates of Maternal Control Style (Sullivan and McGrath, 1999)

Life Histories of Rural Mexican American Adolescents Experiencing Abuse (Champion, 1999)

The Moderator-Mediator Role of Social Support on Early Adolescents (Yarcheski and Mahon, 1999)

Effects of Traumatic Events, Social Support, and Self-Efficacy on Adolescents' Self-Health Assessments (Cheever and Hardin, 1999)

Perceptions About Substance Abuse Among Male Adolescents in Juvenile Detention (Anderson, 1999)

Cross-Cultural Study of Beliefs About Smoking Among Teenaged Females (Hanson, 1999)

Hopefulness and Its Characteristics in Adolescents with Cancer (Hinds et al, 1999)

Applied Nursing Research

Preparing Parents for Their Child's Transfer from the PICU to the Pediatric Floor (Bouve, Rozmus, and Giordano, 1999)

Coping Skills Training for Youths with Diabetes on Intensive Therapy (Grey et al, 1999)

Scholarly Inquiry for Nursing Practice

Evaluating the Outcomes of Parent-Child Family Life Education (Anderson NL et al, 1999)

Image: Journal of Nursing Scholarship

Adolescent Resilience (Hunter and Chandler, 1999)

Religious Faith in Mexican-American Families Dealing with Chronic Childhood Illness (Rehm, 1999)

Clinical Nursing Research

No relevant articles

Nursing Science Quarterly

No relevant articles

A scan revealed 5 relevant articles in *Nursing Research*, 3 articles in *Research in Nursing and Health*, 10 articles in *Western Journal of Nursing Research*, 2 articles in *Applied Nursing Research*, 1 article in *Scholarly Inquiry for Nursing Practice*, and 2 articles from *Image: Journal of Nursing Scholarship*. No relevant articles were found in *Nursing Science Quarterly* or *Clinical Nursing Research*.

Examining the titles of the articles from all the research journals reveals a total of 23 articles. Five of these articles used children as subjects, 4 used mothers or families of children as subjects, 3 used parent-child interaction dyads, and 10 reported on issues affecting adolescents. The *Western Journal of Nursing Research* devoted an entire issue to research on adolescents. You might also recall that several articles reported in Chapter 8 used adolescents as subjects.

Psychological/behavioral issues are addressed (e.g., anger and hopefulness in adolescents, behavior problems in young children, issues of maternal control, coping and resilience in adolescents). Developmental issues are studied (e.g., motor outcomes in preschoolers, development of preterm toddlers), as are spiritual concerns (religious faith and coping with chronic childhood illness). Specific nursing interventions are explored in studies on distraction and pain, preparation of families for pediatric intensive care unit (PICU) transfer, outcomes of parent-child life education, and training in coping skills for diabetic adolescents.

Clinical Nursing Journals

The articles found by scanning the tables of contents of the clinical journals yielded several possibly relevant pediatric research articles as listed in Box 9-4.

Nine clinical journals regularly publish research on care of children and adolescents. Six of these journals publish a wide variety of research results across the pediatric spectrum, while three journals—*Journal of Child and Adolescent Psychiatric Nursing*, *Journal of Pediatric Oncology Nursing*, *Journal of School Nursing*—are highly specialized. Our scan netted six relevant research articles from *Issues in Comprehensive Pediatric Nursing*, six from the *Journal of Child and Adolescent Psychiatric Nursing*, seven from the *Journal of Pediatric Health Care*, four from the *Journal of Pediatric Nursing: Nursing Care of Children and Families*, seven from the *Journal of Pediatric Oncology Nursing*, seven from the *Journal of School Nursing*, four from the *Journal of Society of Pediatric Nurses*, four from *MCN: The American Journal of Maternal Child Nursing*, and eight from *Pediatric Nursing*.

A survey of the titles revealed 17 studies about children; 13 on adolescents; 4 on children and adolescents; 12 on mothers, parents, or families of children or

Box 9-4   Relevant Child and Adolescent Research Articles in Clinical Journals

Issues in Comprehensive Pediatric Nursing

Self-Esteem Changes in Children Enrolled in Weight Management Programs (Cameron, 1999)

The Measurement of Child Characteristics from Infancy to Toddlerhood (Houck, 1999)

"Good Little Girls": Reports of Pregnant Adolescents and Those Who Know Them Best (Ivey, 1999)

Self-Care Agency and Self-Care Practice of Adolescents (Slusher, 1999)

Identification of Nurse-Family Intervention Sites to Decrease Health Related Family Boundary Ambiguity in PICU (Tomlinson, Swiggum, and Harbough, 1999)

Measuring the Compliance Behavior of Adolescents Wearing Orthopedic Braces (Vandal, Rivard, and Bradet, 1999)

Journal of Child and Adolescent Psychiatric Nursing

Childhood Memories About Food: The Successful Dieters Project (Brink, Ferguson, and Sharma, 1999)

Homeless Parents Perceptions of Parenting Stress (Gorzka, 1999)

Self-Protection in Adolescents in Foster Care (Kools, 1999)

Nurse-Parent Relationship Building in Child Psychiatric Units (Scharer, 1999b)

Eating Disorder in a 10-Year-Old Girl (Scharer, 1999a)

Pharmacology in Children and Adolescents with Pervasive Developmental Disorders (Scahill and Koenig, 1999)

Journal of Pediatric Health Care

Maternal Perspectives of Lead Poisoning in Children with Normal and Elevated Lead Levels (Anderson RL et al, 1999)

Playing for Time: Adolescent Perspectives on Lung Transplantation for Cystic Fibrosis (Christian, D'Auria, and Moore, 1999)

School Age Children's Fears, Anxiety, and Human Figure Drawings (Carroll and Ryan-Wenger, 1999)

Children's Responses to Sequential Versus Simultaneous Immunization Injections (Horn and McCarthy, 1999)

Risk Taking in Young Hispanic Children (Kennedy and Rodriguez, 1999)

The Effect of Newborn Early Discharge Follow-Up Program on Pediatric Urgent Care Utilization (Nelson, 1999)

A Descriptive Study of Missed Appointments: Families Perceptions of Barriers to Care (Pesata, Pallija, and Webb, 1999)

Continued

| Box 9-4 | Relevant Child and Adolescent Research Articles in Clinical Journals—cont'd |

Journal of Pediatric Nursing: Nursing Care of Children and Families

An Adolescent and Young Adult Condom Self-Efficacy Scale (Hanna, 1999)

Adolescent Sexuality and Sexually Transmitted Diseases: Attitudes, Beliefs, Knowledge, and Values (Johnson, Rozmas, and Edmisson, 1999)

Mothers' Experiences of Living Worried When Parenting Children with Spina Bifida (Monsen, 1999)

Hispanic Mothers' Knowledge and Care of Their Children with Respiratory Illness: A Pilot Study (Robledo, Wilson, and Gray, 1999)

Journal of Pediatric Oncology Nursing

Venipuncture Versus Central Venous Access: A Comparison of Methotrexate Levels in Pediatric Leukemia Patients (Cash, Schafhauser, and Byers, 1999)

Palatability and Cost Comparison of Five Liquid Corticosteroid Formulations (Hutto and Bratton, 1999)

Leisure-Time Physical Activity and Psychological Well-Being in Adolescents After Cancer Diagnosis (Keats et al, 1999)

Parent Coping and Child Distress Behaviors During Invasive Procedures for Childhood Cancer (LaMontagne et al, 1999)

Preferences for Participation in Treatment Decision Making and Information Needs of Parents of Children with Cancer: A Pilot Study (Pyke-Grimm et al, 1999)

Swimming and Central Venous Catheter-Related Infections on the Child with Cancer (Robbins, Cromwell, and Korones, 1999)

Becoming a Cancer Patient: A Study of Families of Children with Acute Lymphocytic Leukemia (Tarr and Pickler, 1999)

Journal of School Nursing

Giving Voice to Childbearing Teens: Views on Sexuality and the Reality of Being a Young Parent (Clifford and Brykczynski, 1999)

National Survey to Identify the Nursing Interventions Used in School Settings (Cavendish et al, 1999)

Cardiovascular Risk Prevalence Among Diverse School-Age Children: Implications for Schools (Cowell, Warren, and Montgomery, 1999)

Nursing Interventions Used in School Nursing Practice (Pavelka, McCarthy, and Denehy, 1999)

| Box 9-4 | Relevant Child and Adolescent Research Articles in Clinical Journals—cont'd |

Journal of Society of Pediatric Nurses

Examination of Gavage Tube Placement in Children (Ellett and Beckstrand, 1999)

Using Parents' Concerns to Detect and Address Developmental and Behavioral Problems (Glasco, 1999)

Parent Behavior and Child Distress During Urethral Catheterizations (Kleiber and McCarthy, 1999)

Broken Past, Fragile Future: Personal Stories of High Risk Adolescents (Williams and Vines, 1999)

MCN: The American Journal of Maternal Child Nursing

Camp Superteens: An Asthma Education Program for Adolescents (Alaniz and Nordstrand, 1999)

Pregnancy Wantedness in Adolescents Presenting for Pregnancy Testing (Bloom and Hall, 1999)

A Study of Self-Perception in Hyperactive Children (Dumas and Pelletier, 1999)

Assessment of Stature in Children with Orofacial Clefting (Rezvan et al, 1999)

Pediatric Nursing

A Survey of Nursing Practice in the Assessment and Management of Pain in Children (Jacob and Puntillo, 1999)

The Impact of a Chronic Condition on the Families of Children with Asthma (Kurnat and Moore, 1999)

Health Promotion and Injury Prevention Behaviors of Elementary School Children (Polivka and Ryan-Wagner, 1999)

Bibliotherapy: Using Fiction to Help Children in Two Populations Discuss Feelings (Amer, 1999)

School-Age Child and Adolescent Perception of Pain Intensity Associated with Three-Word Descriptors (LaFleur and Raway, 1999)

Accuracy of Tympanic Temperature Readings in Children Under 6 Years of Age (Lanham et al, 1999)

Health Assessment in Child Care Centers: Parent and Staff Perceptions (Alkon and Boyce, 1999)

The Effect of Diabetes on Adolescents' Quality of Life (Faro, 1999) adolescents; and 2 on parent-child interactions. The child studies addressed psychological and behavioral issues, physical issues, and nursing interventions. The adolescent studies were heavily invested in psychological issues, particularly those surrounding sexuality. The studies addressing parent and parent-child issues covered various topics, including parental worry, anxiety, and coping over children with various illnesses and parental perceptions of care and care utilization.

Other Journals

Seven research studies pertinent to the care of children or adolescents were found among various other journals. The results can be viewed in Box 9-5.

Box 9-5   Relevant Pediatric Research Articles from Miscellaneous Nursing Journals

Qualitative Health Research

The Technology-Dependent Child and the Socially Marginalized Family: A Provisional Framework (Cohen, 1999)

Dimensions of Critical Care Nursing

Patterns of Parental Stress in PICU Emergency Admission (Huckabay and Tilem-Kessler, 1999)

Issues in Mental Health Nursing

Depressed Adolescent Mothers' Perceptions of Their Own Maternal Role (Lesser, Koniak-Griffin, and Anderson, 1999)

Optimism and Its Relationship to Depression, Coping, Anger, and Life Events in Rural Adolescents (Puskar et al, 1999b)

AORN

Clinical Impact of Perioperative Respiratory Syncytial Virus Testing (Manworren et al, 1999)

Journal of Advanced Nursing

The Impact of Knowing Your Child Is Critically Ill: A Qualitative Study Of Mothers' Experiences (Noyes, 1999)

Journal of Community Health Nursing

Health Concerns and Risk Behaviors of Rural Adolescents (Puskar et al, 1999a)

Three of the studies addressed various adolescent problems, including sexuality, childbearing, motherhood, depression, coping, anger, and risk behaviors. Three other studies focused on the families or parents of acutely or chronically ill children. The final study focused on the effect of nursing interventions on recovery in children. Four of the studies took place in a community setting and four were in an acute care setting. Three of the studies used qualitative research methodologies, while the remainder employed quantitative methodologies.

These studies are reported in six different journals. The focus of the article was consistent with the focus of the journal, with age as a secondary factor. For example, a study on adolescent depression was reported in *Issues in Mental Health Nursing*, and issues of parental stress in emergency PICU admissions were reported in *Dimensions of Critical Care*. So when you are searching for research for a particular pediatric problem, scan journals that cover specialty issues such as critical care, emergency care, cancer, school health, or community health, as well as the age-specific clinical journals.

Summarizing and Using Scanning Results

Several of the identified research articles have been selected to serve as examples for how research articles might be summarized and the findings used in clinical practice. Several articles tested nursing interventions for effectiveness. They provide concrete data about the effectiveness of certain nursing interventions used in the care of children, adolescents, or their families. We look at several of these articles in more depth.

The first article examined the effects of distraction on children's pain and distress during medical procedures using a meta-analysis* technique (Kleiber and Harper, 1999). A total of 16 studies on distress behavior (491 subjects) and 10 studies on pain (535 subjects) were analyzed. The results showed that distraction had a positive effect on children's distress behavior. These results were influenced by the age of the child and the type of procedure being performed. Children under age 7 were more affected by distraction, and distraction was less effective as the procedure became more painful. The bottom line is distraction is an effective nursing intervention.

*Explanatory note: Meta-analysis is a specialized statistical technique that combines and examines the statistical outcomes of several similar research studies. This allows a better and more objective integration of the findings of existing studies. It helps increase overall sample size and scope of the characteristics of a sample. This technique produces results that provide a sound basis for making changes in clinical practice. So anytime you spot a meta-analysis of multiple nursing studies, take advantage of it.

Another article (Anderson NL et al, 1999) examined the effects of a life education program on parent-child communication and risky sexual behavior for 251 school-aged children and young adolescents (ages 9 to 14) in several diverse communities in Los Angeles County. The study used an experimental longitudinal design as the fundamental design and a qualitative analysis as a secondary approach. (Remember, this use of both qualitative and quantitative methods is known as *triangulation.*) Communication did improve, and sexual behaviors were delayed immediately after the education intervention. However, the effects had disappeared 1 year after the intervention. Results suggest that nurse clinicians who implement family life education programs must do so on an ongoing basis. Other strategies that flowed from the qualitative data were also discussed. Any school or community health nurse who is contemplating the use of such a program would find this study helpful in design, implementation, and evaluation.

A third article (Cameron, 1999) reported on self-esteem levels in obese children enrolled in weight management programs. The quantitative study compared the self-concept of 54 obese children aged 10 to 15 enrolled in a weight management program with 60 children not in the program. The two groups were similar in age, weight, body mass, and self-concept scores at the start of the study. After 12 weeks and the completion of the weight management program by one group, neither group showed a change in weight or body mass. There was no change in self-concept for the control group. However, self-concept in the group that attended the weight management program was significantly decreased. This study suggests that weight management programs may put children at risk for lowered self-concept and may not produce desired weight loss results. Nurses might exercise caution in referring children to weight management programs without proven results that they are effective with children.

Another study (Horn and McCarthy, 1999) used a quantitative experimental approach to see if sequential versus simultaneous injection of immunizations made a difference in distress behaviors and perceived distress in 46 children (4 to 6 years old) getting routine prekindergarten examinations. Subjects were randomly assigned to the sequential or the simultaneous group. Distress perceptions and distress behaviors did not differ for either group. However, parents preferred the simultaneous method. Neither method affected distress behaviors, so nurses might ask parents which method they prefer when giving routine immunizations that can be combined.

Two studies from the *Pediatric Oncology* journal tested interventions for children with cancer. The first of these studies (Cash, Schafhauser, and Byers, 1999) examined whether methotrexate (MTX) levels differed in children with acute lymphocytic leukemia (ALL) when the blood sample was taken from a central venous line (CVC) or via venipuncture. A convenience sample of 33 peak and 33 trough levels were measured using both venipuncture and CVC collection methods for each level measured. Differences in the two collection methods for either the peak or the trough levels were not significant. However, the values of the CVC-drawn trough levels would have altered the clinical management in five of 33 cases. This alteration would not have been made if using the trough levels from a venipuncture. The study recommended that all MTX levels be drawn from the CVC, but trough levels that would alter clinical management should be verified by venipuncture. This method would minimize the number of venipunctures for children with ALL. This study demonstrates a way for nurses to minimize the number of painful venipunctures needed. Results should be used with caution because of the sample size and the convenience sampling technique. However, the study recommendation includes a safety check to ensure proper clinical management. Nurses who work regularly with children with ALL might wish to explore this option in their own clinical setting.

A second cancer study (Hutto and Bratton, 1999) examined the palatability and costs of five commonly used liquid corticosteroid formulations. Corticosteroids are common in cancer treatment of children and are often hard to administer because of the associated bad taste. The study took place in a large cancer center in Dallas. Results showed that the most palatable liquid was also the most cost-efficient. Nurses armed with these results might influence physician-prescribing habits to get the most palatable and cost-efficient liquid formulation.

A final study (Ellett and Beckstand, 1999) examined screening methods for checking placement of gavage tubes in hospitalized children. Tube placement was assessed across time for 39 children. Three screening methods were tested and compared to radiographs. Tube placement errors were made at least once during the observation period in 43.5% of the tubes. The occurrence of error was especially high for initial tube placement. Study results suggest that radiographic methods be used to confirm initial tube placement. Implications for practice suggest that radiography is the only safe way to check gavage tube placements.

Let's examine several of the qualitative studies that I found in the scanning process. A study by Stubblefield and Murray (1999) used a phenomenological approach to investigate 15 parents' perceptions and expectations of health care providers during their children's lung transplant experiences. An unstructured interview technique was used. The study resulted in the identification of two themes: concerned care and collaborative care. Concerned care included the need to be treated as an individual, the need to see familiar faces, a need to feel that their children really mattered, and a fear of feeling abandoned. There was a value placed on continuity of care. Collaborative care included parent desires to be a part of the team and a fear of being caught in the middle between the health care giver and their child. Humanistic nursing theory was used to link study results to nursing practice. This study provides a clear perspective of parental perceptions, fears, and needs, and provides direction for a humanistic approach to nursing care.

A descriptive qualitative study (Ivey, 1999) examined the lives of eight pregnant adolescents (four Caucasian and four African-American) and their mothers using interviews. The mothers viewed the girls as mature and obedient, and they were unaware that the girls were sexually active before the pregnancy. The description of the teens was "good little girls" who were not seen as being at risk for becoming pregnant. These findings might be used for early identification of adolescent girls at risk for becoming pregnant and directing preventive measures appropriately.

A phenomenological study described the lived experience of 13 mothers of adolescents with spina bifida (Monsen, 1999). An unstructured interview was used to collect data. A pattern of "living worried" emerged with two themes. One theme was treating their disabled teens like other nondisabled children. The second theme was to stay in the struggle. The findings of this study show that nurses can use narratives to create supportive relationships with mothers of children with disabilities.

Now that you have seen several examples of how quantitative and qualitative studies might be applied in the care of children and adolescents, practice with some articles of your own by completing the following Student Challenge.

STUDENT CHALLENGE Using Data from Journal Scans

Use the articles that resulted from your journal scan.

1. Read the articles to determine what was studied, who was studied, and what the study results were. Write a brief summary of each article. Use the articles cited as examples in the previous section.

2. Read the discussion sections of articles and make a quick determination about how the results might be used in a clinical practice setting. Write out how the findings might be used and by whom.

How to Read and Evaluate a Research Article on Children

In this section, we examine in more depth one quantitative research article on a pediatric intervention. We again use the research reading strategy and the research study comprehension guidelines discussed in Chapter 7.

STUDENT CHALLENGE Surveying and Examining a Pediatric Research Study

1. Log onto your CD-ROM and find the Survey, Examine, and Critically Read exercise in Chapter 9. Print out the reading strategy and the research article entitled "Children's Responses to Immunization: Lullabies as a Distraction."

2. Take your text, the article, the strategy, and a notepad and pen and find a conducive reading and study environment.

3. Survey the article using the strategy guidelines. Make notes of what you gleaned from your survey.

4. Now go back and read the article paragraph by paragraph and jot down the key idea in each paragraph. Note anything that you don't understand.

5. When you have finished, consult needed references to clarify those things that are unclear.

6. When you have completed these steps, go back to the CD-ROM and complete the rest of the Survey, Examine, and Critically Read exercise, the Study Evaluation exercise, and the Application Visualization exercise for Chapter 9.

ADVENTURE CD 9-1

ADVENTURE CD 9-2

ADVENTURE CD 9-3

These exercises guide you through the critical reading, evaluation, and visualization of the selected research article. When you finish, print out your answers and my responses to the exercises. You should be feeling more confident about reading a research article and pulling out the key ideas.

Resource Kit

Web Sources for Child and Adolescent Research Priorities

Healthy People 2000/2010
National Institute for Nursing Research

Web Sources for Relevant Journal Table of Contents and Abstracts

Nursing Research
Research in Nursing and Health
Issues in Comprehensive Pediatric Nursing
Journal of Child and Adolescent Psychiatric Nursing
Journal of Pediatric Health Care
Journal of Pediatric Oncology Nursing
Journal of Society of Pediatric Nurses
MCN: The American Journal of Maternal Child Nursing
The *Journal of Child and Family Studies* is an excellent source for examples of how research has been used in particular clinical settings.

 Visit the book's MERLIN website at **www.mosby.com/MERLIN/Langford/maze** for further information.

 Check out the exercises on your **CD-ROM.**

References

Alaniz KL, Nordstrand J: Camp superteens: an asthma education program for adolescents, *MCN Am J Matern Child Nurs* 24(3):133, 1999.

Alkon A, Boyce JC: Health assessment in child care centers: parent and staff perceptions, *Pediatr Nurs* 25(4):439, 1999.

Amer K: Bibliotherapy: using fiction to help children in two populations discuss feelings, *Pediatr Nurs* 25(1):91, 1999.

Anderson NLR: Perceptions about substance abuse among male adolescents in juvenile detention, *West J Nurs Res* 21(5):652, 1999.

Anderson NL et al: Evaluating the outcomes of parent-child family life education, *Sch Inq Nurs Pract* 13(3):211, 1999.

Anderson RL et al: Maternal perspectives of lead poisoning in children with normal and elevated lead levels, *J Pediatr Health Care* 13(4):178, 1999.

Bloom KC, Hall DS: Pregnancy wantedness in adolescents presenting for pregnancy testing, *MCN Am J Matern Child Nurs* 24(6):296, 1999.

Bouve LR, Rozmus CL, Giordano P: Preparing parents for their child's transfer from the PICU to the pediatric floor, *Appl Nurs Res* 12(3):114, 1999.

Brink PJ, Ferguson K, Sharma A: Childhood memories about food: the successful dieters project, *J Child Adolesc Psychiatr Nurs* 12(1):17, 1999.

Brooten DA, Youngblut J: Alternate child care, history of hospitalization and preschool child behavior, *Nurs Res* 48(1):29, 1999.

Cameron JW: Self-esteem changes in children enrolled in weight management programs, *Issues Comp Pediatr Nurs* 22(2):75, 1999.

Carroll MK, Ryan-Wenger NA: School age children's fears, anxiety, and human figure drawings, *J Pediatr Health Care* 13(1):24, 1999.

Carroll RM et al: Parent-teen worry about teens contracting AIDS, *West J Nurs Res* 21(2):143, 1999.

Cash M, Schafhauser B, Byers JF: Venipuncture versus central venous access: a comparison of methotrexate levels in pediatric leukemia patients, *J Pediatr Oncol Nurs* 16(4):189, 1999.

Cavendish R et al: National survey to identify the nursing interventions used in school settings, *J Sch Nurs* 15(2):14, 1999.

Champion JD: Life histories of rural Mexican American adolescents experiencing abuse, *West J Nurs Res* 21(5):699, 1999.

Cheever KH, Hardin SB: Effects of traumatic events, social support, and self efficacy on adolescents' self-health assessments, *West J Nurs Res* 21(5):673, 1999.

Christian BJ, D'Auria JP, Moore CB: Playing for time: adolescent perspectives on lung transplantation for cystic fibrosis, *J Pediatr Health Care* 13(3 part 1):120, 1999.

Clifford J, Brykczynski K: Giving voice to childbearing teens: views on sexuality and the reality of being a young parent, *J Sch Nurs* 15(1):4, 1999.

Cohen MH: The technology-dependent child and the socially marginalized family: a provisional framework, *Qual Health Res* 9(5):654, 1999.

Cowell JM, Warren JS, Montgomery AC: Cardiovascular risk prevalence among diverse school-age children: implications for schools, *J Sch Nurs* 15(2):8, 1999.

Dumas D, Pelletier L: A study of self-perception in hyperactive children, *MCN Am J Matern Child Nurs* 24(1):12, 1999.

Ellett MLC, Beckstrand J: Examination of gavage tube placement in children, *J Soc Pediatr Nurses* 4(2):51, 1999.

Faro B: The effect of diabetes on adolescents quality of life, *Pediatr Nurs* 25(3):247, 1999.

Glascoe FP: Using parents' concerns to detect and address developmental and behavioral problems, *J Soc Pediatr Nurses* 4(1):24, 1999.

Gorzka PA: Homeless parents perceptions of parenting stress, *J Child Adolesc Psychiatr Nurs* 12(1):7, 1999.

Grey M et al: Coping skills training for youths with diabetes on intensive therapy, *Appl Nurs Res* 12(1):3, 1999.

Gross D, Sambrook A, Fogg L: Behavior problems among young children in low-income urban day care centers, *Res Nurs Health* 221(1):15, 1999.

Hanna KM: An adolescent and young adult condom self-efficacy scale, *J Pediatr Nurs* 14(1):59, 1999.

Hanson MJS: Cross-cultural study of beliefs about smoking among teenaged females, *West J Nurs Res* 21(5):635, 1999.

Hinds PS et al: Hopefulness and its characteristics in adolescents with cancer, *West J Nurs Res* 21(5):600, 1999.

Horn MI, McCarthy AM: Children's responses to sequential versus simultaneous immunization injections, *J Pediatr Health Care* 13(1):18, 1999.

Houck GM: The measurement of child characteristics from infancy to toddlerhood, *Issues Comp Pediatr Nurs* 22(2):101, 1999.

Huckabay LMD, Tilem-Kessler D: Patterns of parental stress in PICU emergency admission, *DCCN* 18(2):36, 1999.

Hunter AJ, Chandler GE: Adolescent resilience, *Image J Nurs Schol* 31(3):243, 1999.

Hutto CJ, Bratton TH: Palatability and cost comparison of five liquid corticosteroid formulations, *J Pediatr Oncol Nurs* 16(2):74, 1999.

Ivey JB: "Good little girls": reports of pregnant adolescents and those who know them best, *Issues Comp Pediatr Nurs* 22(2):87, 1999.

Jacob E, Puntillo KA: A survey of nursing practice in the assessment and management of pain in children, *Pediatr Nurs* 25(3):278,1999.

Johnson LS, Rozmas C, Edmisson K: Adolescent sexuality and sexually transmitted diseases: attitudes, beliefs, knowledge, and values, *J Pediatr Nurs* 14(3):177, 1999.

Keats MR et al: Leisure-time physical activity and psychological well-being in adolescents after cancer diagnosis, *J Pediatr Oncol Nurs* 16(4):180, 1999.

Kennedy CM, Rodriguez DA: Risk taking in young Hispanic children, *J Pediatr Health Care* 13(3 part 1):126, 1999.

Kleiber C, Harper DC: Effects of distraction on children's pain and distress during medical procedures: a meta-analysis, *Nurs Res* 48(1):44, 1999.

Kleiber C, McCarthy AM: Parent behavior and child distress during urethral catheterizations, *J Soc Pediatr Nurses* 4(3):95, 1999.

Kools S: Self-protection in adolescents in foster care, *J Child Adolesc Psychiatr Nurs* 12(4):139, 1999.

Kurnat EL, Moore CM: Family matters: the impact of a chronic condition on the families of children with asthma, *Pediatr Nurs* 25(3):288, 1999.

LaFleur CJ, Raway B: School-age child and adolescent perception of pain intensity associated with three word descriptors, *Pediatr Nurs* 25(1):45, 1999.

LaMontagne LL et al: Parent coping and child distress behaviors during invasive procedures for childhood cancer, *J Pediatr Oncol Nurs* 16(1):3, 1999.

Lanham DM et al: Accuracy of tympanic temperature readings in children under 6 years of age, *Pediatr Nurs* 25(1):39, 1999.

Ledlie SW: Diagnosis disclosure by family caregivers to children who have perinatally acquired HIV disease: when the time comes, *Nurs Res* 48(3):141, 1999.

Lesser J, Koniak-Griffin D, Anderson NLR: Depressed adolescent mothers' perceptions of their own maternal role, *Issues Mental Health Nurs* 20(2):131, 1999.

Magill-Evans J, Harrison MJ: Parent child interactions and development of toddlers born preterm, *West J Nurs Res* 21(3):292, 1999.

Manworren R et al: Clinical impact of perioperative respiratory syncytial virus testing, *AORN J* 69(5):1003, 1999.

McGrath MM, Sullivan MC: Medical and ecological factors in estimating motor outcomes of preschool children, *Res Nurs Health* 221(2):155, 1999.

McMullen A, Yoos H: Symptom perception and evaluation in childhood asthma, *Nurs Res* 48(1):2, 1999.

Monsen RB: Mothers' experiences of living worried when parenting children with spina bifida, *J Pediatr Nurs* 14(3):157, 1999.

Nelson VR: The effect of newborn early discharge follow-up program on pediatric urgent care utilization, *J Pediatr Health Care* 13(2):58, 1999.

Noyes J: The impact of knowing your child is critically ill: a qualitative study of mothers' experiences, *J Adv Nurs* 29(2):427, 1999.

Pavelka L, McCarthy AM, Denehy J: Nursing interventions used in school nursing practice, *J Sch Nurs* 15(1):29, 1999.

Pesata V, Pallija G, Webb AA: A descriptive study of missed appointments: families perceptions of barriers to care, *J Pediatr Health Care* 13(4):178, 1999.

Polivka BJ, Ryan-Wagner N: Health Promotion and injury prevention behaviors of elementary school children, *Pediatr Nurs* 25(2):127, 1999.

Puskar KR et al: Health concerns and risk behaviors of rural adolescents, *J Community Health Nurs* 16(2):109, 1999a.

Puskar KR et al: Optimism and its relationship to depression, coping, anger, and life events in rural adolescents, *Issues Ment Health Nurs* 20(2):115, 1999b.

Pyke-Grimm KA et al: Preferences for participation in treatment decision making and information needs of parents of children with cancer: a pilot study, *J Pediatr Oncol Nurs* 16(1):13, 1999.

Rehm RS: Religious faith in Mexican-American families dealing with chronic childhood illness, *Image J Nurs Schol* 31(1):33, 1999.

Rezvan I et al: Assessment of stature in children with orofacial clefting, *MCN Am J Matern Child Nurs* 24(5):252, 1999.

Robbins J, Cromwell P, Korones DN: Swimming and central venous catheter-related infections in the child with cancer, *J Pediatr Oncol Nurs* 16(1):51, 1999.

Robledo L, Wilson AH, Gray P: Hispanic mothers' knowledge and care of their children with respiratory illness: a pilot study, *J Pediatr Nurs* 14(4):239, 1999.

Scahill L, Koenig K: Pharmacology in children and adolescents with pervasive developmental disorders, *J Child Adolesc Psychiatr Nurs* 12(1):41, 1999.

Scharer K: Eating disorder in a 10-year-old girl, *J Child Adolesc Psychiatr Nurs* 12(2):79, 1999a.

Scharer K: Nurse-parent relationship building in child psychiatric units, *J Child Adolesc Psychiatr Nurs* 12(4):153, 1999b.

Slusher IL: Self-care agency and self-care practice of adolescents, *Issues Comp Pediatr Nurs* 22(1):49, 1999.

Stubblefield C, Murray RL: Parents call for concerned and collaborative care, *West J Nurs Res* 21(3):356, 1999.

Sullivan MC, McGrath MM: Proximal and distal correlates of maternal control style, *West J Nurs Res* 21(3):313, 1999.

Tarr J, Pickler RH: Becoming a cancer patient: a study of families of children with acute lymphocytic leukemia, *J Pediatr Oncol Nurs* 16(1):44, 1999.

Tomlinson PS, Swiggum P, Harbough BL: Identification of nurse-family intervention sites to decrease health related family boundary ambiguity in PICU, *Issues Comp Pediatr Nurs* 22(1):27, 1999.

U.S. Department of Health and Human Services, Public Health Service: *Healthy People 2000: national health promotion and disease prevention objectives*, Washington, DC, 1991, Author.

Vandal S, Rivard CH, Bradet R: Measuring the compliance behavior of adolescents wearing orthopedic braces, *Issues Comp Pediatr Nurs* 22(2):59, 1999.

Van Riper M: Maternal perceptions of family provider relationships and well-being in families of children with Down Syndrome, *Res Nurs Health* 221(1):15, 1999.

Williams C, Vines SW: Broken past, fragile future: personal stories of high risk adolescent, *J Soc Pediatr Nurses* 4(1):15, 1999.

Yarcheski A, Mahon NE: The moderator-mediator role of social support in early adolescents, *West J Nurs Res* 21(5):685, 1999.

Yarcheski A, Mahon NE, Yarcheski TJ: An empirical test of alternate theories of anger in early adolescents, *Nurs Res* 48(6):317, 1999.

Learning Objectives

1 Identify clinical nursing journals that publish research articles relevant to adults.

2 Discuss clinical and research priorities in the care of adults.

3 Use research literature to clarify identified clinical practice problems for adults.

4 Explore examples of research that has been conducted in various areas of clinical practice with adults.

5 Discuss application of sample research results in clinical practice.

6 Apply the reading strategy to survey, examine, critically read, and evaluate a sample research article on care of adults.

Chapter Outline

What Research Resources Are Available for Adults?

What Approaches Can Be Used for the Review of the Research Literature?
  Addressing clinical and research priorities
  Using issues that arise from clinical practice
  Scanning available resources

What Current Research Is Available?
  Nursing research journals
  Clinical nursing journals
  Summarizing and using scan results
How to Read and Evaluate a Research Article on the Care of Adults

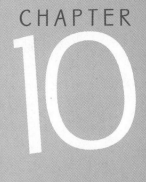

Reading and Using Research in the Care of Adults

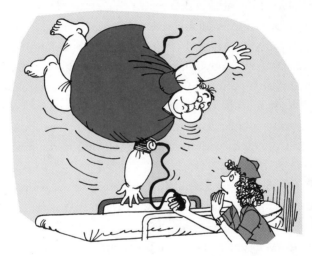

That research article on blood pressure techniques didn't mention anything about what to do when this happens!

Student Quote *"I never even thought about needing updates on basic skills procedures until we did the research survey for class. I've already altered the way I take blood pressures."*

Abstract Several research sources publish articles pertinent to the care of adults. These sources tend to be identified by clinical subspecialty area and can be used to view identified priorities in the care and research for adults, to address identified problems and questions uncovered in clinical practice, or to provide a broad view of currently available research about adults. An abundant number of current research studies are available for use in clinical practice with adults. Samples of current studies are reported and clinical applications are discussed. The use of the research reading strategy is illustrated with one research article on an adult population.

239

In this chapter, we identify periodical publications that contain nursing research on care of adults, explore strategies to simplify the search process and target relevant research articles, and preview sample selections of currently published research. Finally we dissect a sample article using the reading strategy and evaluation criteria presented in Chapter 7.

What Research Resources are Available for Adults?

Several resources are available that report the results of nursing research done with adult subjects. By now the nursing research journals should be familiar to you. Several clinical specialty journals also regularly publish research articles about care affecting adults. You will note that most of these clinical journals are specialty journals that report on a particular segment of nursing care for adults such as mental health, oncology, or critical care, or the care of some specific body system or disease such as the cardiovascular or pulmonary system or cancer. Box 10-1 contains a list of journals most likely to contain research relevant to the practice of nursing care for adults.

You will note no listing for nursing journals that occasionally contain research relevant to the adult population because research studies are scattered among more than 30 different nursing journals. Some of these studies would surface using our search strategy for a specified clinical problem. However, searching for these studies using the journal scan procedure is not a viable option. If you are interested in a listing of nursing journals with information about their function and purpose, check out the Resource Kit at the end of the chapter for a handy website address.

Activity
17

STUDENT CHALLENGE Perusing Specialty Journals

1. If any of the journals listed in Box 10-1 are unfamiliar to you, take time to locate those available in your library. Scan two or three issues of each journal.
2. Note how they are organized. What types of articles are prevalent? Can you readily distinguish research articles from other featured articles? Do you notice a difference in the focus of the various journals?
3. Check out descriptions of the focus or purpose of any unknown journals.
4. Are some journals more readable than others? More helpful?

Box 10-1	Journals Containing Nursing Research Relevant to the Care of Adults

Nursing Research Journals
Nursing Research
Research in Nursing and Health
Western Journal of Nursing Research
Applied Nursing Research
Clinical Nursing Research
Nursing Science Quarterly
Image: Journal of Nursing Scholarship
Scholarly Inquiry for Nursing Practice

Clinical Journals that Regularly Contain Research Articles About the Care of Adults
American Journal of Critical Care
AORN Journal
Cardiovascular Nursing
Heart and Lung: Journal of Critical Care
Issues in Mental Health Nursing
Journal of Community Health Nursing
Journal of Emergency Room Nursing
Oncology Nursing Forum
Public Health Nursing
Rehabilitation Nursing

By now you should begin to notice a difference in the research articles that you see in clinical journals versus the articles reported in research journals. Research reports in research journals tend to be geared to the knowledge and reading level of other researchers. This means they include greater detail about research methodology and statistics and use more technical language. The relevance of the studies to clinical practice may not always be immediately obvious. In short, they require more time and concentration to read and understand.

Research studies in clinical journals are targeted at clinical practitioners. The language is less technical and the methods section and statistical reporting less detailed. The clinical relevance is usually clear cut and easy to ascertain. In short, they are easier to read and apply, but you are less able to ascertain exactly how the research was conducted. However, both serve a useful purpose to you, the research consumer. So keep reading both types. Make note of the journals that provide the most useful information for improving your care to various segments of the adult population.

What Approaches Can Be Used for the Review of Research Literature?

We again explore our three strategies for use of the research literature as it pertains to adults. We explore the relevant clinical and research priorities, identify some sample problems or questions that might arise from clinical practice with an adult population, and we scan the research literature to get a feel for available research that might enhance clinical practice.

Addressing Clinical and Research Priorities

Let's look at the care and research priorities relevant to an adult population. Health maintenance, promotion, and restoration are increasingly important goals in the care of adults, as is combating diseases that carry high morbidity and mortality rates. We view the pertinent *Healthy People 2000* objectives, review research priorities of the National Institute for Nursing Research (NINR), and look at nursing clinical specialty sources for research priorities. *Healthy People 2000* details a number of health care goals and objectives pertinent to adults. These objectives are geared toward health care prevention and are listed in Box 10-2.

The NINR research priorities reveal a number of issues related to care of adults. Preventive care and intervention with HIV/AIDS, management of pain, effective interventions in chronic illness, treatment of traumatic brain injury, and management of cardiovascular risks in special populations were all highlighted in the 1990s. In 2000, the self-management of diabetes and effective sleep interventions topped the list for adults.

A number of clinical specialty areas periodically issue research priority lists. In the 1990s research priorities were generated for such areas as respiratory nursing (American Thoracic Society, 1990), burn nursing (Bayley et al, 1992), long-term care (Haight and Bahr, 1992), public health nursing (Misener et al, 1994), vascular nursing (Hatton and Nunnelee, 1995), oncology nursing (Stetz et al, 1995), orthopedic nursing (Sedlack et al, 1998), mental health nursing (Pullen, Tuck, and Wallace,

Box 10-2 *Healthy People 2000* Objectives

Reduce obesity
Increase physical activity
Improve dietary intake
Reduce periodontal disease and gingivitis
Reduce use of tobacco, alcohol, and drugs
Increase use of seatbelts
Increase helmet use of motorcyclists
Reduce work-related injuries and disease
Reduce incidence of suicide and homicide
Reduce exposure to environmental pollutants
Reduce food-borne infections
Reduce coronary heart disease
Reduce incidence of cancer
Reduce incidence of stroke
Reduce incidence of diabetes
Reduce incidence of HIV infection
Reduce prevalence of STDs

From U.S. Department of Health and Human Services, Public Health Service: *Healthy People 2000: national health promotion and disease prevention objectives*, Washington, DC, 1991, Author.

1999), and nephrology nursing (Lewis et al, 1999). In addition, the World Health Organization established global nursing research priorities (Hirschfeld, 1998). Explore adult care and research priorities by tackling the following Student Challenge.

STUDENT CHALLENGE Checking Adult Care Priorities

1. Check the *Healthy People 2010* goals and objectives. (Refer to the Resource Kit at the end of this chapter to access this website.) Locate the objectives relevant to care for adults. Compare them to the objectives in Box 10-2. Note similarities and differences.

2. Locate the WHO research priorities and see how they compare to the priorities stated by the NINR and *Healthy People 2000*. (Hint: The author is Hirschfeld; check the reference list at end of this chapter.)

3. Locate the latest research priorities of at least two nursing specialty areas of interest relevant to adult care. (Hint: Use MEDLINE or CINAHL and do a search for 1999 to 2001.)

MERLIN
Activity
18

Continued

```
STUDENT CHALLENGE Checking Adult Care Priorities—
                          cont'd

4. Choose one priority area from one of the specialty areas. Run a litera-
   ture search for the year 2000 to present and see what nursing research
   has been conducted in your selected area.
```

Using Issues that Arise from Clinical Practice

In this section, we examine another example of a clinical question that might arise during clinical practice, explore the search process, and examine the search results. We define our problem by parameters that provide guidance in viewing a nursing care problem. Ask yourself the following questions: Who is the target of care (e.g., male, female, young or middle-aged adult, family, or caregiver)? What level of care is involved (e.g., Does the problem require health maintenance or prevention, acute care, or chronic care?)? What aspect of care is involved (e.g., physical, psychological, sociocultural, or spiritual)? What, if any, nursing specialty area is involved (e.g., respiratory, cardiovascular, oncology, rehabilitation, mental health)? Finally, what care setting did the problem arise in (e.g., clinic, physician's office, home, occupational setting, hospital)?

I am a staff nurse in the outpatient clinic of a large cancer treatment center. Regardless of cancer diagnosis or treatment, one theme—being chronically tired—is a constant for all my patients. They use phrases like "tired to the bone," "dead tired," and "beyond exhaustion." They all say they have never felt this tired or experienced this type of tired before. All state they have tried getting more rest, doing less, and eating better, with little effect. I check them for anemia and make sure they see a physician if they are anemic, but I wonder if there is any new wisdom on nursing interventions for this problem. It is obvious that the standard advice to alternate rest and activity, decrease activity, decrease stress, get enough sleep, and eat a balanced diet is not helping much.

I do a CINAHL search using the key words "cancer related fatigue." This sends me to a mapping display that gives me a choice of 10 subject headings. I choose "fatigue" and check the Focus box. (Hint: This means that the search will only consider those articles for which fatigue is a major focus). I choose a second term "cancer patients." With this term I check the Explode box. (Hint: This means that the search will look for articles with this or any related term). Then I combine the terms by selecting the Boolean operator "and" in the box at the top of the mapping display page. This means the search will only look for articles that deal with both "fatigue" and "cancer patients." Finally, I limit the search to the years 1997-1999 and to research articles. I run the search and I get 25 citations.

Fourteen of the citations are immediately eliminated by examining the article titles. Eliminations include articles that focused on testing fatigue scales, fatigue studies with very select populations such as patients undergoing bone marrow transplants, and studies written in a foreign language. Reading available article abstracts and discovering that they were not applicable to my situation eliminated another five studies. Two studies confirmed my patient perceptions about fatigue and its effects, but offered little in the way of solutions. One study confirmed that typical self-help measures such as those tried by my patients were not particularly helpful, but offered no solution other than treating the problem medically with drugs.

However, the final three studies offered me a new strategy. A study by Berger and Farr (1999) provided the first clue. This study examined the circadian activity/rest cycles in relation to cancer-related fatigue for 72 women undergoing chemotherapy for surgically treated breast cancer. Women who were less active, and took more day naps had an increased number of night wakenings (interrupted sleep patterns) and had higher levels of fatigue. Implications for nursing practice were to develop nursing interventions that would promote daytime activity and nighttime rest to help manage fatigue.

The next two articles led the way to a specific intervention. These two studies examined the effects of exercise on cancer-related fatigue. An experimental study by Mock and colleagues (1997) used 46 women who were receiving radiation for early stage breast cancer. Half were randomly assigned to an exercise group and half received the usual care. The exercise group carried out a daily, self-paced, home-based walking exercise program for a 6-week period. The results found that the exercise group had significantly higher levels of physical functioning and significantly lower levels of fatigue and anxiety and less difficulty sleeping. Implications for nursing practice are that a nurse-prescribed and monitored exercise program is an effective, convenient, and low-cost self-care activity.

A study of five cancer patients by Dimeo, Rumberger, and Keul (1998) confirmed that a daily aerobic exercise such as walking could decrease levels of fatigue and increase the ability to carry out normal activities of daily living. Using this data, I clear my plan with the clinic director and decide to try a daily self-paced walking intervention with my patients.

STUDENT CHALLENGE Chasing Adult Challenges

1. Review your experiences in caring for adults and think about a situation you wish to explore in the current research literature.
2. Identify appropriate search parameters for the subject material and conduct a library search for the year 2000 to present. What did you find?
3. If your search was fruitful, retrieve one or two promising articles.
4. Review the articles. How might the results of the studies be helpful in clinical practice?

Activity
19

Scanning Available Resources

Let's explore what is available in the research literature by using our third strategy and scanning the tables of contents and the abstracts of the research and clinical specialty journals listed in Box 10-1. By now you should be developing scanning skills that allow you to do journal scans more efficiently and effectively. For example, some journals and their table of contents and abstracts of articles are available through various websites on the Internet. Those that are available as this book is being published are listed in the Resource Kit. Check the Resource Kit for a handy website that lists links to journals on the Internet. These journals all have descriptive information available on the Web, and many may now offer tables of contents and abstracts. These websites make scanning a particular journal as easy as sitting down with a copy of the journal itself.

How do you scan journals that are not listed on the Web without having actual journals in hand? Make use of CINAHL or MEDLINE electronic search features. Either search mechanism allows you to specify a specific journal or journals and put a limit on the years you are interested in. In MEDLINE, simply make a temporary personalized journal list. List the journal(s) you want searched (e.g., *Applied Nursing Research*). Any search you do uses only those journal(s). Now specify the year you want (e.g., 2000). Then go to the main search page and select Search. (Note: Do not enter any search parameters in the Subject Search box.) The resulting search will retrieve all articles for the specified journals in the specified years (e.g., *Applied Nursing Research* for 2000). You can then do a quick title scan and check those articles that you want to see an abstract for. Pretty neat trick, huh?

CINAHL will let you do the same thing. Just specify the journal(s) and year(s) of interest in the appropriate places and run a search with no specification of subject matter. If you haven't discovered this trick yet, try it out by doing the following Student Challenge.

STUDENT CHALLENGE Scanning Relevant Journals

Select one research journal and two clinical journals from those listed in Box 10-1 that are available in your library and that you have not previously scanned for Chapters 8 or 9.

1. Scan the 2000 table of contents for each of these journals and note those articles that seem relevant to the clinical care of adults.
2. Read the abstracts for the selected articles. Weed out any articles that are not clinically relevant. How long did this take you? Are you getting more proficient? Save these articles. We use them again in the next Student Challenge.

What Current Research Is Available?

The following are specific examples of pertinent research articles for the care of adults that I found by scanning the 1999 tables of contents of the research and clinical journals listed in Box 10-1. Selected articles are briefly summarized and clinical implications are discussed.

Nursing Research Journals

The articles found by scanning the tables of contents of the various research journals yielded the articles listed in Box 10-3. By now, you should be noticing features that allow you to eliminate certain articles as you perform your scan of research journals. For example, the titles should allow you to quickly eliminate articles that focus on tool development and tool reliability and validity or discuss methodological issues. Articles that focus on the education of nurses or nursing administration issues can also be eliminated. Opinion or editorial articles can also be deleted from the scan. More subtle clues also allow elimination of articles from consideration. Articles on children or adolescents are not relevant to an adult

Box 10-3   Relevant Adult Titles in Research Journals

Nursing Research

Unplanned Hospital Readmissions: A Home Care Perspective (Anderson et al, 1999)

Long-Term Nonprogressors with HIV Disease (Barroso, 1999)

The Perimenopausal Transition of Filipino American Midlife Women: Biopsy-chosociocultural Dimensions (Berg, 1999)

The Effects of Sense of Belonging, Social Support, Conflict and Loneliness on Depression (Hagerty and Williams, 1999)

Predicting Intentions to Obtain a Pap Smear Among African American and Latina Women: Testing the Theory of Planned Behavior (Jennings-Dozier, 1999b)

The Effects of Crossed Leg on Blood Pressure Measurement (Marcantonio et al, 1999)

pH and Concentration of Bilirubin in Feeding Tube Aspirates as Predictors of Tube Placement (Metheny et al, 1999)

Adult Emergency Visits for Chronic Cardiorespiratory Disease: Does Dyspnea Matter? (Parshall, 1999)

Caregiving Effectiveness in Families Managing Complex Technology at Home: Replication of a Model (Smith, 1999)

Research in Nursing and Health

Women's Responses to Battering: A Test of the Model (Bunting et al, 1999)

Decision Making Preference and Opportunity in VA Ambulatory Care Patients: Association with Patient Satisfaction (Harvey, Kazis, and Lee, 1999)

Nurses' Judgments Regarding Seclusion and Restraint of Psychiatric Patients: A Social Judgment Analysis (Holzworth and Wills, 1999)

Correlation of Anthropometry with CT in Mexican-American Women (Keller, Chintapalli, and Lancaster, 1999)

Explaining Women's Intentions and Use of Hormones with Menopause (Lauver et al, 1999)

Functional Status from the Patient's Perspective: The Challenge of Preserving Personal Integrity (Leidy and Haase, 1999)

Borderline Personality Disorder: The Voice of the Patients (Nehls, 1999)

The Quality of Life of African American Women with Breast Cancer (Northouse et al, 1999)

Testing a Theory for Health-Related Quality of Life in Cancer Patients: A Structural Equation Approach (Nuamah et al, 1999)

Associations Between Homeless Women's Intimate Relationships and Their Health and Well-Being (Nyamathi et al, 1999)

Box 10-3 Relevant Adult Titles in Research Journals—cont'd

Research in Nursing and Health—cont'd

Describing the Work of Nursing: The Case of Postsurgical Nursing Interventions for Men with Prostate Cancer (Robinson et al, 1999)

Effectiveness of Professional-Peer Group Treatment: Symptom Management for Women with PMS (Taylor, 1999)

Professional Nursing Support for Culturally Diverse Family Members of Critically Ill Adults (Waters, 1999)

Western Journal of Nursing Research

Depressive Symptomatology in Three Latino Groups (Munet-Vilaro, Folkman, and Gregorich, 1999)

Stress, Social Support, and a Sense of Coherence (Wolf and Ratner, 1999)

Applied Nursing Research

Sitting Posture and Prevention of Pressure Ulcers (Defloor and Grypdonck, 1999)

Hope and Anxiety of Individual Family Members of Critically Ill Adults (Fowler and Magarelli, 1999)

Sensations Experienced During Removal of Tubes in Acute Postoperative Patients (Mimnaugh et al, 1999)

Patient Satisfaction with Two Models of Group Therapy for People Hospitalized with Bipolar Disorder (Pollack and Cramer, 1999)

The Effect of Role-Taking Ability on Care Giver-Resident Mealtime Interaction (Schell and Kayser-Jones, 1999)

The Experience of Relapse to Unsafe Behavior Among HIV Positive, Heterosexual, Minority Men (Sherman and Kirton, 1999)

The Quick Relaxation Technique: Effect on Pain Associated with Chest Tube Removal (Houston and Jesurum, 1999)

Effects of Head-of-the-Bed Positioning on the Electrocardiogram (Wright et al, 1999)

Scholarly Inquiry for Nursing Practice

Patterns of Resistance: African-American Mothers and Adult Children with HIV Illness (Boyle, 1999)

Quality of Life for Persons with Developmental Disabilities (Faulkner, 1999)

Image: Journal of Nursing Scholarship

Women Dwelling with Violence (Draucker and Madsen, 1999)

Sleep Patterns of Sheltered Battered Women (Humphreys et al, 1999)

Continued

Box 10-3   Relevant Adult Titles in Research Journals—cont'd

Image: Journal of Nursing Scholarship—cont'd

A Situation-Specific Theory of Korean Immigrant Women's Menopausal Transition (Im and Meleis, 1999)

Effects of Home Care on Caregivers' Psychological Status (Jepson et al, 1999)

Clinical Nursing Research

Culturally Competent Care for Psychiatric Clients Who Have a History of Sexual Abuse (Austin et al, 1999)

Pain, Analgesic Use, and Morbidity in Appendectomy Patients (Cheever, 1999)

Perceived Causes of Urinary Incontinence and Reporting: A Study with Working Women (Hart, Palmer, and Fitzgerald, 1999)

Postoperative Pain after Hospital Discharge (McDonald, 1999)

Ventilated Patients' Self Esteem During Intubation and After Extubation (Menzel, 1999)

Nursing Science Quarterly

Involvement of Relatives in Care of the Dying in Different Care Cultures: Development of a Theoretical Understanding (Andershed and Ternestedt, 1999)

Women's Multiple Role Stress: Testing Neuman's Flexible Line of Defense (Gigliotti, 1999)

The Lived Experience of Serenity (Kruse, 1999)

The Effectiveness of Therapeutic Touch: A Meta-Analytic Review (Peters, 1999)

population. Research done in foreign countries on foreign populations is seldom useful in clinical application. As you refine your scanning techniques, the process becomes more efficient and more productive.

This scan produced a large array of articles as should be expected by the breadth of the population we are using as a search parameter. Examining the titles of the articles among all the research journals reveals a total of 47 articles on the adult population. Nine relevant articles were found in *Nursing Research*, 13 in *Research in Nursing and Health*, 2 in *Western Journal of Nursing Research*, 8 in *Applied Nursing Research*, 2 in *Scholarly Inquiry for Nursing Practice*, 4 in *Image: Journal of Nursing Scholarship*, 5 in *Clinical Nursing Research*, and 4 in *Nursing Science Quarterly*.

This time, it is your job to examine the results of the scan. This will help you make use of the available information just by looking at the study titles. Try the following Student Challenge.

STUDENT CHALLENGE Sorting Out Scan Results

1. Examine the results of the scan of research journals listed in Box 10-3.
2. What patterns do you see in the titles of the research?
3. Which of these articles might be relevant to the adult research priorities we discussed in the previous section?
4. Can you determine which articles are qualitative and which are quantitative?
5. Can you distinguish the target of care, level of care, aspect of care, nursing specialty area, and care setting from the titles?
6. Which studies seem to be research about specific nursing interventions?
7. Which studies do you need to see an abstract of to determine enough about the study to answer the questions raised in this challenge?

Clinical Nursing Journals

The articles found by scanning the tables of contents of the clinical journals yielded a number of possible relevant research articles listed in Box 10-4. Have you been able to distinguish between research and nonresearch articles yet when you are scanning titles in a table of contents? Sometimes it is hard, particularly when the study uses a qualitative methodology. As you become more familiar with the different clinical journals, you will be able to zero in on the research articles more quickly. (Hint: When you are uncertain, take a quick peek at the abstract for the article. If there is no abstract, this is a clue that the article is not a research article.) Look for other clues in CINAHL and MEDLINE citations. Article citations labeled review, editorial, or opinion are not research articles.

Ten clinical journals regularly publish research on care of adults. All of these journals publish research within a confined specialty area. The research articles in the *American Journal of Critical Care* are concerned with critical care usually seen in intensive care and trauma units. Most of the studies primarily target very specific and highly technical nursing interventions. The research articles published in *Heart and Lung* are divided between cardiovascular and pulmonary studies and use

Text continued on p. 257.

| Box 10-4 | Relevant Research Article Titles Using Adult Populations in Clinical Journals |

American Journal of Critical Care

Music: An Intervention for Pain During Chest Tube Removal After Open Heart Surgery (Broscious, 1999)

Achieving Femoral Artery Hemostasis After Cardiac Catheterization: A Comparison of Methods (Schickel et al, 1999)

Change in Quality of Life After Lung Volume Reduction Surgery (Anderson, 1999)

Reliability of an Intravenous Intermittent Access Port for Obtaining Blood Samples for Coagulation Studies (Arrants et al, 1999)

Life with a Left Ventricular Assist Device: The Patient's Perspective (Savage and Canody, 1999)

Effects of Position of Chest Drainage Tube on Volume Drained and Pressure (Schmeltz et al, 1999)

Oral Care in the Adult Intensive Care Unit (Fitch et al, 1999)

Predicting the Risk of Pressure Ulcers in Critically Ill Patients (Carlson, Kemp, and Shott, 1999)

Measurement of Dyspnea in Patients Treated with Mechanical Ventilation (Powers and Bennett, 1999)

Obtaining Blood Samples for Coagulation Studies from a Normal Saline Lock (Powers, 1999)

Effects of Relaxing Music on Cardiac Autonomic Balance and Anxiety after Acute Myocardial Infarction (White, 1999)

The Effects of Earplugs on Sleep Measures During Exposure to Intensive Care Unit Noise (Wallace et al, 1999)

A Survey of Bedside Methods Used to Detect Pulmonary Aspiration of Enteral Formula in Intubated Tube Fed Patients (Metheny, Aud, and Wunderlich, 1999)

Prevalence of Leg Wound Complications After Coronary Artery Bypass Grafting: Determinants of Risk Factors (Goldsborough et al, 1999)

Pain Assessment and Management in Critically Ill Postoperative and Trauma Patients: A Multisite Study (Carroll et al, 1999)

Differences in African American and White Women with Myocardial Infarction: History, Presentation, Diagnostic Methods, and Infarction Type (Griffiths, Pokorny, and Bowman, 1999)

Endotracheal Tube Narrowing after Closed System Suctioning: Prevalence and Risk Factors (Glass, Grap, and Sessler, 1999)

Effects of Injectate Volume on Thermodilution Measurements of Cardiac Output on Patients with Low Ventricular Ejection Fraction (McCloy et al, 1999)

Box 10-4 Relevant Research Article Titles Using Adult Populations in Clinical Journals—cont'd

American Journal of Critical Care—cont'd

A Posthoc Descriptive Study of Patients Receiving Propofol (Kowalski and Rayfield, 1999)

Therapeutic Paralysis of Critically Ill Trauma Patients: Perceptions of Patients and Their Family Members (Johnson et al, 1999)

Use of Backrest Elevation in Critical Care: A Pilot Study (Grap et al, 1999)

AORN Journal

Etiology and Incidence of Pressure Ulcers in Surgical Patients (Schultz AAA, 1999)

Airborne Particulates in the OR Environment (Edmiston et al, 1999)

Ethical Perception and Resulting Action in Perioperative Nurses (Schroeter, 1999)

Clinical Decision-Making Processes in Perioperative Nursing (Parker, Minick, and Kee, 1999)

Clinical Impact of Preoperative Respiratory Syncytial Virus Testing (Manworren et al, 1999)

Heart and Lung: Journal of Critical Care

Frequency of Silent Myocardial Ischemia with 12 Lead ST Segment Monitoring in the Coronary Care Unit: Are There Sex Related Differences? (Adams et al, 1999)

Changes in Cholesterol Levels in Women After Coronary Bypass Surgery (Allen, 1999)

Changes in Health Status and Quality of Life and the Impact of Uncertainty in Patients Who Survive Life Threatening Arrhythmias (Carroll, Hamilton, and McGovern, 1999)

An Evaluation of Facial Expression Displayed by Patients with Chest Pain (Dalton et al, 1999)

Factors Associated with Outcomes 3 Months After Implantable Cardioverter Defibrillator Insertion (Dunbar et al, 1999)

Intradermal Normal Saline Solution, Self Selected Music, and Insertion Difficulty Effects on Intravenous Insertion Pain (Jacobson, 1999)

Symptom Experiences of Lung Transplant Recipients: Comparisons Across Gender, Pretransplantation Diagnosis and Type of Transplantation (Lanuza et al, 1999)

Dyspnea in Patients with Chronic Obstructive Pulmonary Disease: Does Dyspnea Worsen Longitudinally in the Presence of Declining Lung Function? (Lareau et al, 1999)

Continued

Box 10-4 Relevant Research Article Titles Using Adult Populations in Clinical Journals—cont'd

Heart and Lung: Journal of Critical Care—cont'd

How Women Label and Respond to Symptoms of Acute Myocardial Infarction: Responses to Hypothetical Symptom Scenarios (Meischke et al, 1999)

Nursing Intervention and Smoking Cessation: A Meta-Analysis (Rice, 1999)

Readmission of Patients After Coronary Artery Bypass Surgery (Sabourin and Funk, 1999)

Quality of Life Comparisons After Coronary Angioplasty and Coronary Artery Bypass Graft Surgery (Scaggs and Yates, 1999)

Issues in Mental Health Nursing

Why Did She Do That? Issues of Moral Conflict in Battered Women's Decision Making Trauma History of Sheltered Battered Women (Belknap, 1999)

Life Events and Psychological Well Being in Women Sentenced to Prison (Keavney and Zauszniewski, 1999)

Family Functioning in Families Providing Care for a Family Member with Schizophrenia (Saunders, 1999)

Relationship Between Coping Strategies and Depression Among Employed Korean Immigrant Wives (Um and Dancy, 1999)

Effects of Cognitive and Experimental Group Therapy on Self Efficacy and Perceptions of Employability of Chemically Dependent Women (Washington, 1999)

Journal of Cardiovascular Nursing

Effect of Ambient Temperature and Cardiac Stability on Two Methods of Cardiac Output Measurement (Cathelyn and Glenn, 1999)

Preoperative Psychological Predictors of Hospital Length of Stay After Heart Transplantation (Grady, Jalowiec, and White-Williams, 1999)

Women and Cardiac Rehabilitation: Referral and Compliance Patterns (Halm et al, 1999)

Caregiver Satisfaction with the Preparation for Discharge in a Decreased-Length-of-Stay Cardiac Surgery Program (Leske, 1999)

Learning Retention in Patients Receiving Midazolam During Permanent Pacemaker Implantation (Schuster et al, 1999)

Journal of Community Health Nursing

An Analysis of Nurses' Communications in a Shelter Setting (Attala et al, 1999)

Poor Women Living with HIV: Self Identified Needs (Baker, 1999)

| Box 10-4 | Relevant Research Article Titles Using Adult Populations in Clinical Journals—cont'd |

Journal of Community Health Nursing—cont'd

Isolation and Stigmata: The Experience of Patients with Active Tuberculosis (Kelly, 1999)

A Study of Relationship of Caregiving Appraisal to Depressive Symptomology and Home Care Utilization (Schwarz, 1999)

Journal of Emergency Nursing

A Prospective Study of ED Pain Management Practices and the Patient's Perspective (Tanabe and Buschmann, 1999)

Factors Associated with Victimization of Personnel in Emergency Departments (Mayer, Smith, and King, 1999)

The LUNAR Project: A Description of the Population of Individuals Who Seek Health Care at Emergency Departments (MacLean et al, 1999)

Oncology Nursing Forum

The Influence of Daytime Inactivity and Nighttime Restlessness on Cancer-Related Fatigue (Berger and Farr, 1999)

Use of Complementary Therapies in a Rural Cancer Population (Bennett and Lengacher, 1999)

Menopausal Symptoms in Breast Cancer Survivors (Carpenter and Andrykowski, 1999)

Lymphedema Prevention and Management Knowledge in Women Treated for Breast Cancer (Coward, 1999)

The Meaning of Quality of Life in Cancer Survivorship (Dow et al, 1999)

The Role of Protective Clothing in Infection Prevention in Patients Undergoing Autologous Bone Marrow Transplant (Duquette-Petersen et al, 1999)

Breast Cancer Screening in Relation to Access to Health Services (Facione, 1999)

Use of Routine and Breakthrough Analgesia in Home Care (Ferrell, Juarez, and Bornemann, 1999)

Caring for Patients Who Experience Chemotherapy-Induced Side Effects: The Meaning for Oncology Nurses (Fall-Dickson and Rose, 1999)

Perceptual Determinants of Pap Test Up-To-Date Status Among Minority Women (Jennings-Dozier, 1999a)

The Effects of Guided Imagery on Comfort of Women with Early Stage Breast Cancer Undergoing Radiation Therapy (Kolcaba and Fox, 1999)

Engagement in Breast Screening Behaviors (Lauver et al, 1999)

Anxiety and Directed Attention in Women Awaiting Breast Cancer Surgery (Lehto and Cimprich, 1999)

Continued

Box 10-4 Relevant Research Article Titles Using Adult Populations in Clinical Journals—cont'd

Oncology Nursing Forum—cont'd

Side-Effects Burden, Psychological Adjustment, and Life Quality in Women with Breast Cancer: Pattern of Association over Time (Longman, Braden, and Mishel, 1999)

Relationship Between Fatigue and Quality of Life in Patients with Glioblastoma Multiformae (Lovely, Miakowski, and Dodd, 1999)

The Effect of Nutritional Supplements on Food Intake in Patients Undergoing Radiotherapy (McCarthy and Weihofen, 1999)

Comparison of Sleep Quality in Patients with Cancer and Healthy Subjects (Owen, Parker, and McGuire, 1999)

Catheter Port Cleansing Techniques and the Entry of Povidone-Iodine into the Epidural Space (Paice, DuPen, and Schwertz, 1999)

Breast Cancer Screening and African American Women: Fear, Fatalism, and Silence (Phillips, Cohen, and Moses, 1999)

The Husband's Untold Account of His Wife's Breast Cancer: A Chronologic Analysis (Samms, 1999)

Chemotherapy Medication Errors: Descriptions, Severity and Contributing Factors (Schulmeister, 1999)

Cervical Cancer Screening Knowledge, Behaviors and Beliefs in Vietnamese Women (Schulmeister and Lifsey, 1999)

Does Emotional Expression Make a Difference in Reactions to Breast Cancer? (Walker, Nail, and Croyle, 1999)

Taste Changes Experienced by Patients Receiving Chemotherapy (Wickham et al, 1999)

Public Health Nursing

A Cholesterol Intervention Program for Public Health Nurses in the Rural Southeast: Description of the Intervention, Study Design, and Baseline Results (Keyserling et al, 1999)

An Explanatory Model of Variables Influencing Health Promotion Behaviors in Smoking and Non-Smoking College Students (Martinelli, 1999)

African American Women's Experiences with Physical Activity in Their Daily Lives (Nies, Vollman, and Cook, 1999)

Wellness Profile of Midlife Women with a Chronic Illness (Paul and Weinert, 1999)

Surveillance of Suicidal Behavior in Kitsap County, Washington (Simmons, Peterson, and Hale, 1999)

Box 10-4 | Relevant Research Article Titles Using Adult Populations in Clinical Journals—cont'd

Rehabilitation Nursing

Nurses' Assessment of Patients' Cognitive Orientation in a Rehabilitation Setting (Alverzo and Galski, 1999)

Using the Functional Independence Measure Instrument to Predict Stroke Rehabilitation Outcomes (Black, Soltis, and Bartlett, 1999)

Social Problem Solving Partnerships with Family Caregivers (Grant, 1999)

Outcomes of Nurse Caring as Perceived by Individuals with Spinal Cord Injury During Rehabilitation (Lucke, 1999)

Personal Perceptions and Women's Participation in Cardiac Rehabilitation (Missik, 1999)

Cardiac Rehabilitation: Participating in an Exercise Program in a Quest to Survive (Mitchell, Muggli, and Sato, 1999)

Research Supporting the Congruence Between Rehabilitation Principles and Home Health Nursing Practice (Neal, 1999)

Music Therapy as a Treatment Method for Improving Respiratory Muscle Strength in Patients with Advanced Multiple Sclerosis: A Pilot Study (Wiens, Relmer, and Guyn, 1999)

both quantitative and qualitative methodologies. Many are related to stated research priorities (e.g., the study on smoking cessation, the study on pain interventions, the studies targeted at sex-related differences).

The *Journal of Cardiovascular Nursing*, as you might expect, publishes studies on cardiovascular nursing. The *Journal of Community Health Nursing* and *Public Health Nursing* publish research conducted in the community and addressing community health issues. The *Journal of Emergency Nursing* researches issues of interest to nurses in emergency care centers. The articles in *Issues in Mental Health* address such diverse mental health concerns as abuse, well-being in prison, depression, and the effects of mental illness on family functioning. *AORN Journal* has studies relevant to the perioperative experience.

The *Oncology Forum* is a prolific source of research on cancer and cancer care. Many of the studies target and test highly specific nursing interventions (e.g., the role of protective clothing, use of routine and breakthrough analgesia, the effects of guided imagery, effects of nutritional supplements, and catheter port cleansing). Others examine the larger picture of what it is like to have a diagnosis of cancer (e.g., the meaning of the quality of life, life quality in women with breast cancer, anxiety while awaiting surgery). Still others examine issues central to cancer patients such as fatigue, pain, side effects, and quality of sleep. There are studies that address psychological, physical, and sociocultural aspects of the cancer experience. Some studies examine screening activities such as Pap smears or breast self-examination or mammogram.

Rehabilitation Nursing studies target long-term care issues and chronic illness or disability. Most of the journals listed in Box 10-4 devote at least 50% of their journal space to research articles. The *Journal of Community Health Nursing, Journal of Emergency Nursing,* and *American Operating Room Nurses Journal* publish fewer research articles but still serve as excellent resources.

Try a quick analysis of the clinical research titles using the following Student Challenge.

STUDENT CHALLENGE Sorting Out Clinical Scan Results

1. Examine the results of the scan of clinical journals listed in Box 10-4.
2. What patterns do you see in the titles of the research?
3. Which of these articles might be relevant to the adult research priorities we discussed ?
4. Can you determine which articles are qualitative and which are quantitative?
5. Can you distinguish the target of care, level of care, aspect of care, nursing specialty area, and care setting from the titles?
6. Which studies seem to be research about specific nursing interventions?
7. Which studies do you need to see an abstract of to determine enough about the study to answer the questions raised in this challenge?

Summarizing and Using Scan Results

Several of the identified research articles have been selected to serve as examples for how research articles might be summarized and the findings used in clinical practice. A number of articles in both the research and clinical journals examined aspects of nursing care. They provide concrete data about the effectiveness of certain nursing interventions used in the care of adult populations. We look at several of these articles in more depth.

The first article (Metheny et al, 1999) examined whether pH readings and spectrographic bilirubin levels could be used instead of radiographs (x-rays) to accurately predict whether a feeding tube was in the stomach rather than in the lungs or the intestine. Aspirates of GI contents were taken from acutely ill adults with new feeding tubes in the stomach ($n = 209$) and with feeding tubes in the intestine ($n = 228$) as visualized on radiograph. One hundred fifty respiratory aspirates were taken. Bilirubin and pH levels were taken on all samples. Results showed that mean levels of pH in the lungs and intestine were significantly higher than in the stomach; mean bilirubin levels in the lung and stomach were significantly lower than in the intestine. A decision rule was made based on data overlap. A pH of greater than 5 and bilirubin of less than 5 mg/dl correctly identified all respiratory cases. A pH of greater than 5 and a bilirubin of greater than or equal to 5 mg/dl identified 75% of the intestine placements and a pH of less than or equal to 5 and a bilirubin of less than 5 mg/dl correctly identified 67% of the stomach placements. These preliminary results indicate that these measurements could be used to reduce the number of radiographs used to exclude respiratory placement and to distinguish between gastric and intestinal placement.

This study provides evidence that nurses could verify tube placement at the bedside with simple laboratory tests and prevent the use of radiographs. Don't be surprised if this becomes standard nursing practice in the not-too-distant future. However, because this nursing intervention issue involves a possible life-threatening event if a tube is incorrectly placed and not discovered, the study results are considered preliminary, and follow-up studies are needed.

A second study (Taylor, 1999) using a quasi-experimental longitudinal design examined the effectiveness of a PMS symptom management program in relieving the distress of women with PMS. A sample of 91 women with severe PMS were randomly assigned to treatment and control groups. Three pen and paper scales were used to measure menstrual symptom severity, personal demands (e.g., anxiety, distress, anger, depression) and personal resources (e.g., self-esteem, well-being). These measurements were taken twice before treatment to serve as baseline measures and at 3, 6, 12, and 18 months after treatment. A PMS symptom management program with "nonpharmacologic strategies involving self-monitoring, self-regulation and self/environmental guidance" with peer support and nurse guidance was used in a group format for a total of 12 hours. The results showed this intervention strategy to be extremely effective in relieving PMS symptoms and personal distress and in strengthening personal resources. These changes were enduring over the 18-month period of the study. The strategies were spelled out well in the article.

Nurses in primary care settings such as clinics or physician offices could apply the symptom management strategies detailed in this article in a group or individual format to help women manage their PMS. These strategies might also be tested with other stress-related health problems such as heart disease, arthritis, or autoimmune disorders. This study provides a detailed set of nursing interventions that when used could have broad implications for general health promotion in women.

A third study (Defloor and Grypdonck, 1999) examined sitting posture and its effect on the pressure exerted on the tissue at the seat surface. Fifty-six healthy volunteers were tested in eight different postures for four different types of specialty pressure relief cushions. The posture that caused the least amount of pressure was a sitting back posture with the lower legs on a rest. The next lowest pressure was caused by an upright position in the chair with the feet flat on the ground. The two postures causing the greatest pressure readings were a slouched posture and a posture where the person slid down in the chair. Of the four cushion types, all had pressure-reducing effects. However the cushion with the lowest pressure readings while the individual is slouching or sliding down was a thick air cushion.

This study gives evidence that regular monitoring of posture and use of a pressure reducing seat cushion should be a part of any protocol designed to prevent decubitus ulcers in patients at risk. This information is useful to all nurses who provide care to individuals at risk for decubitus ulcer formation. This includes the critically ill, the neurologically impaired, the frail elderly, and those with long-term or permanent disabilities that impair sensation. Nurses in rehabilitation facilities, nursing or residential care facilities, or home care should find this study particularly helpful.

A fourth study (Kolcaba and Fox, 1999) examined whether guided imagery would increase comfort for women with early stage breast cancer undergoing radiation treatment. Fifty-three women were randomly assigned to treatment and control groups. The treatment group listened to a guided imagery tape daily during radiation treatments. A comfort scale was used to measure comfort in both groups before, during, and after a course of radiation treatments. The results demonstrated that the guided imagery group had higher comfort levels than the control group. So guided imagery is an effective nursing intervention to enhance comfort levels for women undergoing radiation therapy for early stage breast cancer. This intervention could prove a useful and cost-effective strategy to increase patient comfort when confronted with a variety of noxious treatments. Nurses in a number of settings might want to consider trying and evaluating a guided imagery intervention for various medical treatments.

We also examine several of the qualitative studies uncovered in the scanning process. The first study (Nehls, 1999) used a phenomenological approach to explore the experience of living with the psychiatric diagnosis of borderline personality disorder. Thirty individuals who were receiving care at public sector mental health care settings were interviewed using an unstructured interview technique. Analysis identified three predominant themes: "living with the label," "living with self-destructive behavior perceived as manipulation," and "living with limited access to care." The findings indicate that we could improve mental health care to those with borderline personality disorders by confronting our own prejudices as nurses, better understanding the concept of self-harm, and better use of opportunities to establish a trusting relationship and generate effective dialogue. The results of this study are particularly useful for any nurse who has daily contact with patients with mental health disorders. It highlights the need for an effective therapeutic nurse-patient relationship in caring for these individuals.

A second qualitative study (Nies, Vollman, and Cook, 1999) examined African-American women's experiences with physical activity. Focus groups of women 35 to 50 years of age were used to discuss physical activity and its place in their lives. Transcripts of the group interactions were coded and analyzed. Certain barriers and facilitators to the use of exercise were identified. Facilitators included such things as daily routine, convenient and affordable activities, personal safety, childcare, enjoyment, and family and peer support. Barriers included such things as competing responsibilities, lack of convenient facilities, lack of home space, fatigue, unsafe neighborhood, lack of childcare, and lack of motivation. Results of this study could be used as data in generating new strategies to reduce a sedentary lifestyle in African-American women. Nurses in clinics, home care, and physician offices who have regular contact with this population can make use of this knowledge when offering interventions aimed at increasing physical activity.

A third study (Kelly, 1999) examined the experiences of 28 individuals with active tuberculosis who were being treated in public health clinics. A semi-structured interview technique was used to gather data. Analysis showed that patients viewed themselves as disease vectors and pariahs whose family and friends avoided or shunned them. The patients responded by isolating themselves and becoming secretive about their disease or trying to pretend it didn't exist. Nurses that treat tuberculosis patients in the community setting could use the information in this study to better understand behaviors that may be labeled as noncompliant and to design interventions that better address those behaviors, thus enhancing overall effectiveness of treatment. The community health nurse might also use this knowledge to address community attitudes and behaviors.

Now that you have seen several examples of how quantitative and qualitative studies might be applied in the care of adults, practice with some articles of your own by completing the following Student Challenge.

STUDENT CHALLENGE Using Data from Journal Scans

Use the articles that resulted from your journal scan.
1. Read the articles to determine what was studied, who was studied, and what the study results were. Write a brief summary of each article. Use the articles previously cited as examples.
2. Read the discussion sections of articles and make a quick determination about how the results might be used in a clinical practice setting. Write out how the findings might be used and by whom.

How to Read and Evaluate a Research Article on the Care of Adults

In this section, we examine one quantitative research article on a clinical intervention in more depth. We again use our research reading strategy, research comprehension, and research evaluation guidelines.

ADVENTURE CD
10-1

STUDENT CHALLENGE Surveying, Examining, and Critically Reading an Adult Research Study

1. Log on to your CD-ROM and look for the Survey, Examine, and Critically Read exercise in Chapter 10. Print out the reading strategy and the research article entitled "Intradermal Normal Saline Solution, Self-Selected Music, and Insertion Difficulty Effects on Intravenous Insertion Pain."

STUDENT CHALLENGE Surveying, Examining, and Critically Reading an Adult Research Study—cont'd

2. Take your text, the article, the strategy, and a notepad and pen and find a conducive reading and study environment.
3. Survey the article using the strategy guidelines. Make notes of what you gleaned from your survey.
4. Now go back and read the article paragraph by paragraph and jot down the key idea in each paragraph. Note anything that you don't understand.
5. When you have finished, consult needed references to clarify those things that are unclear.
6. When you have completed these steps, go back to the CD-ROM and complete the Survey, Examine, and Critically Read exercise, the Study Evaluation exercise, and the Application Visualization exercise for Chapter 10.

These exercises guide you through the critical reading, evaluation, and visualization of the selected research article. When you finish, print out your answers and my responses to the exercises. You should be feeling more confident about reading a research article and pulling out the key ideas.

Resource Kit

Web Sources for Adult Research Priorities

Healthy People 2000 and *Healthy People 2010*
National Institute for Nursing Research

Web Sources for Relevant Journal Table of Contents and Abstracts

AORN Journal
Journal of Emergency Nursing
Nursing Research
Research in Nursing and Health
Heart and Lung
Issues in Mental Health Nursing

Resource Kit—cont'd

Miscellaneous Web Resources

Want to check out other nursing journals on-line? Check MERLIN for a site that lists web links to 162 nursing journals. Many are in the process of making tables of contents available. Check the journals in Box 10-1 and see if any more of them are now scannable on-line.

Visit the book's MERLIN website at
www.mosby.com/MERLIN/Langford/maze
for further information.

Check out the exercises on your **CD-ROM.**

References

Adams MG et al: Frequency of silent myocardial ischemia with 12 lead ST segment monitoring in the coronary care unit: are there sex related differences? *Heart Lung* 28(2):81, 1999.

Allen J: Changes in cholesterol levels in women after coronary bypass surgery, *Heart Lung* 28(4):270, 1999.

Alverzo JP, Galski T: Nurses' assessment of patients' cognitive orientation in a rehabilitation setting, *Rehab Nurs* 24(1):7, 1999.

American Thoracic Society Section on Nursing: Research priorities in respiratory nursing, *Am Rev Respir Dis* 142:1459, 1990.

Andershed B, Ternestedt B: Involvement of relatives in care of the dying in different care cultures: development of a theoretical understanding, *Nurs Science Q* 12(1):45, 1999.

Anderson KL: Change in quality of life after lung volume reduction surgery, *Am J Crit Care* 8(6):389, 1999.

Anderson MA et al: Unplanned hospital readmissions: a home care perspective, *Nurs Res* 48(6):299, 1999.

Arrants J et al: Reliability of an intravenous intermittent access port for obtaining blood samples for coagulation studies, *Am J Crit Care* 8(5):344, 1999.

Attala JM et al: An analysis of nurses' communications in a shelter setting, *J Community Health Nurs* 16(1):29, 1999.

Austin W et al: Culturally competent care for psychiatric clients who have a history of sexual abuse, *Clin Nurs Res* 8(1):5, 1999.

Baker SK: Poor women living with HIV: self identified needs, *J Community Health Nurs* 16(1):41, 1999.

Barroso J: Long-term nonprogressors with HIV disease, *Nurs Res* 48(5):242, 1999.

Bayley EW et al: Research priorities for burn nursing: rehabilitation, discharge planning and follow up care, *J Burn Rehab* 13:471, 1992.

Belknap RA: Why did she do that? Issues of moral conflict in battered women's decision making, *Issues Ment Health Nurs* 20(4):387, 1999.

Bennett M, Lengacher C: Use of complementary therapies in a rural cancer populations, *Oncol Nurs Forum* 26(8):1287, 1999.

Berg JA: The perimenopausal transition of Filipino American midlife women: biopsychosociocultural dimensions, *Nurs Res* 48(2):71, 1999.

Berger AM, Farr L: The influence of daytime inactivity and nighttime restlessness on cancer-related fatigue, *Oncol Nurs Forum* 26(10):1663, 1999.

Black TM, Soltis T, Bartlett C: Using the functional measure instrument to predict stroke rehabilitation independence outcomes, *Rehab Nurs* 24(3):109, 1999.

Boyle JS: Patterns of resistance: African-American mothers and adult children with HIV illness, *Sch Inq Nurs Pract* 13(2):111, 1999.

Broscious SK: Music: an intervention for pain during chest tube removal after open heart surgery, *Am J Crit Care* 8(6):410, 1999.

Bunting SM et al: Women's responses to battering: a test of the model, *Res Nurs Health* 22(1):49, 1999.

Carlson EV, Kemp MG, Shott S: Predicting the risk of pressure ulcers in critically ill patients, *Am J Crit Care* 8(4):262, 1999.

Carpenter JS, Andrykowski MA: Menopausal symptoms in breast cancer survivors, *Oncol Nurs Forum* 26(8):1311, 1999.

Carroll DL, Hamilton GA, McGovern BA: Changes in health status and quality of life and the impact of uncertainty in patients who survive life threatening arrhythmias, *Heart Lung* 28(4):251, 1999.

Carroll KC et al: Pain assessment and management in critically ill postoperative and trauma patients: a multisite study, *Am J Crit Care* 8(2):105, 1999.

Cathelyn J, Glenn LL: Effect of ambient temperature and cardiac stability on two methods of cardiac output measurement, *J Cardiovasc Nurs* 13(3):93, 1999.

Cheever KH: Pain, analgesic use, and morbidity in appendectomy patients, *Clin Nurs Res* 8(3):267, 1999.

Coward DD: Lymphedema prevention and management knowledge in women treated for breast cancer, *Oncol Nurs Forum* 26(6):1047, 1999.

Dalton JA et al: An evaluation of facial expression displayed by patients with chest pain, *Heart Lung* 28(3):168, 1999.

Defloor T, Grypdonck MHK: Sitting posture and prevention of pressure ulcers, *Appl Nur Res* 12(3):136, 1999.

Dimeo F, Rumberger BG, Keul J: Aerobic exercise as therapy for cancer fatigue, *Med Sci Sports Exerc* 30(4):475, 1998.

Dow KH et al: The meaning of quality of life in cancer survivorship, *Oncol Nurs Forum* 26(3):519, 1999.

Draucker CB, Madsen C: Women dwelling with violence, *Image J Nurs Schol* 31(4):327, 1999.

Dunbar SB et al: Factors associated with outcomes 3 months after implantable cardioverter defibrillator insertion, *Heart Lung* 28(5):303, 1999.

Duquette-Petersen L et al: The role of protective clothing in infection prevention in patients undergoing autologous bone marrow transplant, *Oncol Nurs Forum* 26(8):1319, 1999.

Edmiston CE et al: Airborne particulates in the OR environment, *AORN J* 69(6):1169, 1999.

Facione NC: Breast cancer screening in relation to access to health services, *Oncol Nurs Forum* 6(4):689, 1999.

Ferrell BR, Juarez G, Bornemann T: Use of routine and breakthrough analgesia in home care, *Oncol Nurs Forum* 26(10):1655, 1999.

Fall-Dickson JM, Rose L: Caring for patients who experience chemotherapy-induced side effects: the meaning for oncology nurses. *Oncol Nurs Forum* 26(5):901, 1999.

Faulkner MS: Quality of life for persons with developmental disabilities, *Sch Inq Nurs Pract* 13(3):239, 1999.

Fitch JA et al: Oral care in the adult intensive care unit, *Am J Crit Care* 8(5):314, 1999.

Fowler TJ, Magarelli K: Hope and anxiety of individual family members of critically ill adults, *Appl Nur Res* 12(3):121, 1999.

Gigliotti E: Women's multiple role stress: testing Neuman's flexible line of defense, *Nurs Science Q* 12(1):36, 1999.

Glass C, Grap MJ, Sessler CN: Endotracheal tube narrowing after closed system functioning: prevalence and risk factors, *Am J Crit Care* 8(2):93, 1999.

Goldsborough MA et al: Prevalence of leg wound complications after coronary artery bypass grafting: determinants of risk factors, *Am J Crit Care* 8(3):149, 1999.

Grady KL, Jalowiec A, White-Williams C: Preoperative psychological predictors of hospital length of stay after heart transplantation, *J Cardiovasc Nurs* 14(1):12, 1999.

Grant JS: Social problem solving partnerships with family caregivers, *Rehab Nurs* 24(6):254, 1999.

Grap MJ et al: Use of backrest elevation in critical care: a pilot study, *Am J Crit Care* 8(1):475, 1999.

Griffiths DH, Pokorny ME, Bowman JM: Differences in African American and white women with myocardial infarction: history, presentation, diagnostic methods, and infarction type, *Am J Crit Care* 8(2):101, 1999.

Hagerty BM, Williams RA: The effects of sense of belonging, social support, conflict and loneliness on depression, *Nurs Res* 48(4):215, 1999.

Haight BK, Bahr ST: Setting an agenda for clinical nursing research in long term care, *Clin Nurs Res* 1(2):144, 1992.

Halm M et al: Women and cardiac rehabilitation: referral and compliance patterns, *J Cardiovasc Nurs* 13(3):83, 1999.

Hart KJ, Palmer MH, Fitzgerald S: Perceived causes of urinary incontinence and reporting: a study with working women, *Clin Nurs Res* 8(3):267, 1999.

Harvey RM, Kazis L, Lee AF: Decision making preference and opportunity in VA ambulatory care patients: association with patient satisfaction, *Res Nurs Health* 22(1):39, 1999.

Hatton JM, Nunnelee JD: Research priorities in vascular nursing, *J Vasc Nurs* 13(1):1, 1995.

Hirschfeld MJ: WHO priorities for a common nursing research agenda, *Image J Nurs Schol* 30(2):114, 1998.

Holzworth RJ, Wills CE: Nurses judgments regarding seclusion and restraint of psychiatric patients: a social judgment analysis, *Res Nurs Health* 22(3):189, 1999.

Houston S, Jesurum J: The quick relaxation technique: effect on pain associated with chest tube removal, *Appl Nurs Res* 12(4):196, 1999.

Humphreys J et al: Trauma history of sheltered battered women, *Issues Mental Health Nurs* 20(4):319, 1999.

Humphreys JC et al: Sleep patterns of sheltered battered women, *Image J Nurs Schol* 31(2):139, 1999.

Im E, Meleis A: A situation-specific theory of Korean immigrant women's menopausal transition, *Image J Nurs Schol* 31(4):333, 1999.

Jacobson AF: Intradermal normal saline solution, self selected music, and insertion difficulty effects on intravenous insertion pain, *Heart Lung* 28(2):114, 1999.

Jennings-Dozier K: Perceptual determinants of Pap test up-to-date status among minority women, *Oncol Nurs Forum* 26(8):1327, 1999a.

Jennings-Dozier K: Predicting intentions to obtain a Pap smear among African American and Latina women: testing the theory of planned behavior, *Nurs Res* 48(4):198, 1999b.

Jepson C et al: Effects of home care on caregivers' psychological status, *Image J Nurs Schol* 31(2):115, 1999.

Johnson KL et al: Therapeutic paralysis of critically ill trauma patients: perceptions of patients and their family members, *Am J Crit Care* 8(1):490, 1999.

Keavney ME, Zauszniewski JA: Life events and psychological well being in women sentenced to prison, *Issues Mental Health Nurs* 20(1):73, 1999.

Keller C, Chintapalli K, Lancaster J: Correlation of anthropometry with CT in Mexican-American women, *Res Nurs Health* 22(2):145, 1999.

Kelly P: Isolation and stigmata: the experience of patients with active tuberculosis, *J Community Health Nurs* 16(4):233, 1999.

Keyserling TC et al: A cholesterol intervention program for public health nurses in the rural southeast: description of the intervention, study design, and baseline results, *Public Health Nurs* 16(3):156, 1999.

Kolcaba K, Fox C: The effects of guided imagery on comfort of women with early stage breast cancer undergoing radiation therapy, *Oncol Nurs Forum* 26(1):67, 1999.

Kowalski SD, Rayfield CA: A posthoc descriptive study of patients receiving propofol, *Am J Crit Care* 8(1):507, 1999.

Kruse BG: The lived experience of serenity, *Nurs Sci Q* 12(2):143, 1999.

Lanuza DM et al: Symptom experiences of lung transplant recipients: comparisons across gender, pretransplantation diagnosis and type of transplantation, *Heart Lung* 28(6):429, 1999.

Lareau SC et al: Dyspnea in patients with chronic obstructive pulmonary disease: does dyspnea worsen longitudinally in the presence of declining lung function? *Heart Lung* 28(1):65, 1999.

Lauver DR et al: Engagement in breast screening behaviors, *Oncol Nurs Forum* 26(5):545, 1999.

Lauver DR et al: Explaining women's intentions and use of hormones with menopause, *Res Nurs Health* 22(4):309, 1999.

Lehto RH, Cimprich B: Anxiety and directed attention in women awaiting breast cancer surgery, *Oncol Nurs Forum* 26(4):767, 1999.

Leidy NK, Haase JE: Functional status from the patient's perspective: the challenge of preserving personal integrity, *Res Nurs Health* 22(1):67, 1999.

Leske JS: Caregiver satisfaction with the preparation for discharge in a decreased-length-of-stay cardiac surgery program, *J Cardiovasc Nurs* 14(1):35, 1999.

Lewis SL et al: Research priorities for nephrology nursing, *ANNA J* 26(2):215, 1999.

Longman AJ, Braden CJ, Mishel MH: Side-effects burden, psychological adjustment, and life quality in women with breast cancer: pattern of association over time, *Oncol Nurs Forum* 26(5):909, 1999.

Lovely MP, Miakowski C, Dodd M: Relationship between fatigue and quality of life in patients with glioblastoma multiformae, *Oncol Nurs Forum* 26(5):921, 1999.

Lucke KT: Outcomes of nurse caring as perceived by individuals with spinal cord injury during rehabilitation, *Rehab Nurs* 24(6):247, 1999.

MacLean SL et al: The LUNAR project: a description of the population of individuals who seek health care at emergency departments, *J Emerg Nurs* 25(4):269, 1999.

Manworren RC et al: Clinical impact of preoperative respiratory syncytial virus testing, *AORN J* 69(5):1003, 1999.

Marcantonio R et al: The effects of crossed leg on blood pressure measurement, *Nurs Res* 48(2):105, 1999.

Martinelli AM: An explanatory model of variables influencing health promotion behaviors in smoking and nonsmoking college students, *Public Health Nurs* 16(4):263, 1999.

Mayer BW, Smith FB, King CA: Factors associated with victimization of personnel in emergency departments, *J Emerg Nurs* 25(5):361, 1999.

McCarthy D, Weihofen D: The effect of nutritional supplements on food intake in patients undergoing radiotherapy, *Oncol Nurs Forum* 26(5):897, 1999.

McCloy K et al: Effects of injectate volume on thermodilution measurements of cardiac output in patients with low ventricular ejection fraction, *Am J Crit Care* 8(2):86, 1999.

McDonald DD: Postoperative pain after hospital discharge, *Clin Nurs Res* 8(4):355, 1999.

Meischke H et al: How women label and respond to symptoms of acute myocardial infarction: responses to hypothetical symptom scenarios, *Heart Lung* 28(4):261, 1999.

Menzel LK: Ventilated patients' self esteem during intubation and after extubation, *Clin Nurs Res* 8(1):51, 1999.

Metheny NA, Aud MA, Wunderlich RJ: A survey of bedside methods used to detect pulmonary aspiration of enteral formula in intubated tube fed patients, *Am J Crit Care* 8(3):160, 1999.

Metheny NA et al: pH and concentration of bilirubin in feeding tube aspirates as predictors of tube placement, *Nurs Res* 48(4):189, 1999.

Mimnaugh L et al: Sensations experienced during removal of tubes in acute postoperative patients, *Appl Nur Res* 12(2):78, 1999.

Misener TR, Watkins JG, Ossege J: Public health nursing research priorities, *Public Health Nurs* 11(1):66, 1994.

Missik E: Personal perceptions and women's participation in cardiac rehabilitation, *Rehab Nurs* 24(4):158, 1999.

Mitchell R, Muggli M, Sato A: Cardiac rehabilitation: participating in an exercise program in a quest to survive, *Rehab Nurs* 24(6):236, 1999.

Mock V et al: Effects of exercise on fatigue, physical functioning, and emotional distress during radiation therapy for breast cancer, *Oncol Nurs Forum* 24(6):991, 1997.

Munet-Vilaro F, Folkman S, Gregorich S: Depressive symptomatology in three Latino groups, *West J Nurs Res* 21(2):209, 1999.

Neal LJ: Research supporting the congruence between rehabilitation principles and home health nursing practice, *Rehab Nurs* 24(3):115, 1999.

Nehls N: Borderline personality disorder: the voice of the patients, *Res Nurs Health* 22(4):285, 1999.

Nies MA, Vollman M, Cook T: African American women's experiences with physical activity in their daily lives, *Public Health Nurs* 16(1):23, 1999.

Northouse LL et al: The quality of life of African American women with breast cancer, *Res Nurs Health* 22(6):435, 1999.

Nuamah IF et al: Testing a theory for health-related quality of life in cancer patients: a structural equation approach, *Res Nurs Health* 22(3):231, 1999.

Nyamathi A et al: Associations between homeless women's intimate relationships and their health and well-being, *Res Nurs Health* 22(6):486, 1999.

Owen DC, Parker KP, McGuire DB: Comparison of sleep quality in patients with cancer and healthy subjects, *Oncol Nurs Forum* 26(10):1649, 1999.

Paice PA, DuPen A, Schwertz D: Catheter port cleansing techniques and the entry of povidone-iodine into the epidural space, *Oncol Nurs Forum* 26(3):603, 1999.

Parker CB, Minick P, Kee CC: Clinical decision-making processes in perioperative nursing, *AORN J* 70(1):45, 1999.

Parshall M: Adult emergency visits for chronic cardiorespiratory disease: does dyspnea matter? *Nurs Res* 48(2):62, 1999.

Paul L, Weinert C: Wellness profile of midlife women with a chronic illness, *Public Health Nurs* 16(5):341, 1999.

Peters RM: The effectiveness of therapeutic touch: a meta-analytic review, *Nurs Science Q* 12(1):52, 1999.

Phillips JM, Cohen MZ, Moses G: Breast cancer screening and African American women: fear, fatalism, and silence, *Oncol Nurs Forum* 26(3):561, 1999.

Pollack LE, Cramer RD: Patient satisfaction with two models of group therapy for people hospitalized with bipolar disorder, *Appl Nurs Res* 12(3):143, 1999.

Powers J, Bennett SJ: Measurement of dyspnea in patients treated with mechanical ventilation, *Am J Crit Care* 8(4):254, 1999.

Powers JM: Obtaining blood samples for coagulation studies from a normal saline lock, *Am J Crit Care* 8(4):250, 1999.

Pullen L, Tuck I, Wallace DC: Research priorities in mental health nursing, *Issues Mental Health Nurs* 20(3):217, 1999.

Rice VH: Nursing intervention and smoking cessation: a meta-analysis, *Heart Lung* 28(6):438, 1999.

Robinson L et al: Describing the work of nursing: the case of postsurgical nursing interventions for men with prostate cancer, *Res Nurs Health* 22(4):321, 1999.

Sabourin CB, Funk M: Readmission of patients after coronary artery bypass surgery, *Heart Lung* 28(4):243, 1999.

Samms MC: The husband's untold account of his wife's breast cancer: a chronologic analysis, *Oncol Nurs Forum* 26(8):1351, 1999.

Saunders JC: Family functioning in families providing care for a family member with schizophrenia, *Issues Mental Health Nurs* 20(2):95, 1999.

Savage LS, Canody C: Life with a left ventricular assist device: the patient's perspective, *Am J Crit Care* 8(5):340, 1999.

Scaggs BG, Yates BC: Quality of life comparisons after coronary angioplasty and coronary artery bypass graft surgery, *Heart Lung* 28(6):409, 1999.

Schell ES, Kayser-Jones J: The effect of role-taking ability on care giver-resident mealtime interaction, *Appl Nurs Res* 12(1):38, 1999.

Schickel SI et al: Achieving femoral artery hemostasis after cardiac catheterization: a comparison of methods, *Am J Crit Care* 8(6):406, 1999.

Schmeltz JO et al: Effects of position of chest drainage tube on volume drained and pressure, *Am J Crit Care* 8(5):319, 1999.

Schroeter K: Ethical perception and resulting action in perioperative nurses, *AORN J* 69(5):991, 1999.

Schulmeister L: Chemotherapy medication errors: descriptions, severity and contributing factors, *Oncol Nurs Forum* 26(6):1033, 1999.

Schulmeister L, Lifsey DS: Cervical cancer screening knowledge, behaviors and beliefs in Vietnamese women, *Oncol Nurs Forum* 26(5):879-887, 1999.

Schultz AAA et al: Etiology and incidence of pressure ulcers in surgical patients, *AORN J* 70(3):434, 1999.

Schuster MM et al: Learning retention in patients receiving midazolam during permanent pacemaker implantation, *J Cardiovasc Nurs* 14(1):27, 1999.

Schwarz KA: A study of relationship of caregiving appraisal to depressive symptomology and home care utilization, *J Community Health Nurs* 16(2):95, 1999.

Sedlak C et al: Orthopedic nursing research priorities, *Orthop Nurs* 17(2):51, 1998.

Sherman DW, Kirton CA: The experience of relapse to unsafe behavior among HIV positive, heterosexual, minority men, *Appl Nur Res* 12(2):91, 1999.

Simmons NA, Peterson JW, Hale C: Surveillance of suicidal behavior in Kitsap County, Washington, *Public Health Nurs* 16(5):337, 1999.

Smith CE: Caregiving effectiveness in families managing complex technology at home: replication of a model, *Nurs Res* 48(3):120, 1999.

Stetz KM et al: Oncology nursing society research priorities survey, *Oncol Nurs Forum* 22(4):785, 1995.

Tanabe P, Buschmann MB: A prospective study of ED pain management practices and the patient's perspective, *J Emerg Nurs* 25(3):171, 1999.

Taylor D: Effectiveness of professional-peer group treatment: symptom management for women with PMS, *Res Nurs Health* 22(6):496, 1999.

Um CC, Dancy BL: Relationship between coping strategies and depression among employed Korean immigrant wives, *Issues Ment Health Nurs* 20(5):485, 1999.

U.S. Department of Health and Human Services, Public Health Service: *Healthy People 2000: national health promotion and disease prevention objectives*, Washington, DC, 1991, Author.

Walker BL, Nail LM, Croyle RT: Does emotional expression make a difference in reactions to breast cancer? *Oncol Nurs Forum* 26(6):1025, 1999.

Wallace CJ et al: The effects of earplugs on sleep measures during exposure to intensive care unit noise, *Am J Crit Care* 8(4):210, 1999.

Washington O: Effects of cognitive and experimental group therapy on self efficacy and perceptions of employability of chemically dependent women, *Issues Mental Health Nurs* 20(3):181, 1999.

Waters CM: Professional nursing support for culturally diverse family members of critically ill adults, *Res Nurs Health* 22(2):107, 1999.

White JM: Effects of relaxing music on cardiac autonomic balance and anxiety after acute myocardial infarction, *Am J Crit Care* 8(4):220, 1999.

Wickham RS et al: Taste changes experienced by patients receiving chemotherapy, *Oncol Nurs Forum* 26(4):697, 1999.

Wiens ME, Relmer MA, Guyn HL: Music therapy as a treatment method for improving respiratory muscle strength in patients with advanced multiple sclerosis: a pilot study, *Rehab Nurs* 24(2):74, 1999.

Wolf AC, Ratner PA: Stress, social support, and a sense of coherence, *West J Nurs Res* 21(2):182, 1999.

Wright C et al: Effects of head-of-the-bed positioning on the electrocardiogram, *Appl Nurs Res* 12(3):163, 1999.

Learning Objectives

1   Identify clinical nursing journals that publish research articles relevant to older adults.

2   Discuss clinical and research priorities in the care of older adults.

3   Use research literature to clarify identified clinical practice problems for older adults.

4   Explore examples of research conducted in various areas of clinical practice with older adults.

5   Discuss application of sample research results in clinical practice.

6   Apply the reading strategy to survey, examine, critically read, and evaluate a sample research article on older adults.

Chapter Outline

What Research Resources Are Available for the Care of Older Adults?

What Approaches Can Be Used for Review of the Research Literature?
  Addressing clinical and research priorities
  Using issues that arise from clinical practice
  Scanning available resources

What Current Research Is Available?
  Nursing research journals
  Clinical nursing journals
  Summarizing and using scan results
How to Read and Evaluate a Research Article on the Care of Older Adults

Reading and Using Research in the Care of Older Adults

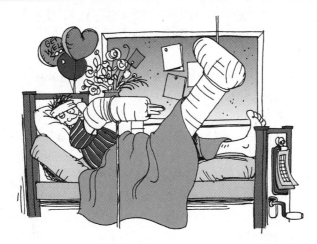

Obviously no one in this institution has read the latest research on fall prevention.

Student Quote   *"I never connected with old people until I read a study [qualitative] that told it their way [from their perspective]. It really opened my eyes."*

Abstract   Several research sources publish articles pertinent to the care of older adults. Many of the research articles on older adults focus on the clinical specialty issues identified for adults and can be distinguished only by looking at the age of the sample. Other articles address specific clinical issues unique to the aging population. These sources are used to demonstrate the research available on identified priorities for the aging and sample problems and questions arising from clinical practice and to examine a cross-section of current research about older adults. Samples of current studies are summarized, and clinical applications are discussed. The use of the research reading strategy is illustrated with one qualitative research article on an older adult population.

In this chapter, we identify periodicals that contain nursing research on care of older adults, target relevant research articles, and preview sample selections of currently published research. Finally we dissect a sample article using the reading strategy and evaluation criteria presented in Chapter 7.

> An older adult is defined as anyone 65 years of age or older.

What Research Resources Are Available for the Care of Older Adults?

Many of the resources available for reporting nursing research relevant to older adults are the same as those we identified for the adult population. One clinical journal currently available, the *Journal of Gerontological Nursing,* focuses on research relevant to the older adult. Box 11-1 contains a list of journals most likely to contain research relevant to the practice of nursing for older adults.

The last category of journals listed in Box 11-1 are journals that specialize in nursing issues related to the care of the older adult. Although *Geriatric Nursing* does not regularly print nursing research articles, it does occasionally have such articles. It does review current research on the older adult and uses current research to illustrate specified clinical examples. As with adults, studies on the older adult are scattered across a wide range of journals other than those listed in Box 11-1. Try the following Student Challenge one last time.

STUDENT CHALLENGE Perusing Specialty Journals

1. If any journals left on the list in Box 11-1 are unfamiliar, take time to locate and scan two or three issues of each journal.
2. Locate a description of the journal's purpose and evaluate its readability.

What Approaches Can Be Used for Review of the Research Literature?

We again explore our three strategies for use of the research literature as it pertains to older adults. We explore the relevant clinical and research priorities, iden-

| Box 11-1 | Journals Containing Nursing Research Relevant to Care of Older Adults |

Nursing Research Journals

Nursing Research
Research in Nursing and Health
Western Journal of Nursing Research
Applied Nursing Research
Clinical Nursing Research
Nursing Science Quarterly
Image: Journal of Nursing Scholarship
Scholarly Inquiry for Nursing Practice

Clinical Journals that Regularly Contain Research Articles About the Care of Older Adults

Cardiovascular Nursing
Heart and Lung: Journal of Critical Care
Issues in Mental Health Nursing
Journal of Community Health Nursing
Journal of Emergency Nursing
Journal of Gerontological Nursing
Oncology Nursing Forum
Public Health Nursing
Rehabilitation Nursing

Gerontological Journals that Occasionally Contain Research on the Care of Older Adults

Geriatric Nursing
Elderly Care

tify some sample problems or questions that might arise from clinical practice with an aging population, and we scan the research literature to get a feel for available research that might enhance clinical practice.

Addressing Clinical and Research Priorities

Let's look at the care and research priorities relevant to an adult population. Slowing age-related changes such as visual or hearing impairment; loss of bone and muscle mass; maintaining functional independence in primary and secondary activities of daily living; coping with impairment, reduced function, and disability; and death with dignity are important goals in the care of older adults. We view the pertinent *Healthy People 2000* objectives, review research priorities of the National Institute for Nursing Research (NINR), and look at available nursing clinical specialty sources for research priorities.

Healthy People 2000 details several health care goals and objectives aimed specifically at the older adult. The objectives for adults listed in Chapter 10 are also relevant to older adults. Those objectives focused specifically on the older adult are listed in Box 11-2.

The NINR research priorities reveal several issues related to care of older adults. Long-term care; management of chronic neurological conditions such as stroke, Parkinson's disease, and Alzheimer's disease; and end-of-life care including palliation, management of pain, maintaining quality of life and choices during end-stage care were all priorities in the 1990s. In 2000, enhancing end-of-life care remained a top priority.

Specialty organizations have established or enumerated other research priorities in the 1990s. The *Journal of Gerontological Nursing* explored priority issues for nursing care of the older adult in 1995 (Gueldner et al). A long-term care research agenda was outlined in *Clinical Nursing Research* in 1992 (Haight and Bahr). *Elderly*

Box 11-2   *Healthy People 2000* Objectives

Improve nutrition through increased home delivery of meals
Reduce loss of natural teeth
Increase skin, oral, and rectal examinations and examinations for occult
    blood and use of sigmoidoscopy
Reduce loss of abilities to perform activities of daily living
Reduce hearing impairment
Reduce visual impairment
Reduce hip fractures
Increase routine screenings for urinary incontinence, sensory impairments,
    and functional status
Reduce incidence of pneumonia and influenza and increase pneumonia and
    influenza immunization
Increase use of community-based health promotion programs
Increase monitoring of prescription and over-the-counter drugs

From U.S. Department of Health and Human Services, Public Health Service: *Healthy People 2000: national health promotion and disease prevention objectives*, Washington, DC, 1991, Author.

Care reported on a way to develop a user-focused agenda in gerontological nursing research (McCormack and Ford, 1999).

Try the following Student Challenge to discover the very latest in research priorities for the older adult.

STUDENT CHALLENGE Checking Research Priorities for Older Adults

1. Check the *Healthy People 2010* goals and objectives. (Refer to the Resource Kit at the end of this chapter to access this website.) Locate the objectives relevant to care for older adults. Compare them to the objectives in Box 11-2. Note similarities and differences.
2. Check to see if any research priorities for the older adult have been reported by specialty journals after 1999. (Hint: Run a CINAHL search using the key words "nursing research priorities.")
3. Choose one of the research priorities previously listed or that you have uncovered in your search. Run a literature search for the years 2000 to present and see what nursing research has been conducted in your selected area.

MERLIN
Activity
20

Using Issues that Arise from Clinical Practice

In this section, we examine another example of a clinical question that might arise during clinical practice, explore the search process, and examine the search results. When we look at problems that arise in our practice with older adults, we need to first ask what function age plays in the identified problem. Is age a primary focus (i.e., a major factor in the cause of the problem), or is the problem one that could occur at any age. If the answer is the latter, then ask whether you are focusing on how the problem uniquely impacts the older adult. Remember the other parameters we've used to help define problems (i.e., the target of care, level of care, aspect of care, and care setting).

I am a nurse who works in a residential care setting for the elderly. There has been increased concern regarding several residents who have fallen lately. We are getting ready to adopt a risk factors checklist. I have been asked to come up with additional ideas to help decrease the number of falls. I head for the literature with an interest in the current research available on the subject of falls and how they might be prevented or reduced. I do a CINAHL search, entering the key word "falls." This sends me to a mapping display with two subject headings. I choose "accidental falls" and check the Explode box. I am then given the option of 10 subheadings under accidental falls. Because I am unsure which might be useful, I check the box to include all of the headings. I now decide to place several limits on my search by clicking on the "Limit" heading at the top of the search screen. I then limit my search to United States nursing journals for the years 1997 through 1999 that reported research on falls for those aged 65 to 79. I get a total of 20 articles from the search. I later run a second search to include those aged 80 and above. It yields one additional study. So I have a total of 21 studies to look at.

I pull the abstracts for all 21 articles. Eight articles are quickly eliminated; one because falls were not a primary focus of the study, another because it studied subjects in Japan, two because they were testing reliability and validity of instruments, and four because they were not research studies. One of these four is, in fact, a review of the research literature on falls from 1992 to 1994. This leaves me with 12 articles. Seven of these examined various risk factors for falls. Four articles tested various nursing interventions for fall prevention. One article was a qualitative study. It examined the experience of falling from the perspective of the person falling. All of these studies provide helpful information.

The risk factor articles (Resnick, 1999; Mentes et al, 1999; Arbesman and Wright, 1999; Tsai et al, 1998; Topp et al, 1997; Isberner et al, 1998; Fortin et al, 1998) used subjects drawn from retirement communities, long-term care facilities, hospitals, and home environments. Likely risk factors included physiological factors (e.g., atrial fibrillation, neurosensory impairment, dehydration, infection, hypoxia, generalized muscle weakness, postural control, frequent urinary voiding urgency), organic factors (e.g., degree of alertness and attention, confusion, dementia, delirium), environmental factors (e.g., use of restraints, availability of hand holds, footing and walking surfaces, use of assistive walking devices), and demographic factors (e.g., age, gender, marital status, history of falls). Although many of the factors cited were expected, some were new to me. These served to confirm the risk factors checklist we were getting ready to adopt at the facility.

The intervention-based studies (Mosley et al, 1998; Ash, MacLeod, and Clark, 1998; Abreu et al, 1998; Schoenfelder and Van Why, 1997) used subjects from hospitals, a community-based senior citizens center, and private homes. Only one intervention strategy produced a significant reduction in falls (Mosley et al, 1998). This intervention strategy was based on data from research studies, expert opinion, and a pilot study. It showed that 72% of the hospital units that implemented the strategy had significantly fewer falls. The research also demonstrated that the majority of those who did fall were at risk for falling according to their fall assessment scores. I decide to take this strategy back to the director of nursing for my facility and discuss using a modified version tailored for our institution.

The qualitative studies (Porter, 1999; Turkoski et al., 1997) provided valuable information about the experience of falling from the patient's perspective and the clinical knowledge nurses use to assess risk and prevent falls. (Check out the article evaluation section for a better picture of the fall experience article). I decide to use these two articles for reading for the staff and to help in constructing a staff-training program. Now you try the following Student Challenge.

STUDENT CHALLENGE Chasing the Challenges of Aging

1. Review your experiences in caring for older adults and think about a situation that you wish to explore in the current research literature.
2. Identify appropriate search parameters for the subject material and conduct a library search for the year 2000 to present. What did you find?
3. If your search was fruitful, retrieve one or two promising articles.
4. Review the articles. How might the results of the studies be helpful in clinical practice?

Scanning Available Resources

Let's explore what was available in the research literature by using our third strategy and scanning the table of contents and the abstracts of the research and clinical specialty journals listed in Box 11-1.

STUDENT CHALLENGE Scanning Relevant Journals

Select one research journal and one clinical journal from those listed in Box 11-1 that are available in your library.
1. Scan the 2000 table of contents for each of these journals and note those research articles that seem relevant to the care of older adults.
2. Read the abstracts for the selected articles. Weed out any articles that are not clinically relevant. How long did this take you? Are you getting more proficient?

Save these articles. We use them again in the next Student Challenge.

What Current Research Is Available?

The following are specific examples of pertinent research articles for the care of older adults that I found by scanning the 1999 tables of contents of the research and clinical journals listed in Box 11-1. Selected articles are briefly summarized and clinical implications are discussed.

Nursing Research Journals

The articles found by scanning the tables of contents of the various research journals yielded the article titles listed in Box 11-3.

This scan produced a total of 21 articles on the older adult population. The *Western Journal of Nursing Research* devoted most of an issue to research on caregiving issues with the elderly. Some titles identify older adults as the target population. For other studies, the population is not evident until you read the abstract.

Box 11-3   Relevant Titles for the Aging in Research Journals

Nursing Research

Mood and Blood Pressure Responses in Black Female Caregivers and Non-caregivers (Picot et al, 1999)

Cognitive-Behavioral Intervention for Homebound Caregivers of Persons with Dementia (Chang, 1999)

Problem-Solving Counseling for Caregivers of the Cognitively Impaired: Effective for Whom? (Roberts et al, 1999)

Research in Nursing and Health

Acute Confusion Indicators: Risk Factors and Prevalence Using MDS Data (Mentes et al, 1999)

Mediation Effect of Social Support Between Ethnic Attachment and Loneliness in Older Korean Immigrants (Kim, 1999)

Appropriateness of Self-Care Responses to Symptoms Among Elders: Identifying Pathways of Influence (Edwardson and Dean, 1999)

Initiation of Physical Restraint in Nursing Home Residents Following Restraint Reduction Efforts (Sullivan-Marx et al, 1999)

Functional Status from the Patient's Perspective: The Challenge of Preserving Personal Integrity (Leidy and Haase, 1999)

Box 11-3   Relevant Titles for the Aging in Research Journals—cont'd

Western Journal of Nursing Research

Grief in Child and Spouse Caregivers of Dementia Patients (Lindgren, Connelly, and Gaspar, 1999)

Fatigue Among Elders in Caregiving and Noncaregiving Roles (Teel and Press, 1999)

Is There a Difference Between Family Caregiving of Institutionalized Elders with or Without Dementia? (Levesque, Ducharme, and LaChance, 1999)

Respite—A Coping Strategy for Family Caregivers (Strang and Haughey, 1999)

Applied Nursing Research

Mutuality and Preparedness of Family Caregivers for Elderly Women After Bypass (Kneeshaw, Considine, and Jennings, 1999)

Depression Among Nursing Home Elders: Testing an Intervention Strategy (McCurren, 1999)

Nurses' Perceptions of Chemical Restraint Use in Long Term Care (Thurmond, 1999)

Scholarly Inquiry For Nursing Practice

No relevant articles

Image: Journal of Nursing Scholarship

Depression, Social Support, and Quality of Life in Older Adults with Osteoarthritis (Blixen and Kippes, 1999)

Persistence of Self in Advanced Alzheimer's Disease (Tappen et al, 1999)

Ethnomethodologic Analysis of Accounts of Feeding Demented Residents in Long Term Care Facilities (Pierson, 1999)

Clinical Nursing Research

Falls in a Community of Older Adults (Resnick, 1999)

A Typology of Consumers of Institutional Respite Care (Smyer and Chang, 1999)

Adherent and Nonadherent Medication-Taking in Elderly Hypertensive Patients (Johnson, Williams, and Marshall, 1999)

Nursing Science Quarterly

No relevant research

An examination of the titles of the articles listed in Box 11-3 reveals several patterns. Eight of the 21 articles focus on caregivers of the elderly as the target population. Issues of primary importance in an older population are clearly evident by the article topics, including dementia, confusion, and depression; and falls, preserving personal integrity, and maintaining functional status. Nursing issues such as restraint use, medication-taking, and feeding are also addressed.

Clinical Nursing Journals

The articles found by scanning the tables of contents of the clinical journals yielded several relevant research articles listed in Box 11-4.

Eight clinical journals regularly publish research on care of older adults. All of these journals publish that research within a confined specialty area. The *Journal of Gerontological Nursing* publishes articles in the area of gerontological nursing, and many of these articles are research studies. A total of 32 relevant articles surfaced, most of which are found in the *Journal of Gerontological Nursing*. As expected, the articles in the specialty journals focus on the specialty topic (e.g., can-

---

Box 11-4   Relevant Research Article Titles for Older Adults in Clinical Journals

Heart and Lung: Journal of Critical Care

Effects of Age on Activity Patterns After Coronary Artery Bypass Surgery (Redeker and Wykpisz, 1999)

The Meaning of Hospital Care as Narrated by Elderly Patients with Chronic Heart Failure (Ekman, Lundman, and Norgerg, 1999)

Issues in Mental Health Nursing

Psychological Correlates of Subjective Health in Sexagenarians, Octogenerians and Centarians (Quinn et al, 1999)

Use of the Cognitive Abilities Screening Instrument to Assess Elderly Persons with Schizophrenia in Long Term Care Settings (Sherrell et al, 1999)

Quality of Life and Successful Aging in Long Term Care: Perceptions of Residents (Guse and Masesar, 1999)

Effect of Self Care ADLs on Self Esteem of Intact Nursing Home Residents (Blair, 1999)

| Box 11-4 | Relevant Research Article Titles for Older Adults in Clinical Journals—cont'd |

Journal of Cardiovascular Nursing

The Effects of Discharge Planning and Home Follow Up Intervention on Elders Hospitalized with Common Medical and Surgical Cardiac Conditions (Naylor and McCauley, 1999)

Dysrhymthia Update: Differential Diagnosis of Supraventricular Tachycardia in an Elderly Man (McCauley, Lloyd, and Doherty, 1999)

Prosthetic Valve Endocarditis Leading to Valve Replacement: A Case Study (Hubner, 1999)

Journal of Community Health Nursing

Caregivers of Chronically Ill Elderly: Perceived Burden (Faison, 1999)

A Study of the Relationship of Caregiving Appraisal to Depressive Symptomatology and Home Care Utilization (Schwarz, 1999)

Journal of Emergency Nursing

Adding Medications in the Emergency Department: Effect on Knowledge of Medications in Older Adults (Hayes, 1999)

Elderly Patients' Perceptions of Care in the Emergency Department (Watson, Marshall, and Fosbinder, 1999)

Journal of Gerontological Nursing

A Comparative Study of Nurses and Elderly Patients Ratings of Pain and Pain Tolerance (Bergh and Szostrom, 1999)

Institutionalized Older Adults' Perceptions of Nursing Caring Behaviors. A Pilot Study (Marini, 1999)

The Effectiveness of Slow-Stroke Massage in Diffusing Agitated Behaviors in Individuals with Alzheimer's Disease (Rowe and Alfred, 1999)

Comparison of Caregivers', Residents', and Community-Dwelling Spouses' Opinions about Expressing Sexuality in an Institutional Setting (Gibson et al, 1999)

Communicating with Individuals with Dementia: The Impaired Person's Perspective (Acton et al, 1999)

Interventions for Disruptive Behaviors: Use and Success (Bair, 1999)

Comparison of Three Instruments in Predicting Accidental Falls in Selected Inpatients in a General Teaching Hospital (Eagle et al, 1999)

An Intervention Study to Enhance Medication Compliance in Community Dwelling Elderly Individuals (Fulmar et al, 1999)

Continued

| Box 11-4 | Relevant Research Article Titles for Older Adults in Clinical Journals—cont'd |

Journal of Gerontological Nursing—cont'd

Developing Individualized Care in Nursing Homes: Integrating the Views of Nurses and Certified Nurses Aides (Walker et al, 1999)

Assessing Patients in the Early Stages of Irreversible Dementia: The Relevance of Patient Perspectives (Burgener and Dickerson-Putman, 1999)

Moments of Excellence: Nurses Response to Role Redesign in Long-Term Care (Turkel, Tappen, and Hall, 1999)

Water Intake of Nursing Home Residents (Gasper, 1999)

Oncology Nursing Forum

An Intervention to Decrease Cancer Fatalism Among Rural Elders (Powe and Weinrich, 1999)

The Effect of an Educational Intervention on Decreasing Pain Intensity in Elderly People with Cancer (Clotfelter, 1999)

Public Health Nursing

A Model for Building Collective Capacity in Community-Based Programs: The Elderly in Need Project (Moyer et al, 1999)

Rehabilitation Nursing

Continuity and Discontinuity: The Quality of Life Following Stroke (Secrest and Thomas, 1999)

Getting Up from Here: Frail Older Women's Experiences After Falling (Porter, 1999)

Mechanical Restraints, Rehabilitation Therapies, and Staffing Adequacy as Risk Factors for Falls in an Elderly Hospitalized Population (Arbesman and Wright, 1999)

A Decentralized Admission Screening Protocol for a Geriatric Rehabilitation Program: Does It Make a Difference? (Touranbeau, Prentice, and Costello, 1999) cer or cardiovascular or public health). However, themes are once again evident as we review the titles. Elder issues such as self-care, quality of life, and pain are evident. Diseases and conditions common to the older adult such as dementia, Alzheimer's, and stroke are addressed. Nursing intervention issues such as falls, medication compliance, hydration, activity patterns, and general nursing interventions are apparent. There is also another report on caregivers. What other trends or patterns do you see when scanning the titles in Box 11-4?

Summarizing and Using Scan Results

Several of the identified research articles have been selected to serve as examples for how research articles might be summarized and the findings used in clinical practice. Several articles in both the research and clinical journals examined aspects of nursing care. They provide concrete data about the effectiveness of certain nursing interventions used in the care of adult populations. We look at several of these articles in more depth.

The first study (Roberts et al, 1999) tested the effectiveness of a nurse counseling strategy in helping family caregivers of homebound cognitively impaired elders to cope. An experimental study randomly assigned 77 caregivers to a treatment or control group. The treatment group received problem-based nurse counseling. All subjects were measured for their psychological adjustment to the relative's illness and for the variables of psychological distress, perceived caregiver burden, and coping skills. These measurements were made after 6 months and again after 1 year. On the whole, subjects in the counseling intervention showed no significant improvement on psychological adjustment, distress, or burden. However, they reported perceiving the counseling as helpful.

A subset of the counseling group (those who tested as having limited coping skills in the use of logical analysis) had significantly decreased psychological distress and improved psychological adjustment. Caregivers in both groups whose relatives were admitted to a nursing home showed improvements in their psychological adjustments, whereas caregivers in both groups whose relative remained in the home showed declines in their psychological adjustments. Counseling was perceived as helpful by caregivers. Caregivers with poor logical analysis coping abilities significantly benefited from counseling. The most psychological benefit came from removal of the relative from a home care situation.

A related experimental study (Chang, 1999) randomly assigned 65 caregivers to a treatment group who received a specific 2-week cognitive behavioral intervention and a control group who received phone call follow-up. Variables of coping strategies, caregiver burden, caregiver satisfaction, and emotional and physical health were measured at baseline and at 4, 8, and 12 weeks. Both groups showed a significant reduction in anxiety and decrease in satisfaction over time. Both groups also showed a decreased use of emotion-focused coping strategies. The treatment group showed less depression over time than the control group. The intervention thus proved effective for preventing progression of depression in caregivers.

Both of these studies indicate some promise in the use of specific nursing interventions with family caregivers. Additional research is needed to examine various strategies across several variables.

Another pilot study examined variables that might predict the application of restraints for older adults in a nursing home setting (Sullivan-Marx et al, 1999). Data were collected for a large number of resident characteristics and environmental factors for 335 residents of three nursing homes. The incidence of restraint use was also collected. All homes had just had various programs aimed at reduction of the use of restraints. The incidence of restraint use was low with just 23 occurrences. Seventeen of these were in one facility, indicating a probable lack in their restraint reduction program. Findings indicated that only the cognitive status of the resident and the staff-mix ratios were predictive of restraint use. Restraints were used more frequently on the cognitively impaired and when more licensed personnel were available for care. The use of such a large number of variables and such a small sample size severely limit these results and indicate need for further study before any practice recommendations are made.

Another experimental study (Blair, 1999) involved two units of nursing home residents. Ten residents on one unit received routine task-oriented nursing care while 10 residents on a second unit received an educative-supportive system of nursing care. This nursing strategy was designed to foster autonomy and control among the residents. All residents were cognitively and physically intact and able to perform independent activities of daily living. The group who received the supportive educative nursing intervention approach performed significantly more self-care behaviors and had significantly higher self-esteem levels than those in the routine nursing care group. Implications for nursing support the need for an environment in which nursing care enhances opportunities for autonomy and personal control and a sense of competence. This study demonstrates that such nursing care interventions are taught relatively easily to staff and are easy to implement.

Another study (Naylor and McCauley, 1999) examined 202 patients aged 65 or older with common cardiac conditions who were randomly assigned to control or treatment groups. The treatment group received comprehensive discharge planning and follow-up by an advanced practice nurse for 4 weeks after discharge. The control group received the usual level of nursing care. The functional status of both groups was comparable. The intervention group had significantly fewer readmissions and a reduced number of hospital days on readmission. This study supports the use of discharge planning and home follow-up care that includes telephone and home visits by an advanced practice nurse.

A study by Clotfelter (1999) examined the effect of an educational intervention on the pain intensity of 36 elderly outpatients with cancer. One group was shown a video and given a pamphlet on ways to manage their cancer pain. Control group members received the usual routine information from the office staff. The group who received the intervention showed significantly lower levels of pain intensity than those in the control group. This study supports that nurses can effectively design and use interventions to help elderly individuals more effectively manage their cancer pain.

Several qualitative investigations were done on elder and elder care experiences. We review some of these. The first was a study done with 10 caregivers for elders with dementia (Strang and Haughey, 1999). It examined how family caregivers viewed the experience of respite (temporary relief from responsibilities of care). The respite experience was described as a process of "getting out" and was seen as a coping strategy. Three phases were identified: recognizing the need to get out, giving oneself permission to get out temporarily, and having available social support resources to facilitate getting out. This information can be of value to the nurse who works with long-term family caregivers to assist caregivers in identifying when respite care is needed, to help them give themselves permission to use respite care, and to have mechanisms in place to readily access respite care.

A qualitative study (Tappen et al, 1999) was done with 23 residents of two urban nursing homes who were in the middle or late stages of Alzheimer's disease. Thirty-minute conversations were held with the residents about their recent activities, the immediate environment, their families, their health, and their past experiences. These conversations were taped and analyzed for evidence that supported or countered the notion of a persistence of self (personal identity).

Findings indicated the respondents were aware of themselves and their cognitive changes. This runs counter to the prevailing theme that the self is diminished in the late stages of Alzheimer's disease. Holding such a belief might lead to task-oriented care and low expectations for therapeutic intervention. A better understanding of the concept of self and evidence that it persists in the face of declining cognition should lead nurses to think about ways to care that avoid dehumanization and encourage therapeutic relationships. Taking the time and effort to converse with and use questioning as a technique to draw Alzheimer's patients into the conversation facilitate therapeutic interaction.

Another qualitative study (Acton et al, 1999) reported on communications with individuals with dementia and demonstrated that individuals with dementia were able to send and receive meaningful communication. This study enhances the implications of the previous study and reiterates the need for client-centered interventions and interactions with persons who have cognitive impairments. Now complete the following Student Challenge.

STUDENT CHALLENGE Using Data from Journal Scans

Use the articles that resulted from your journal scan.

1. Read the articles to determine what was studied, who was studied, and what the study results were. Write a brief summary of each article. Use the previously cited articles as examples.
2. Read the discussion sections of articles and make a quick determination about how the results might be used in a clinical practice setting. Write out how the findings might be used and by whom.

How to Read and Evaluate a Research Article on the Care of Older Adults

In this section, we examine one qualitative research article on a clinical intervention in more depth. We again use our research reading strategy, research comprehension, and research evaluation guidelines.

STUDENT CHALLENGE Surveying, Examining, and Critically Reading an Adult Research Study

1. Log onto your CD-ROM and look for the Survey, Examine, and Critically Read exercise in Chapter 11. Print out the reading strategy and the research article entitled "'Getting Up from Here': Frail Older Women's Experiences After Falling."
2. Take your text, the article, the strategy, and a notepad and pen, and find a conducive reading and study environment.
3. Survey the article using the strategy guidelines. Make notes of what you gleaned from your survey.
4. Now go back and read the article paragraph by paragraph and jot down the key idea in each paragraph. Note anything that you don't understand.
5. When you have finished, consult needed references to clarify those things that are unclear.
6. When you have completed these steps, go back to the CD-ROM and complete the Survey, Examine, and Critically Read exercise, the Study Evaluation exercise, and the Application Visualization exercise for Chapter 11.

ADVENTURE CD
11-1

ADVENTURE CD
11-2

ADVENTURE CD
11-3

These CD-ROM exercises guide you through the critical reading, evaluation, and visualization of the selected research article. When you finish, print out your answers and my responses to the exercises. You should be feeling pretty good about your abilities to read and summarize a research article about now.

Resource Kit

Web Sources for Older Adult Research Priorities
  Healthy People 2000 and *Healthy People 2010*
  National Institute for Nursing Research

Web Sources for Relevant Journal Table of Contents and Abstracts
  Nursing Research
  Research in Nursing and Health

MERLIN
Activity
21

Continued

Activity

22

Resource Kit—cont'd

Web Sources for Relevant Journal Table of Contents
and Abstracts—cont'd

Geriatric Nursing

Journal of Gerontological Nursing

Miscellaneous Web Resources

Go to MERLIN and link to the 162-journal site to see if any journals are
relevant to care of the older adult.

Visit the book's MERLIN website at
www.mosby.com/MERLIN/Langford/maze
for further information.

References

Abreu N et al: Effect of group versus home visit safety education and prevention strategies for falling in community-dwelling elderly persons, *Home Health Care Manage Pract* 10(4):57, 1998.

Acton GJ et al: Communicating with individuals with dementia. The impaired person's perspective, *J Gerontol Nurs* 25(2):6, 1999.

Arbesman MC, Wright C: Mechanical restraints, rehabilitation therapies, and staffing adequacy as risk factors for falls in an elderly hospitalized population, *Rehab Nurs* 24(3):122, 1999.

Ash KL, MacLeod P, Clark L: A case control study of falls in a hospital setting, *J Gerontol Nurs* 24(12):7, 1998.

Bair B et al: Interventions for disruptive behaviors. Use and success, *J Gerontol Nurs* 25(1):13, 1999.

Bergh I, Szostrom: A comparative study of nurses and elderly patients ratings of pain and pain tolerance, *J Gerontol Nurs* 25(5):30-36, 1999.

Blair CE: Effect of self care ADLs on self esteem of intact nursing home residents, *Issues Ment Health Nurs* 20(6):559, 1999.

Blixen CE, Kippes C: Depression, social support, and quality of life in older adults with osteoarthritis, *Image J Nurs Schol* 31(3):221, 1999.

Burgener SC, Dickerson-Putman J: Assessing patients in the early stages of irreversible dementia: the relevance of patient perspectives, *J Gerontol Nurs* 25(2):33, 1999.

Chang BL: Cognitive behavioral intervention for homebound caregivers of persons with dementia, *Nurs Res* 48(3):173, 1999.

Clotfelter CE: The effect of an educational intervention on decreasing pain intensity in elderly people with cancer, *Oncol Nurs Forum* 26(1):27, 1999.

Eagle DJ et al: Comparison of three instruments in predicting accidental falls in selected inpatients in a general teaching hospital, *J Gerontol Nurs* 25(7):40, 1999.

Edwardson SR, Dean KJ: Appropriateness of self-care responses to symptoms among elders: identifying pathways of influence, *Res Nurs Health* 22(4):329, 1999.

Ekman I, Lundman B, Norgerg AP: The meaning of hospital care as narrated by elderly patients with chronic heart failure, *Heart Lung* 28(3):203, 1999.

Faison KJ: Caregivers of chronically ill elderly: perceived burden, *J Community Health Nurs* 16(4):243, 1999.

Fortin JD et al: An analysis of risk assessment tools for falls in the elderly, *Home HealthC Nurse* 16(9):624, 1998.

Fulmar TT et al: An intervention study to enhance medication compliance in community dwelling elderly individuals, *J Gerontol Nurs* 25(8):6, 1999.

Gasper PM: Water intake of nursing home residents, *J Gerontol Nurs* 25(4):23, 1999.

Gibson MC et al: Comparison of caregivers', residents, and community-dwelling spouses' opinions about expressing sexuality in an institutional setting, *J Gerontol Nurs* 25(4):30, 1999.

Gueldner S et al: Gerontological nursing issues and demands beyond the year 2000, *J Gerontol Nurs* 21(6):6, 1995.

Guse LW, Masesar MA: Quality of life and successful aging in long term care: perceptions of residents, *Issues Ment Health Nurs* 20(6):527, 1999.

Haight BK, Bahr SRT: Setting an agenda for clinical nursing research in long term care, *Clin Nurs Res* 1(2):144, 1992.

Hayes KS: Adding medications in the emergency department: effect on knowledge of medications in older adults, *J Emerg Nurs* 25(3):178, 1999.

Hubner C: Prosthetic valve endocarditis leading to valve replacement: a case study, *J Cardiovasc Nurs* 13(2):82, 1999.

Isberner F et al: Falls of elderly rural home health clients, *Home Health Care Serv Q* 17(2):41, 1998.

Johnson MJ, Williams M, Marshall ES: Adherent and nonadherent medication-taking in elderly hypertensive patients, *Clin Nurs Res* 8(4):318, 1999.

Kim O: Mediation effect of social support between ethnic attachment and loneliness in older Korean immigrants, *Res Nurs Health* 22(2):169-175, 1999.

Kneeshaw MF, Considine R, Jennings J: Mutuality and preparedness of family caregivers for elderly women after bypass, *Appl Nurs Res* 12(3):128, 1999.

Leidy NK, Haase JE: Functional status from the patient's perspective: the challenge of preserving personal integrity, *Res Nurs Health* 22(1):67, 1999.

Levesque L, Ducharme F, LaChance L: Is there a difference between family caregiving of institutionalized elders with or without dementia? *West J Nurs Res* 21(4):473, 1999.

Lindgren CL, Connelly CT, Gaspar HL: Grief in child and spouse caregivers of dementia patients, *West J Nurs Res* 21(4):521, 1999.

Marini B: Institutionalized older adults' perceptions of nursing caring behaviors: a pilot study, *J Gerontol Nurs* 25(5):10, 1999.

McCauley KN, Lloyd CT, Doherty JU: Dysrhymthia update: differential diagnosis of supraventricular tachycardia in an elderly man, *J Cardiovasc Nurs* 13(2):97, 1999.

McCormack B, Ford P: Gerontological nursing research: developing a user-focused agenda, *Elderly Care* 11(5):33, 1999.

McCurren C: Depression among nursing home elders: testing an intervention strategy, *Appl Nurs Res* 12(4):185, 1999.

Mentes J et al: Acute confusion indicators: risk factors and prevalence using MDS data, *Res Nurs Health* 22(2):95, 1999.

Mosley A et al: Initiation and evaluation of a research-based fall prevention program, *J Nurs Care Qual* 13(2):38, 1998.

Moyer A et al: A model for building collective capacity in community-based programs: the elderly in need project, *Public Health Nurs* 16(3):205, 1999.

Naylor MD, McCauley KM: The effects of discharge planning and home follow up intervention on elders hospitalized with common medical and surgical cardiac conditions, *J Cardiovasc Nurs* 14(1):44, 1999.

Picot SJ et al: Mood and blood pressure responses in black female caregivers and noncaregivers, *Nurs Res* 48(3):150, 1999.

Pierson CA: Ethnomethodologic analysis of accounts of feeding demented residents in long term care facilities, *Image J Nurs Schol* 31(2):127, 1999.

Porter EJ: Getting up from here: frail older women's experiences after falling, *Rehab Nurs* 24(5):201, 1999.

Powe BD, Weinrich S: An intervention to decrease cancer fatalism among rural elders, *Oncol Nurs Forum* 26(3):583, 1999.

Quinn ME et al: Psychological correlates of subjective health in sexagenarians, octogenerians and centarians, *Issues Ment Health Nurs* 20(2):151, 1999.

Redeker NS, Wykpisz E: Effects of age on activity patterns after coronary artery bypass surgery, *Heart Lung* 28(1):5, 1999.

Resnick B: Falls in a community of older adults, *Clin Nurs Res* 8(3):251, 1999.

Roberts J et al: Problem-solving counseling for caregivers of the cognitively impaired: effective for whom? *Nurs Res* 48 (3):162, 1999.

Rowe M, Alfred D: The effectiveness of slow-stroke massage in diffusing agitated behaviors in individuals with Alzheimer's disease, *J Gerontol Nurs* 25(6):22, 1999.

Schoenfelder DP, Van Why K: A fall prevention education educational program for community dwelling seniors, *Public Health Nurs* 14(6):383, 1997.

Schwarz KA: A study of the relationship of caregiving appraisal to depressive symptomatology and home care utilization, *J Community Health Nurs* 16(2):95, 1999.

Secrest JA, Thomas SP: Continuity and discontinuity: the quality of life following stroke, *Rehab Nurs* 24(6):240, 1999.

Sherrell K et al: Use of the cognitive abilities screening instrument to assess elderly persons with schizophrenia in long term care settings, *Issues Ment Health Nurs* 20(6):541, 1999.

Smyer T, Chang BL: A typology of consumers of institutional respite care, *Clin Nurs Res* 8(1):26, 1999.

Strang VR, Haughey M: Respite—a coping strategy for family caregivers, *West J Nurs Res* 21(4):450, 1999.

Sullivan-Marx EM et al: Initiation of physical restraint in nursing home residents following restraint reduction efforts, *Res Nurs Health* 22(5):369, 1999.

Tappen RM et al: Persistence of self in advanced Alzheimer's disease, *Image J Nurs Schol* 31(2):121, 1999.

Teel CS, Press AN: Fatigue among elders in caregiving and noncaregiving roles, *West J Nurs Res* 21(4):498, 1999.

Thurmond JA: Nurses' perceptions of chemical restraint use in long term care, *Appl Nurs Res* 12(3):159, 1999.

Topp R et al: Postural control and strength and mood among older adults, *Appl Nurs Res* 10(1):11, 1997.

Touranbeau A, Prentice D, Costello S: A decentralized admission screening protocol for a geriatric rehabilitation program: does it make a difference? *Rehab Nurs* 24(2):62, 1999.

Tsai Y et al: Falls in a psychiatric unit, *Appl Nurs Res* 11(3):115, 1998.

Turkel M, Tappen RM, Hall R: Moments of excellence: nurses response to role redesign in long-term care, *J Gerontol Nurs* 25(1):7, 1999.

Turkoski B et al: Clinical nursing judgment related to reducing the incidence of falls by elderly patients, *Rehabil Nurs* 22(3):124, 1997.

U.S. Department of Health and Human Services, Public Health Service: *Healthy People 2000: national health promotion and disease prevention objectives*, Washington, DC, 1991, Author.

Walker L et al: Developing individualized care in nursing homes: integrating the views of nurses and certified nurses aides, *J Gerontol Nurs* 25(3):30, 1999.

Watson WT, Marshall ES, Fosbinder D: Elderly patients' perceptions of care in the emergency department, *J Emerg Nurs* 25(2):88, 1999.

Learning Objectives

1 Discuss research utilization and its component categories.

2 Cite examples of instrumental, conceptual, and persuasive use of research findings.

3 Describe the responsibilities of researchers, practitioners, administrators, and educators in the use of research.

4 Review approaches for exploration of research literature.

5 Describe the criteria for determining whether research findings are useable.

6 Discuss strategies to promote development and retention of research utilization skills.

Chapter Outline

What Is Research Utilization?
  Conceptual utilization
  Instrumental utilization
  Persuasive utilization
Who Is Involved in Research Utilization?
  Researcher
  Practitioner
  Administrator
  Educator
How Is Research Used in Practice?
  Approaches for research utilization
  Criteria for research utilization
    Relevance
    Merit and applicability
    Implementation

Strategies to strengthen your utilization potential
  Maintain ties with library resources
  Exploit additional research learning opportunities
  Plan for timely perusal of research literature
  Assess your clinical environment
  Get other nurses involved
  Explore institutional research support systems

Use It or Lose It: Putting Research into Action

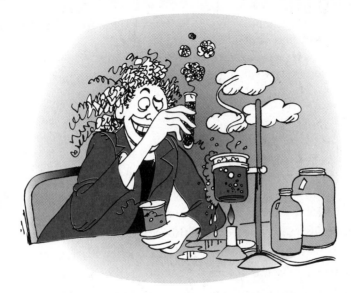

Whadda ya mean this is not what you meant by putting research into practice?

Student Quote   *"I've been a nurse for awhile, but I sort of never thought of research as being part of my responsibilities before."*

Abstract   Research utilization is the mechanism used to translate research into practice. The utilization approach may be formal or informal and can be classified as conceptual, instrumental, or persuasive. All nurses share responsibility for research utilization through the enacting of different roles. The goal is for the practicing nurse to be a research consumer who uses relevant research findings to define and enhance his or her clinical practice. This can be done by using a variety of approaches, criteria, and strategies to find, read, evaluate, and implement research findings.

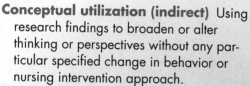

KEY TERMS

Utilization Explanations

Conceptual utilization (indirect) Using research findings to broaden or alter thinking or perspectives without any particular specified change in behavior or nursing intervention approach.

Instrumental utilization (direct) Concrete application of the research findings to institute new nursing interventions or alter or delete existing interventions.

Persuasive utilization (symbolic) Use of research findings as a tool to advocate for a certain practice or intervention.

Replication Conduct of additional research studies on an identified problem to determine whether consistent results can be achieved.

Research utilization Process of translating research findings into practice.

Utilization criteria Criteria used to evaluate whether research findings can be adapted for use in the clinical arena.

You should now be feeling more at ease with your abilities to find and read research studies. These abilities will continue to develop if you make a habit of using them on a regular basis. The next step is to incorporate these research results into your clinical practice. Research-based care promotes a practice environment in which you use research findings and critical thinking skills to make informed patient care decisions. When you use research findings as a foundation for nursing care, you become a true research consumer. As a research consumer, you have added another tool that allows you to regularly evaluate, update, and improve your nursing care. This chapter is designed to assist you in integrating your newly found skills into the regular conduct of your clinical practice. This is the final step needed to become a research consumer.

What Is Research Utilization?

Research utilization is the mechanism used to translate the knowledge that has been generated by research into clinical practice. This may be viewed as an informal or a formal process. For example, I might read a study, think it's a neat approach, and decide to try it out with my next patient. This is an informal approach to research utilization. Most individually instituted research utilizations are informal in nature. A research-based intervention protocol that replaces the previous protocol in the institution's procedure manual is a formal approach to research utilization. Research utilization efforts that are systematically introduced within an organization or institution are formal.

When we first begin to read and attempt to integrate research findings into practice, most of our utilization efforts tend to be informal. However, the ultimate goal is to formalize research utilization to promote research-based policies, procedures, and clinical practice guidelines. Ultimately, only when research findings are used in a systematic and structured way will we ensure the promotion of consistent, cost-effective, and high quality nursing care.

Use of research has also been categorized as conceptual, instrumental, or persuasive (Caplan and Rich, 1975; Beyer and Trice, 1982). A research study by Estabrooks (1999) was conducted to examine whether these theoretical categorizations were viable. Her research findings provided evidence that these three categories did indeed exist and could be measured and tested. We use these categories in our discussion.

Conceptual Utilization

Conceptual utilization, also known as indirect utilization, is when research consumers use research results to broaden or alter their thinking or perspectives without any particular specified change in behavior. When we use research findings in a conceptual manner, we use the findings to provide us with a more complete picture or to enhance our knowledge base. We then draw on this expanded knowledge base when making clinical decisions. These findings may provide evidence to confirm things we already know or believe. They may provide rationale to support clinical protocols already in place. However, while they may produce changes in our general approach to patients, they do not lead to specific documentable changes in patient interventions. Qualitative research findings are often used in this conceptual manner.

The findings of several research articles we previewed in Chapters 8 to 11 probably contribute to conceptual utilization. For example, the study about postpartum maternal fatigue (Troy, 1999) might cause us as nurses to reformulate our thinking about fatigue in the postpartum period and to extend the time frame in which we expect or assess new mothers for fatigue. The article on self-esteem levels in obese children who enroll in structured weight loss (Cameron, 1999) might reinforce our opinions that these programs do more harm than good, and we might continue to exercise caution in referral to such programs. The qualitative study about the experiences of living with a diagnosis of borderline personality disorder (Nehls, 1999) may reinforce the importance of the therapeutic nurse-patient relationship and help us persist in this approach amid environmental pressures to "perform the tasks and get the job done."

Instrumental Utilization

In **instrumental utilization,** also known as direct utilization, there is a concrete application of the research findings. We use the particular study findings to alter our nursing interventions. Specific nursing actions are implemented, changed, or stopped as a result of the research study outcomes. These research findings may even translate into a complete change in protocol. We also reviewed research results in Chapters 8 to 11 that could be used to alter our nursing intervention approach. The study about the use of pacifiers to reduce pain in low-birth-weight infants (Stevens et al, 1999) might lead us to use a pacifier when subjecting an infant to a painful procedure such as a heel stick for drawing blood. The meta-analysis study on distraction procedures to decrease pain in small children (Kleiber and Harper, 1999) might lead us to try such techniques when performing painful procedures such as giving an injection. The study that demonstrated that blood pressure measurements are increased when the patient crosses his or her legs during the procedure (Marcantonio, 1999) might lead us to be sure that our patients are flat footed when we take a sitting blood pressure.

Persuasive Utilization

In **persuasive utilization,** also known as symbolic utilization, research findings are used as a tool to advocate for a certain practice or intervention. It might be used informally to convince colleagues to alter some aspect of their clinical practice or formally to persuade an organization or institution to change a particular policy, procedure, or prevailing practice. In Chapter 11, in the clinical practice problem section (see pages 277 and 278), we viewed a scenario in which a residential care nurse combed the research literature for ways to prevent falls. An intervention protocol was discovered that had reduced falls significantly in the reported study (Mosley et al, 1998). If the nurse were to take these results back to the director of nursing and advocate that the institution adopt the intervention strategy, this would be an example of persuasive utilization.

If you review the three definitions and the cited examples, you should note that these definitions are not mutually exclusive of one another. Uses might overlap or vary from nurse to nurse. For example, we might use findings from a particular study in both an instrumental and a persuasive manner. Or I might use the results from a particular study in a conceptual manner, and you might use them in an instrumental manner. While some studies inherently lend themselves to a particular mode of utilization, the same set of study results can be used differently. The use of study findings is often influenced by the readers' prevailing knowledge, expertise, and clinical setting.

For example, suppose that you are a discharge-planning nurse in an acute facility and that I am a home care nurse. We both read the study cited in Chapter 11 by Naylor and McCauley (1999) that examined the effectiveness of comprehensive discharge planning in reducing hospital readmissions for elderly cardiac patients. You might take that information and use it as confirmation that discharge planning is helpful and that what you do is valuable. This is a conceptual use of the results. You might integrate some of the specific techniques from the study used in your own approach to discharge planning. This is instrumental. You might take the results to your supervisor to advocate for in-home follow-up of the discharge planning that you do. This is a persuasive use of the findings.

I might read the results in my position as a home care nurse and use them as confirmation of my own observations that my patients who have had discharge planning seem better prepared to function in the home environment (conceptual). I might decide to coordinate my follow-up home care with the discharge planning nurses in the various acute care facilities from which my patients are drawn (instrumental). I might convince my home care agency that we need to establish a formal protocol to collaborate with discharge planning nurses to facilitate the implementation and evaluation of the discharge planning instructions received by our clients (persuasive).

12-3

Who Is Involved in Research Utilization?

All nurses share responsibility for the utilization of clinical research findings. However the responsibilities vary with the role or position of the nurse. We now look at some of the differences for the researcher, the practitioner, the administrator, and the educator. Pay particular attention to those responsibilities that you shoulder as a practitioner.

Researcher

Researchers conduct the research that will ultimately form the foundation for clinical practice. As such they have several responsibilities. First, they must choose research topics that address identified priorities and critically defined problem areas in the clinical arena. Collaboration with clinical practitioners can keep researchers in better touch with clinical issues and can assist in more relevant and timely problem identification. Researchers must conduct quality research that is scientifically grounded and clearly builds on previous knowledge. Research must be replicated to provide a broader base for clinical utilization. **Replication** is when more than one research study is conducted on an identified research problem to see whether the same results can be achieved. Results must be disseminated (communicated) in clinical nursing journals that are widely read by practitioners and at nursing conferences that are attended by practitioners. The study should be presented in a clear, organized, and easily read format. The general process and bottom-line results should be readily graspable by any intelligent reader. Clinical implications should be clearly spelled out with concrete examples given. The researcher should identify the study's limitations and fully discuss the generalizability of the results.

Practitioner

Clinical practitioners are the front line in research utilization. If they do not regularly read, evaluate, and incorporate research results into their daily practice regimens, then the work of the researcher and the outcomes of the research are lost. Thus practitioners bear many responsibilities for research utilization as well. First, practitioners must regularly search and read the available research literature. They also need to avail themselves of ongoing educational opportunities that boost research utilization skills. These include attendance at professional and clinical conferences where research papers and presentations are featured. Applicable research findings should be regularly gleaned and conceptually or instrumentally integrated into clinical practice and shared with colleagues. Practitioners need to be attuned to problems and questions that arise in the clinical area that might be addressed by research. Relationships with researchers should be cultivated and administrative support mechanisms explored. Finally, practitioners should exploit opportunities to be involved in clinical research projects and formal research utilization projects.

Administrator

Administrators are key players in formalizing research utilization in the clinical area. They play a pivotal role in ensuring that research utilization is a systematic process used to promote the delivery of consistently effective and scientifically grounded nursing care. As such, administrators must foster a climate that supports and rewards the use of research in practice. This includes provision of adequate resources, personnel, and a positive emotional climate. This means providing formalized mechanisms for the promotion of research utilization. Such mechanisms might include an institutional research utilization committee with regular review of current clinical research, regular review and revision of institution policies, and procedures and prevailing practices that reflect use of research literature. Mechanisms should also be in place to conceive, carry out, and evaluate formal utilization projects and clinical protocols. Administrators should foster relationships with researchers and encourage the conduct of research in the institution. Finally, administrators should systematically evaluate and reward clinicians for research utilization and clinical innovation.

Educator

Educators are responsible for ensuring that all the other nurses (researcher, practitioner, administrator) are adequately prepared for their roles in the research utilization process. This includes designing course offerings and learning packages at all levels (undergraduate, graduate, continuing education) that articulate effective approaches and strategies to research utilization. Because the level of focus for this text is undergraduate education, I will use it as an illustrative example.

Undergraduate students must be given ample opportunity to develop and practice the requisite skills for use of research results in the clinical practice arena. If educators have any hope that their students will continue to incorporate research into practice as graduates, they must cultivate such utilization as a habit. They are also responsible for incorporating current relevant research results into their clinical teaching content. This incorporation should be openly articulated and demonstrated to students. In this way, teachers serve as role models to students. Teachers must require that students demonstrate the use of relevant research in the preparation of clinical care plans and in the care given. Research findings and their utilization should be included as expected discussion in clinical practice conferences.

STUDENT CHALLENGE Exploring Roles and Responsibilities

Let's explore how serious your clinical institution is about research in nursing. If you are currently employed, use that institution for the exercise. If not, select an institution where you've had clinical experiences while in school.

1. Interview two to three staff nurses. Ask them whether the institution supports nursing research (e.g., Is the institution involved in nursing research? In research utilization projects/protocols?).
2. Are clinical nurses evaluated and rewarded for utilizing nursing research in their practice?
3. Is support readily available (e.g., research and clinical journals in library, nursing research department or committee, nurse researcher on staff, time and funding to attend clinical and research conferences, in-services on research utilization, available research journal clubs)?

How Is Research Used in Practice?

Helping you as a research consumer to translate research into practice is the ultimate goal of this book. Although organizations can use many formal strategies and processes, the focus here is on you—the individual consumer—and how you can incorporate what you read into your real-world practice of nursing. This section examines three basic approaches to searching the research literature, discusses criteria that can be used to judge use of various research findings, and then illustrates strategies you can use to enhance your abilities to integrate research findings into your practice.

Approaches for Research Utilization

We used three approaches in exploring the research literature for use in the clinical area in Chapters 8 to 11. These three approaches form the backbone of research utilization. They are as follows:

1. Identification and review of the clinical and research priorities in a defined area of clinical practice
2. Identification of problems routinely confronted in clinical practice
3. Identification of useful research findings through scanning pertinent published research resources

All three of these approaches are valuable. We examined several sources for clinical and research priorities: the public policy arena (*Healthy People 2000* and *Healthy People 2010*), the National Institute for Nursing Research (NINR), and professional clinical specialty organizations. Timely review of these priorities keeps you on top of what is happening in your practice area and alerts you to what is viewed as important at a national level.

The second approach of identifying problems from your own clinical practice requires that you stay actively engaged in questioning what you do and why you do it. In fact, finding and raising questions that are answerable with research findings are possible at every point in the nursing process. Research can help you focus on better ways to collect and use data. For example, you might find alternate collection formats that improve data accuracy; or you might discover what data should be collected about certain types of clients with certain types of problems in various clinical settings. Research on nursing diagnoses helps you distinguish frequently occurring from rarely occurring defining characteristics and often leads to better validation of various diagnoses. In this way you can use that particular diagnosis with more confidence. Research can also make planning more effective. It can look at a patient problem, identify which nursing actions are needed, when they are needed, and who is most likely to benefit. We have seen how helpful research is in testing the effectiveness of nursing interventions. Research also helps you document whether the outcomes of specified nursing interventions are helpful to the patient.

The third approach of scanning the available current literature may be the most valuable approach for novice clinical nurses and research consumers. It keeps you in contact with the relevant research being conducted in your area of clinical practice. As you read these studies and struggle with how you might use the findings in your own clinical area, it should trigger additional questions in your mind about your practice. This then feeds back into approach number 2 and helps you identify additional clinical questions and problems.

Criteria for Research Utilization

After you have located and surveyed a research study, you must determine whether it is relevant to your clinical area, whether the results have merit and are applicable to your area, and how to implement relevant and applicable results. We have addressed these **utilization criteria** in a number of places in this text. However, we now group and identify the criteria for deciding whether to use research findings in your clinical setting.

RELEVANCE

The first issue you must address is relevance. You are trying to determine whether the findings from a particular research study are useful or helpful to your clinical practice. You begin to address this issue when you first evaluate the title of a re-search study and make a decision about whether to call up the abstract. You make further judgments about relevance when you evaluate the abstract and decide whether to survey the article itself. Your final evaluation of relevance comes when you determine whether the stated findings of the study apply to your clinical situation. To determine relevance you might ask yourself the series of questions that appear in Box 12-1. An answer of "no" to any of the proposed questions calls the relevance of the study into question for your particular situation.

MERIT AND APPLICABILITY

The second issue you want to address concerns the merit and applicability of the study. Here you are trying to decide whether the study results are accurate, be-lievable, and meaningful and whether they can be applied to your clinical set-ting. When you evaluated the studies in Chapters 7 to 11 using Step 4 of your reading strategy, you were examining merit. You were asking how well the re-searcher used the research process and whether the study was a good study. As stated in Chapter 7, you don't yet have the skills to address the theoretical and methodological merits of a study, but you can make beginning judgments about the quality of a study. To help determine the study's merit you might ask yourself the questions in Box 12-2.

Box 12-1   Criteria for Determining Clinical Relevance

- Is the study a clinical study?
- Are the sample/participants in the study similar to patients that you work with in clinical settings?
- Is the setting used in the study similar to the setting you work in?
- Is the problem being studied one that you have seen in your clinical area?
- Do the study findings address issues that nursing has the power to change (e.g., Can you identify which step in the nursing process would be altered by implementing the findings?)?
- Are the study findings helpful to your clinical routine?
- Do they add to your knowledge base?

If the answer to any of the questions is "no," then the merit might need further consideration. Merit is particularly important if you are considering using the study findings to alter an existing nursing intervention (instrumental utilization). If you wish to use the study results to support a formal change in intervention protocols (formal persuasive utilization), proof of merit is crucial, and you may need a resource person with research critique skills to evaluate the study from a theoretical and methodological point of view.

IMPLEMENTATION

The third issue that must be addressed is whether the findings from a particular study can be effectively implemented in your practice setting. This involves looking at such issues as importance, feasibility, cost, and risk versus benefit. To help determine the study's potential for implementation, try asking the questions found in Box 12-3. Assessing implementation is important for instrumental utilization that requires a change in the prevailing procedures or policies in an institution.

These criteria usually become important if you are trying a formal persuasive utilization. These are the kinds of questions the administration or utilization committee are likely to evaluate before deciding to try out an intervention or care protocol that changes standing policies, procedures, or practices. If you are

---

Box 12-2 Criteria for Determining Clinical Merit

- Are key elements of the study easily identified?
- Are the steps of the research process followed?
- Are ideas concisely and comprehensively identified?
- Do the results make sense?
- Do quantitative studies use reliable and valid instruments?
- Do qualitative studies address issues of accuracy, comprehensiveness, and credibility of data?
- In qualitative studies, does the final picture of the phenomena under study flow logically from the data?
- In quantitative studies, does the discussion section clearly identify who the results could be applied to? Were the findings clearly tied to existing knowledge?
- In quantitative studies, have other studies been done that address the identified problem (i.e., Are there replications, meta-analysis, or evidence in the literature of similar findings?)?

Box 12-3   Criteria for Determining Implementation Possibilities

- Who will be affected and in what numbers?
- What are the advantages of implementation?
- What are the risks of implementation?
- What are the risks of no implementation?
- Do the advantages outweigh the risks?
- How complex is the change (e.g., a simple intervention, or a lengthy protocol that requires extensive retraining of personnel)?
- How much will it cost (e.g., needed staff training, equipment, supplies)?
- Who is affected by the change besides nursing? (e.g., physicians, pharmacy, housekeeping, billing, patient services)
- What are the tangible observable outcomes of the utilization (e.g., Will it save money? Make the staff function better? Decrease patient complications?)?

ADVENTURE
CD
12-4

integrating study results as apart of your nursing knowledge base (conceptual utilization), an implementation review is unnecessary. If you decide to informally try a research-based intervention in your practice and this intervention fits within standard practices of the institution (i.e., it violates no protocol or procedure guideline) and requires no resource expenditures or risk to the patient, an implementation review is unnecessary. Examples of this informal implementation might include expanding the questions asked about assessing a certain patient problem such as pain, or using music as a distraction technique during a painful procedure.

The following is an example of an intervention that would require a formal change in institutional practice. Let's imagine for a minute that your institution uses heparin to irrigate and flush peripheral intravenous locks. You have just come across a meta-analysis (Goode et al, 1991) that analyzed 17 different research studies conducted in the late 1980s and early 1990s. These studies compared the effectiveness of saline to heparin as an irrigant for peripheral intravenous locks. After analysis of the studies Goode and colleagues (1991) concluded that saline was just as effective as heparin at maintaining patency, preventing phlebitis, and keeping the line in place. In addition, saline costs less and eliminates potential patient complications associated with the use of anticoagulants.

You are excited about this news and want to use it in your intermediate care unit. When you talk to your unit manager, she thinks it is a good idea and asks you to make a presentation at a nurse manager's meeting. You use the three sets of criteria above and come prepared to show that the study results are relevant, the study had merit, and the intervention has high implementation potential in the institution. The bottom line is that it is a simple intervention change that requires no new resources and little staff training, and it will save money and decrease potential patient complications. The nurse managers take the idea up the administrative chain of command and the decision is to try it out on your unit and evaluate its effectiveness.

You will probably not initiate such persuasive utilization approaches as a novice practitioner and beginning research consumer. However, as you gain experience and confidence in your research reading and informal utilization skills, you may find that you can be an effective force in advocating for research-based changes in your institution.

Strategies to Strengthen Your Utilization Potential

You can cultivate many practical ideas and strategies to ensure that the knowledge generated from research becomes a part of your clinical practice. We examine some of these in the following sections.

MAINTAIN TIES WITH LIBRARY RESOURCES

Upon graduation many students lose touch with the library. This may be because they move, or simply because they associate the library with being in school. Don't let this happen to you.

- Continue using your academic library. Most universities extend library privileges to their alumni. Take advantage of this perk.
- If your school library is not accessible, explore other library resources in your community that carry nursing materials.
- Explore the library resources available in your employing institution. Find out how you can make requests that they carry relevant journals in your practice area.
- Remember to maximize use of electronic resources. Use your home computer to log onto the Internet and to do literature searches and read journals on-line.

■ Subscribe to key nursing journals that regularly publish articles relevant to your clinical area (particularly research articles). You might choose one clinical research journal and one or two clinical specialty journals.

EXPLOIT ADDITIONAL RESEARCH LEARNING OPPORTUNITIES

Look beyond your formal education for experiences that will reinforce and enhance your research consumer skills.

■ Maintain membership in your professional associations, including clinical specialty associations. Subscriptions to certain journals are often provided as a part of the membership package.

■ Attend professional conferences and take advantage of research presentations and research poster sessions. Talk to the researchers, ask them questions about how they see their results being used in the real world of nursing practice.

■ Take advantage of research opportunities that come your way. Volunteer to be a data collector on a research project in your institution.

■ Pay attention to journal articles that describe research utilization projects or highlight the application of research findings to solve a specified clinical problem.

■ Avail yourself of emerging journals that focus on use of research findings in practice and the synthesis of research knowledge. (Check out the Resource Kit for journal listings.)

PLAN FOR TIMELY PERUSAL OF RESEARCH LITERATURE

You have learned and practiced a valuable strategy for scanning available research in various clinical areas. Make this scanning process a habit.

■ Make a list of journals that regularly contain research articles relevant to your clinical area.

■ Perform an electronic search of these journals at least twice a year. Schedule time in your calendar. When you find relevant studies, retrieve them.

■ Read the articles using your systematic reading strategy.

■ Critically read and evaluate the studies.

■ Deliberately determine how you will use the findings in your practice.

ASSESS YOUR CLINICAL ENVIRONMENT

Be aware of what is happening in your practice environment. Ask questions about standard procedures and practices. Why is it done this way? What is the rationale? Is it based on a scientific foundation or is it just because it's always been done that way?

Merlin
Activity
23

- Identify gaps, inefficiencies, and problems in clinical practice.
- Review the literature for research-based solutions or for findings that will enhance your knowledge base or supply rationale for nursing decisions.

GET OTHER NURSES INVOLVED

Don't keep your new-found consumer skills a secret.

- Share your research discoveries with your co-workers and your supervisors. Let them know what you find in the literature.
- Get other nurses involved in reading and interpreting research articles.
- Start a journal club where a group of nurses share their insights on research articles. (Check the Resource Kit for more information.)
- Bring examples of research utilization projects that have been tried in other institutions and ask about trying them in your setting.

EXPLORE INSTITUTIONAL RESEARCH SUPPORT SYSTEMS

It is much easier to use research findings in the clinical area if you work in an institution that values and rewards such behavior.

- Ask questions about the institution's commitment to research-based nursing practice before you are employed. (e.g., Do they have a research utilization committee? Are nurses evaluated for use of research in their practice? Is nursing research occurring in the institution? Are the nurses in the facility encouraged to participate? What nursing resources are available in the library?)
- If possible choose an employing institution that demonstrates its value for the implementation of nursing research. (Hint: They are likely to be progressive in other areas of nursing as well).
- If support for utilization of nursing research is lagging, investigate what you might do to contribute to increasing it. (Hint: Enthusiastic sharing with your co-workers and supervisor can often spark a wave of interest)

The use of the approaches, criteria, and strategies that have been discussed to enhance research utilization will help you grow, develop, and mature in the clinical practice arena. As you keep expanding your knowledge base and insist on using a scientifically based foundation for practice, you will ensure that you are providing your patients with the best nursing care possible.

NOW GO FORTH AND BECOME RESEARCH CONSUMERS.

Resource Kit

Journal Clubs

A journal club provides a way to receive support and confirmation of newly developing research consumer skills. It allows you to critically read and explore various research articles with a group of your peers. If you are interested in starting such a club and need guidance, check out the following articles:

Shearer J: The nursing research journal club, *J Nurs Staff Dev* 11(2):104, 1995.

Speers AT: An introduction to nursing research through an OR nursing journal club, *AORN J* 69(6):1232, 1999.

Tibbles L, Sanford R: The research journal club: a mechanism for research utilization, *Clin Nurs Spec* 8(1):23, 1994.

More Journals

Several journals provide examples of research that has been translated into practice or describes research utilization projects. You have been introduced to many of them in the lists of clinical journals that report research studies presented in Chapters 8 to 11. Check out your specialty area for journals that report on use of nursing research and give clinical examples of application of research findings.

And More Journals

Remember the two new electronic journals that provide resources for translating research to practice. You might want to check them out on the Internet.

Research for Nursing Practice publishes examples of research that has been carried out in nursing practice settings.

The Online Journal of Knowledge Synthesis for Nursing is sponsored by Sigma Theta Tau and provides critical reviews of research literature on a topic and implications for practice.

 Visit the book's MERLIN website at **www.mosby.com/MERLIN/Langford/maze** for further information.

 Check out the puzzles, mazes, and games on your **CD-ROM.**

References

Beyer J, Trice H: The utilization process: a conceptual framework and the synthesis of empirical findings, *Adm Science Q* 27:591, 1982.

Cameron JW: Self-esteem changes in children enrolled in weight management programs, *Issues Comp Pediatr Nurs* 22(2):75, 1999.

Caplan N, Rich R: *The use of social science knowledge in policy decisions at the national level*, Ann Arbor, Mich, 1975, University of Michigan.

Estabrooks CA: The conceptual structure of research utilization, *Res Nurs Health* 22(3):203, 1999.

Goode CJ et al: A meta-analysis of effects of heparin flush: quality and cost implications, *Nurs Res* 40(6):324, 1991.

Kleiber C, Harper DC: Effects of distraction on children's pain and distress during medical procedures: a meta-analysis, *Nurs Res* 48(1):44, 1999.

Marcantonio R et al: The effects of crossed leg on blood pressure measurement, *Nurs Res* 48(2):105, 1999.

Mosley A et al: Initiation and evaluation of a research-based fall prevention program, *J Nurs Care Qual* 13(2):38, 1998.

Naylor MD, McCauley KM: The effects of discharge planning and home follow up intervention on elders hospitalized with common medical and surgical cardiac conditions, *J Cardiovasc Nurs* 14(1):44, 1999.

Nehls N: Borderline personality disorder: the voice of the patients, *Res Nurs Health* 22(4):285, 1999.

Stevens B et al: The efficacy of developmentally sensitive interventions and sucrose for relieving procedural pain in very low birth weight neonates, *Nurs Res* 48(1):35, 1999.

Troy NW: A comparison of fatigue and energy levels at six weeks and 14 to 19 months postpartum, *Clin Nurs Res* 8(2):135, 1999.

GLOSSARY

A

Abstract A summary of the essential characteristics of something more extensive (e.g., a summary of a research article).

Abstracts Special indexes that include citations and summaries of articles.

Accuracy Conformity to existing facts and the truth as we know it.

Adequacy Sufficient scope and depth of information presented for a specific audience.

Advance organizers Preselected mental landmarks that serve to organize materials as you read. They are often provided by bold headings, outlines, and so on.

Applied research Quantitative research directed at solving a practical problem.

Archives A collection of older materials that have some historical value.

Audit trails (decision trails) Validity check used in qualitative research to ensure that adequate documentation is available about the process data collection and analysis.

Authority Knowledge gleaned from the expertise of others.

B

Balance Presentation of competing points of view.

Basic (pure) research Quantitative research done to establish or extend concepts or theories.

Basic social process A social or psychological process identified as enduring over time regardless of environmental conditions (e.g., stages of death and dying).

Bias Any influence that may alter the outcomes of a research study.

Biophysical instrument Used to measure physiological characteristics of a subject (e.g., glucometer).

Book (monograph) A volume about a single subject or related subjects published once (later editions may update material).

Bookmark A way to mark and easily access a favorite or easily used website.

Bracketing A process used by the qualitative researcher to identify and set aside personal beliefs about the phenomenon under study.

Browser A program that opens and displays pages on the World Wide Web.

C

Call number (classification number) A number or letter and number combination assigned to each book and/or journal to indicate where it is shelved in a library.

313

Case study An in-depth research study of an individual unit (e.g., a person, family, group, or other identified social unit).

Catalog A list of all books owned by the library with a citation and call number for each book.

CD-ROM A compact disk containing one or more electronic databases, programs, or images.

Circulating Materials that may be checked out of the library.

Citation Bibliographic information about books or journals (e.g., author, title, source, date of publication).

Clinical nursing research Nursing research that has direct impact on nursing interventions with clients.

Cluster sample Multistage probability sampling where larger clusters (groups) are randomly selected first and then smaller clusters are randomly chosen (e.g., patients).

Coding Process by which data are categorized and conceptualized.

Collection All materials owned by a library.

Collective case study A series of case studies that examine similar patterns about identified phenomena.

Comprehension Ability to perceive and understand concepts or ideas.

Concept A mental picture of an object or phenomenon. Concepts may be concrete or abstract.

Conceptual definition Statement attaching a specified meaning to a word (e.g., what the word means for a particular research study).

Conceptual framework A loosely related collection of concepts that have not yet been tested.

Conceptual utilization (indirect) Research findings used to broaden or alter thinking or perspectives without any particular specified change in behavior or nursing intervention approach.

Constant A characteristic that does not vary for a particular research study.

Constant comparative method Method of analysis used in grounded theory where categories of meaning are derived by comparing collected data incidents to one another until concepts emerge.

Construct validity Validity that is assessed using a combination of logic and statistical measures.

Content validity Validity that is assessed by a logical evaluation and judgment of whether the instrument reflects the content of the concept.

Control Mechanisms used by the researcher to reduce the influence of extraneous variables.

Control group The group of subjects in an experimental study that do not receive the treatment.

Convenience (accidental) sample Nonprobability sample that selects the most convenient subjects at hand.

Credibility An examination of the validity or quality of the data in a qualitative research study.

Criterion (concurrent/predictive) validity Validity that is assessed using statistical measures.

Critical case sampling Selection of subjects identified as demonstrating what has been identified by the researcher as a "critical incident" during data collection.

Critically read Step 3 of the research reading strategy; designed to focus on key steps in the research process.

Cross-sectional study Quantitative research in which data are collected at one point in time.

Currency Addresses the immediacy of presented information.

D

Data Measurable bits of information collected for purposes of analysis.

Database A collection of related information such as a catalog, index, or abstract.

Data collection Gathering the information necessary to address the research problem.

Data immersion data to become familiar with the content, feeling, and tone of the data.

Deductive reasoning A logical system of thinking that starts with the whole and breaks it down into its component parts.

Dependent variable Variable that is affected by the action of the independent variable.

Descriptive statistics Statistics used to describe and summarize data.

Descriptive study Quantitative research that describes the concepts under study.

Dissertation (thesis) A research paper written by a graduate student as part of the degree requirement.

Download Transferring a file from the Internet to a computer.

E

Effective reading rate The number of words that can be read in a minute while maintaining a high level of comprehension.

Electronic database A database accessed for a search by computer.

E-mail Electronic mail; postage-free messages that are sent via the Internet from one computer to another.

Equivalence Assessment of reliability is by correlating two different forms of the same instrument (parallel forms) or the scores of two or more raters (interrater reliability).

Ethnography Qualitative research design that focuses on the world view of an identified cultural group.

Evaluate Step 4 in the research reading strategy; designed to judge the quality of the article.

Examine Step 2 of the research reading strategy; designed to identify key ideas and sort out the meaning of the article.

Experimental design A research design characterized by three factors: (1) manipulation, (2) use of a control group, and (3) random assignment.

Experimental research Quantitative research in which one concept (independent variable) is manipulated to determine whether another concept (dependent variable) is affected.

Explanatory study Quantitative research that attempts to uncover why certain concepts occur and/or how they interact.

Exploratory study Quantitative research that explores the dimensions of concept(s) under study.

Extraneous variable Variable that interferes with the relationship of the independent and dependent variables in a specified study.

Extreme (deviant) sampling Selection of subjects who exemplify the phenomena to be studied.

F

Field A natural setting where investigation and data collection takes place in a qualitative study.

Field notes Written accounts of what a researcher sees, hears, experiences, and thinks during the course of data collection in a qualitative study.

File attachment A file that is added to an E-mail message.

File transfer protocol (FTP) A program that allows you to transfer files from the Internet to your computer.

Findings Results of the statistical analysis of study data.

Frequency The number of times that scores or categories of a variable occur.

Frequency distribution An ordered graphic display or plot of the frequencies for an interval or ration level variable.

G

Generalization The ability to apply study results from the sample to the population.

Grounded theory Qualitative research that develops theoretical propositions about identified social-psychological processes from collected data.

H

Historical method Qualitative analysis of historical events to draw additional insights or inferences about how past events impact the present.

Holdings The specific volumes or issues of periodicals owned by the library

Home page The first or base page for a website. It often serves as a map and directs you to places of interest on the site

HTML (HyperText Markup Language) The codes and instructions used to control the appearance and function of a website. It inserts links, graphics, and other multimedia objects on the web page.

HTTP (HyperText Transfer Protocol) The language used to transfer web pages over an Internet connection. The first letters in a URL for a site on the WWW.

Hypertext An electronic document format that permits links to other web pages or other related websites. The link is underlined and can be accessed by a mouse click on the link.

Hypothesis Statement of predicted relationship or difference between two or more variables.

I

Implications Inferences drawn about the results of a research study.

Independent variable Variable that causes a change in the dependent variable.

Index A list of periodical citations arranged by subject or author. Indexes are usually organized around a specific subject area or field of study.

Inductive reasoning A logical system of thinking that begins with the component parts and builds them into a whole.

Inferential statistics Statistics used to study relationships or differences among variables in a sample and infer the results back to the population.

Information rich sample Sample that provides a powerful picture of the phenomena under study in qualitative research.

Informed consent An agreement by a research subject to voluntarily participate in a study after being fully informed about the study and the inherent risks and benefits of participation.

Institutional review board (IRB) Committee responsible for review of research proposals to ensure that human subjects are protected from harm.

Instrument Device or technique used to collect data in a research study (e.g., biophysical instruments, such as glucometers; psychological instruments, such as questionnaires or interviews; behavioral instruments, such as observation).

Instrumental utilization (direct) Concrete application of the research findings to institute new nursing interventions or alter or delete existing interventions.

Intensity sampling Selection of subjects who are experiential experts or authorities on a selected phenomenon.

Interlibrary loan A library service that allows books and copies of articles to be borrowed from other libraries for use.

Internal consistency Assessment of reliability using correlation statistics to measure whether the subparts of an instrument all measure the same thing.

Internet service provider (ISP) A company that provides a connection to the Internet (e.g., AT&T Worldnet, Microsoft Internet, Sprint Earthlink).

Interval Level of measurement where categories of a variable are made up of "real" numbers that allow us to order the numbers and to know the distance between those numbers.

Interview Instrument used to collect self-reported psychologic data using oral question-and-answer format. The interview may be structured or nonstructured.

Intuition Insight into the whole of a situation without possessing readily supportable or confirming data.

K

Knowledge Essential information about the world around us that allows us to function more effectively.

Kurtosis The height of the distribution.

L

Limitations Identified problems or weaknesses in a research study.

Listserver (listserv) An electronic mailing list.

Literature review A critical summary of available theoretical and research literature on the selected research topic. It places the research problem for a particular study in context of what is currently known about the topic.

Lived experience Some dimension of daily experience for a particular set of individuals.

Log off Disconnecting from the Internet.

Log on Connecting to the Internet.

Longitudinal study A quantitative study that collects data at several points over a period of time.

M

Manipulation An intervention or treatment introduced by the researcher in an experimental study.

Maximum variety sampling The deliberate selection of subjects who are different, who come from different backgrounds, for the purpose of observing commonalties of experience.

Mean The average of all the scores.

Measurement A set of rules used to assign numbers to variables.

Measures of central tendency Statistical tests that describe how data for a variable tend to cluster together in a distribution (e.g., mode, median, mean).

Measures of dispersion Statistical tests that describe how data for a variable tends to spread out in a distribution (e.g., range, variance, standard deviation).

Measures of shape Statistical tests that describe the shape of the distribution for a variable (e.g., skewness, kurtosis).

Median The middle value in a frequency distribution of numbers.

Member checks Validity measures used in qualitative research. They are made by having study participants review the material once it has been analyzed and interpreted.

Meta-analysis A specialized statistical technique that combines and examines the statistical outcomes of several similar research studies.

Microform Materials that have been reduced and placed on photographic film (e.g., microfiche, microfilm).

Mode The numerical value that occurs most often for a particular variable.

N

Navigate Moving from site to site on the Internet.

Newsgroup Discussion via posting on an electronic bulletin board.

Nominal Level of measurement where variable is broken into two or more categories and assigned arbitrary numbers.

Noncirculating Materials that cannot be checked out of the library.

Nonexperimental design A research design for which there is no treatment or manipulation of the independent variable.

Nonexperimental research Quantitative research where concepts are not manipulated. They are examined as they occur naturally.

Nonparticipant observation The researcher is a bystander or passive participant in the activities being observed.

Nonprobability sampling Selection of a sample using nonrandom techniques.

Nursing research Use of the research process to gain knowledge that is important to nurses and the practice of nursing.

O

Observation Data collection method using the researcher as the instrument to gather behavioral data from subjects by watching and/or interacting with them. May be structured or nonstructured and participant or nonparticipant.

On-line (1) Computerized materials that are accessed by other computers (e.g., a computer network); (2) an active connection to the Internet.

On-line service A commercial network that provides a wide range of on-line services, including access to the Internet, news, games, travel information, and so on (e.g., CompuServe, AOL, Prodigy).

Operational definition Specifies how a variable is to be measured.

Ordinal Level of measurement that reflects a rank order among the categories of a variable

P

Participant observation The researcher is an active part of the activities or behaviors engaged in by the participants being observed.

Periodical A journal or magazine.

Personal experience Knowledge derived from the cumulative experiences of living.

Persuasive utilization (symbolic) Use of research findings as a tool to advocate for a certain practice or intervention.

Phenomenology The qualitative study of lived experience to understand and attach meaning to that experience.

Population All known subjects that possess common characteristic of interest to a researcher.

Predictive study Quantitative research that attempts to predict the occurrence of explained events.

Presentation Manner in which information is displayed.

Probability (random) sampling Selection of a sample using techniques to ensure that each subject in the population has an equal chance of being selected.

Probes Questions used to elicit more detailed information from a respondent when using a nonstructured interview approach.

Problem statement Interrogative or declarative statement that describes the purpose of a research study, identifies key concepts, and sets study limits.

Prospective study Quantitative research that collects data as the events occur.

Purposive sample Nonprobability sample in which subjects are hand picked by the researcher based on a set of defined criteria.

Q

Qualitative research An objective way to study the subjective human experience using nonstatistical methods of analysis.

Qualitative (categorical) variable Variable that changes in terms of the presence or absence of a specified trait.

Quantitative research Systematic process used to gather and statistically analyze information that has been measured by an instrument and converted to numerical data.

Quantitative (continuous) variable Variable that changes in terms of amount or degree (e.g., income, height, weight).

Quasi-experimental design A type of experimental design in which there is neither a control group nor random assignment.

Questionnaire Instrument used to collect self-reported psychological data from study subjects using pen and paper.

Quota sample Nonprobability sample that is conveniently selected according to prespecified characteristics (e.g., gender or ethnicity).

R

Random assignment Placement of subjects into treatment or control groups using techniques that ensure each subject had an equal chance of being in either group.

Range The distance between the highest and lowest scores for a variable

Ratio Level of measurement where variable possesses same properties as interval data plus a meaningful zero.

Reading level The readability of a specific piece of written material.

Reading rate The number of words that can be read in a minute.

Reading strategy (method) A system that breaks a reading assignment down into manageable parts that are more readily processed.

Reasoning Use of logical thought patterns to solve problems. May be inductive or deductive in nature.

Recommendations Statements derived from a research study to guide future research about a specified topic.

Reference collection Noncirculating materials meant to be used as reference rather than read through (e.g., indexes, encyclopedias, dictionaries).

Reliability (general definition) Dependability and trustworthiness of information.

Reliability (as used in quantitative research) A characteristic of a good instrument; the assessed degree of consistency and dependability of that instrument.

Reliability (as used in qualitative research) Concern with the accuracy and comprehensiveness of collected data.

Replication Conduct of additional research studies on an identified problem to determine whether consistent results can be achieved.

Research A systematic process using both inductive and deductive reasoning to confirm and refine existing knowledge and to build new knowledge.

Research critique A detailed critical examination and evaluation of the theoretical and methodological merits of a given research study.

Research design The overall plan for collecting data in a research study.

Research process An orderly series of phases and steps that allow the researcher to move from asking a question to finding an answer.

Research question Use of an interrogative format to identify the variables to be studied and possible relationships or differences between those variables.

Research reading strategy A five-step process designed to increase comprehension and application of research studies. The steps are survey, examine, critically read, evaluate, and visualize.

Research utilization Process of translating research findings into practice

Retrospective study Quantitative research that collects data on events that have already occurred.

S

Sample A subset of a population selected to participate in a research study.

Sampling The process used to select the sample.

Saturation Point at which sampling and data collection are stopped in a grounded theory study because the information being collected is redundant and repetitive.

Search Use of indexes, abstracts, and catalogs to find information about a specified subject.

Search engine Tools to find and retrieve specific information on the World Wide Web (e.g., Yahoo!, Lycos, Infoseek, Altavista, Excite).

Server (host) A computer that offers an information service over the Internet.

Setting The physical location and conditions under which a research study takes place.

Significance The likelihood that the study results are meaningful (i.e., not due to chance). The statistical p value is used to report significance.

Simple random sample Probability sample in which all subjects in a population are numbered, and a sample is selected using a lottery or table of random numbers.

Skewness Degree of symmetry or asymmetry of the distribution curve.

Speed reading Reading at an increased rate through techniques that encourage fewer eye fixations on the page.

Stability Assessment of reliability by correlating the scores obtained when an instrument is administered twice to the same group of subjects over a period of time.

Stacks Library bookshelves.

Standard deviation The average distance of spread in a frequency distribution.

Stratified random sample Probability sample in which the subjects are subdivided into groups according to some characteristic. The subsets are then randomly sampled.

Structured observation Specified behaviors are predetermined and listed on a checklist to be counted or checked off during observation period.

Summary A concise recapitulation of previously stated information that captures the main ideas.

Survey Step 1 of the research reading strategy; designed to provide a general overview and feel for the article.

Systematic sample Probability or nonprobability sample in which every k^{th} (e.g., every fifth, or seventh, or twentieth) subject is selected. If the list is in random order, the sample selected is a probability sample. If the list is ordered (e.g., alphabetical), the sample selected is nonprobable.

T

Telnet Software that allows users to log onto another computer from a remote site. It will show only the text, no graphics or pictures.

Theory Integrated and interrelated set of concepts used to explain some phenomenon.

Theoretical framework The theoretical foundation or frame of reference for a research study.

Theoretical sampling Procedure used in grounded theory to gather additional data about emerging concepts.

Tradition The handing down of knowledge from one generation to the next.

Treatment The intervention in an experimental study that is being manipulated.

Treatment group The group of subjects in an experimental study that receive the treatment

Trial and error Trying a succession of alternative solutions until one solves the problem at hand.

Triangulation The use of both quantitative and qualitative research methodologies in a study or series of studies.

U

Uniform resource locator (URL) The address system used by the Internet to assist in locating a web page or file.

Unstructured observation Behaviors are described and recorded as or after they occur using a journal, diary, or field notes.

Upload Transfer of a file from your computer to another computer, using the Internet.

User A client that communicates via computer and uses Internet services offered by servers or hosts.

User name The name you use to identify your computer to another computer or computer system.

Utilization criteria Criteria used to evaluate whether research findings can be adapted for use in the clinical arena.

V

Validity (as used in quantitative research) A characteristic of a good instrument; the extent of an instrument's ability to measure what it purports to measure.

Validity (as used in qualitative research) Concern with the credibility of the study. For example, does the interpretation of data match the recorded description of the data.

Variable A concept, characteristic, or trait that varies (e.g., takes on measurably different values) within an identified population in a research study.

Variance The average area of spread under a frequency distribution curve.

Visualize Step 5 in the research reading strategy; designed to apply research results to practice.

Volume A single book or a bound sequence of issues of a periodical.

W

Web page One screen on a website.

Website A sequence of web pages created by an organization or an individual for conveying information.

World Wide Web (www) A collection of computers on the Internet that are interconnected by hypertext and store websites.

INDEX

Internet—cont'd
   services on, 29-31
   use of, 31-49
      communicating and, 38-42
      navigating and, 31-38
      for professional purposes, 43-49
      traditional tools and, 42-43
Internet Explorer, 31-32
   E-mail and, 39
Internet Grateful Med, 44
Internet Public Library, 37
Internet service provider, 31
   definition of, 26
   finding, 48-49
Interpretation of results in quantitative re-
      search, 131-132
Interrogative form of problem statement, 103
Intervals in quantitative research, 125, 126
Intervention-based studies on older adult care,
      278-279
Interviews
   in qualitative research, 153-155
   in quantitative research, 118, 120
Introduction of research article, 169-170
   qualitative studies and, 174, 185
   quantitative studies and, 173, 180
Intuition
   definition of, 72
   knowledge derived from, 78-79
IRB; *see* Institutional review board
ISP; *see* Internet service provider
Issues in Comprehensive Pediatric Nursing, 225
Issues in Mental Health Nursing
   adult care and, 254
   child and adolescent care and, 228
   maternal-infant care and, 205, 206
   older adult care and, 282

J

Journals
   clinical nursing; *see also* Clinical nursing
      journals
   electronic, 45, 47
   in information search, 19

Journals—cont'd
   nursing research, 90; *see also* Nursing
      research journals
   research reported in, 166-171
Journal for Society of Pediatric Nurses, 206
Journal of Advanced Nursing, 228
Journal of Cardiovascular Nursing
   adult care and, 254, 257
   older adult care and, 283
*Journal of Child and Adolescent Psychiatric
      Nursing*, 225
Journal of Community Health Nursing
   adult care and, 254-255, 257
   child and adolescent care and, 228
   maternal-infant care and, 205, 206
   older adult care and, 283
Journal of Emergency Nursing
   adult care and, 255, 257
   older adult care and, 283
Journal of Gerontological Nursing, 274, 276, 282,
      283-284
Journal of Nurse Midwifery, 206
*Journal of Obstetric, Gynecologic, and Neonatal
      Nursing*, 203-204, 205
Journal of Pediatric Health Care
   child and adolescent care and, 225
   maternal-infant care and, 206
*Journal of Pediatric Nursing: Nursing Care of
      Children and Families*, 226
Journal of Pediatric Oncology Nursing, 226,
      231
Journal of School Nursing
   child and adolescent care and, 216, 226
   maternal-infant care and, 205, 206
Journal of Society of Pediatric Nurses, 227
Journal of Transcultural Nursing, 206

K

Knowledge, 72, 74-81
Kurtosis in quantitative research, 129

L

Learning, distance, 48
Learning-related reading, 53